PUBLIC HEALTH *DIS*-SERVICE

The Perveted Pandemic Legacy of the
Public Health Service

by

S. H. Shakman

INSTITUTE OF SCIENCE
InstituteOfScience.com

INSTITUTE OF SCIENCE

P.O. Box 3234

Santa Monica, CA 90408

http://www.InstituteOfScience.com
email: mail@InstituteOfScience.com

phone: 424-248-5635

Published by the INSTITUTE OF SCIENCE

First Printed 2014; updates 2018

Warning and Disclaimer: Although every possible effort has been made to assure the accuracy and correctness of information herein, the publisher hereby: apologizes and disclaims liability for any errors which have escaped editing; and disclaims any and all medical or legal liability in the event the contents of this book are utilized as a direct source of any dental or medical advice. The reader is encouraged to access original works discussed herein to assure accuracy of information, particularly on such critical matters as vaccine preparation, etc., and to refer any medical questionsconcerning discussions herein and related medical treatment to appropriate professionals. A proper professional assessment of all of a person's medical conditions must always be taken into account prior to development of a treatment plan. In this regard, as differing professional opinions abound, a "second opinion" (or more) is highly recommended.

Printed in the United States of America

CONTENTS

INTRODUCTION

This volume is a by-product of the process of reprinting, in book form, E.C. Rosenow's detailed eleven part series of articles on the pandemic of 1918-1919, as originally published in the 1919 *Journal of the American Medical Association* (Parts 1-4) and the 1920 *Journal of Infectious Diseases* (Parts 5-11). That work is currently available in print and digital formats at Amazon.com and Kindle books as "*Studies in Influenza and Pneumonia*" by E.C. Rosenow, comprising Rosenow's comprehensive and essential study of the 1918-1919 Influenza/Pneumonia pandemic. Portions of the "Foreword" of that volume are incorporated herein as background and introduction to Rosenow's relevant work and legacy.

In order to document and assess the modern view of Rosenow's contribution, the writer conducted a review of modern and historical articles on the pandemic. Particularly prominent among modern items was a 2010 *J Infect Dis* article, referred to herein as Chien 2010 (Y.W. Chien, K.P. Klugman, D.M. Morens, *J Infect Dis* 2010 Vol. 202, 11, "Efficacy of Whole-Cell Killed Bacterial Vaccines in Preventing Pneumonia and Death during the 1918 Influenza Pandemic"; Appendix A). **The importance of Chien 2010 to the perception, history and future of influenza and pneumonia research cannot be overly emphasized.**

One of the co-authors of Chien 2010, David M. Morens, is Senior Scientific Advisor to Anthony Fauci of the National Institutes of Health (NIH), with whom Morens has also co-authored other Pandemic-related articles. And another co-author, Keith P. Klugman, heads up pneumonia research for the Bill and Melinda Gates Foundation. As such this article may easily be considered to represent an, if not **the**, authoritative NIH view.

Moreover, while not specifically so stated but nonetheless confirmed within the Chien 2010 article, most (about 80%) of the total of historical vaccines listed and assessed therein were actually from Rosenow (his and ¾ of Cadham's civilian vaccines [see Table 2, page 12, below & Appendix D – Cadham (p. 886)]. These vaccines were specifically intended to reduce severity and fatalities due to pneumonia and were remarkably successful in doing so. Coincidentally they also reduced the incidence of influenza.

But whereas Chien 2010 claimed to assess the effectiveness of these vaccines in "preventing pneumonia and death", it grossly misrepresented and undervalued them. Chien 2010 explicitly obscured the fact that these anti-pneumonia vaccines also reduced the incidence of influenza – simply dismissing this fact because it is "not consistent with our understanding of influenza etiology". This fundamental design flaw is inherently and blatantly unscientific.

This design flaw and its implications are discussed in detail in Chapter 3 below. A preview:

As shown in Table 2 for Rosenow (p. 12), unvaccinated persons were in fact far more likely to suffer Influenza (2.96), Pneumonia (4.21), and Death (4.45) than vaccinated.

However, in essence, Chien 2010 divided Pneumonia and Death data by the Influenza data, thus misrepresenting Pneumonia and Death among unvaccinated persons as only about 1½ times more likely than those vaccinated.

In possible defense of Chien 2010 co-authors Morens (of Fauci/NIH) and Klugman (of B&M Gates), it may be noted that the primary co-author of Chien 2010 was an Emory U. graduate student, Y.W. Chien. Chien's 2011 Phd thesis, on which Klugman was faculty advisor, features and incorporates the Chien 2010 article in entirety. In this article, Chien constructed an intricate hypothesis – at best grossly misleading and fundamentally incorrect (see particularly Chapter 3 for further details). However, this does not absolve Morens and Klugman, as well as their esteemed sponors/associates Fauci/NIH, B&M Gates, and Emory University, as well as the *J Infect Dis*, from taking proper corrective action to the extent possible.

Beyond this fundamental and pervasive design flaw, Chien 2010 was particularly and heavily influenced by 2009 and 2010 articles by Public Health Service (PHS) essayist John M. Eyler (Appendices B & C), as discussed in detail in Chapter 4.

Probably the most damaging of numerous inaccuracies put forth by Eyler, and adopted ("hook, line, and sinker") by Chien 2010, was Eyler's assertion that most of the anti-pandemic vaccinations came late in the pandemic. This was absolutely not correct, as discussed below in Chapter 2, pp. 17, 19. Eyler's error was seemingly based on his having misread George McCoy's 1919 reference to **"a vaccine made from the influenza [Pfeiffer's] bacillus alone"** (G.McCoy, *JAMA* **73**, p.402; Appendix L.*).* Eyler wrongly attributed this to all of the other anti-penumonia pandemic vaccines, which mistake became a primary assumption permeating and mortally undercutting what was a fundamental premise of Chien 2010.

And beyond their own respective critical "unforced errors", the works of Eyler and Chien 2010 were heavily influenced by G. McCoy's arguably-intentionally deceptive presentations. McCoy seems to have been engaged in particular efforts to discredit Rosenow, as well as others, as discussed and illustrated herein (see particularly Chapter 5 and Appendices A-L). Chien 2010 and Eyler 2009-2010 have brought this sad legacy into the 21st Century.

> During the Pandemic, McCoy served as Director of Public Service's Hygienic Laboratory. Later, in 1930 when McCoy was still serving as its Director, this Laboratory was renamed as the National Institute of Health. Thus, McCoy became the first so-named NIH Director (although the title was also retroactively given to McCoy's three predecessors at the Hygienic Laboratory).

There are even broader scientific and medical implications. Prior to the pandemic, medical science was continuing along proven historical lines underlying the greats of immunology, Koch, Henle, Ehrlich, etc. The importance of satisfying criteria set forth in the works of Henle and Koch (aka "Koch's Postulates") for the causation of disease was preeminent. But a century later, broad swaths of modern medical science seem to have abandoned these unimpeachable criteria.

For example, Eyler 2010, referring to the possible culpability of a (discredited) microbe, e.g. the so-called influenza or Pfeiffer's bacillus, in the 1918-9 pandemic, claimed *"The failure to satisfy Koch's Postulates by producing an experimental disease in animals by the inoculation of pure culture was not in itself damning."* On the contrary, it actually was and is, in and of itself, absolutely damning. The failure of investigators, then and now, to satisfy Koch's Postulates simply indicates that they had not / have not isolated the correct organism.

In accord with principles established by Koch and Henle, Rosenow did properly satisfy requirements for proving causation with an organism isolated during the pandemic (as he had done for a wide range of conditions over his five-plus decades of active research and publications). In the case of pandemic influenza, this was definitively discussed as early as the second of his eleven-part series on the Pandemic. [*JAMA* 1919, **72**, 1604-7, II. "The experimental production of symptoms and lesions …."]

Moreover, Rosenow's exhaustively-documented work over the decades clearly shows that the diversionary "modern" concept of an "animal model" for a given disease is simply unnecessary, and incredibly wasteful in the course of implemenation. The true "model" for a given disease is a previously healthy lab animal, purposely infected with the correct causative organism. [We shall decline here to address relative merits and morals of experiments on lab animals versus humans].   Rosenow and others, before and since, had used healthy animals of various types, all of which were successfully infected with the indicated ailments and passed them on to subsequent generations – when inoculated with the properly-identified organism – thereby fulfilling Koch's Postulates.

Searching medical history for an explanation as to what may have befallen the great traditions of medicine's late-19th-Century pioneers, we may find a measure of twisted truth in a statement made by Eyler 2010: *"If anything, the experience of 1918-1919 served to deconstruct existing biomedical knowledge."* Rather, it may be offered that the misrepresentations of George McCoy and others with whom he was closely associated (arguably and prominently JAMA Editor George Simmons) diverted attention from bottom-line, irrefutable, historical biochemical knowledge – and continue to do so through the ill-advised works of Eyler, Chien 2010, and their presumably-unwitting agents, i.e., the likes of Anthony Fauci of NIH and the Bill and Melinda Gates Foundation.

The bottom line is:
– There were in fact a number of very effective vaccines against both pandemic influenza and pandemic pneumonia in 1918-1919.
– The vaccines developed by Rosenow and others were far more efficacious against pandemic pneumonia than pneumonia vaccines available today (e.g., Pneumovax).

The writer offers apologies in advance for any seemingly-excessive duplications and/or otherwise-deficient editing, inclusion of which within this compilation will hopefully nonetheless provide valuable perspectives on the themes discussed herein. As time and circumstance allows, various sections may be revisited and revised. In any case, hopefully these sections may serve as guides for further exploration of the literature. (Please note that portions of selected articles have been quoted below; subsequently it was decided to include the full articles in entirety within Appendices A-L to facilitate more adequate review, resulting in reduncies in text.)

S. H. Shakman
InstituteOfScience.com / I-o-S.org
2014; as augmented February 20, 2018.

Chapter 1: Rosenow on Pneumonia, the Pneumococcus, etc.

The writer was already somewhat familiar with E.C. Rosenow's involvement with the 1918-9 pandemic when he came across a discussion of **a modern pneumonia vaccine with "the potential to prevent an estimated** *one-third of pneumonia deaths* linked to swine flu." [LA Times, 8/4/2009].

This sparked the recollection that Rosenow, through the Mayo Foundation, had reported a much larger reduction in pneumonia deaths during the 1918-1919 pandemic with a vaccine he had developed at that time, as compared to the modern pneumonia vaccines. The mortality rate in a group inoculated three times with Rosenow's mixed vaccine was less than 1/4 (1.00/4.45) that of un-inoculated persons. Thus, **Rosenow's vaccine had prevented more than an estimated** *three-fourths of pneumonia deaths* **(in persons receiving his vaccine, versus those not)** linked to the 1918-9 Influenza Pandemic (see last column in Table 2, below.) – much better than the mere potential one-third anticipated for the modern pneumonia vaccine!

This was the initial impetus for putting together a book comprised of Rosenow's complete series of pandemic articles. These original 1919-1920 articles are available in print form or online through most medical libraries; nonetheless, publication in a single combined and much more easily accessible book form seemed to make sense. And as the world keeps a watchful eye on the 21st Century threat of the likes of so-called Severe Acute Respiratory Syndrome (SARS) and whatever comes next, it is clear that Rosenow's work may be as germane as ever. Having studied, written about, and occasionally lectured on the significance of Rosenow's monumental (six-decade-spanning) body of works over the prior decade-plus (unfortunately without gaining notable traction in the general public arena), to the writer this seemed like a unique opportunity to get the word out on the incomparable E.C. Rosenow legacy.

Rosenow had joined the Mayo Foundation at its inception in 1915, after working closely with the likes of Frank Billings and Charles Mayo for more than a decade prior; and he went on to serve as head of the Division of Experimental Bacteriology at the Mayo Foundation for nearly three decades (1915-1944). Thus he was already well established with the Mayo brothers and with the Mayo Foundation when the pandemic of 1918-9 occurred, and was Mayo's primary investigator during the crisis.

Rosenow's truly monumental body of work overall, more than 300 published articles in mainstream medical journals, spanned more than a half century (1902-1958), and over the decades his work garnered considerable support both within the Mayo Foundation and the medical community at large. At the same time, this work had understandingly evoked considerable resistance by numerous members within the authoritative dental and medical communities – in particular his exhaustive and arguably-irrefutable documentation of the relation of oral infections (e.g. infected teeth and/or tonsils) to a wide range of systemic disease(s). While some critics were expressing understandable skepticism of Rosenow's controversial body of work, others arguably may have been moreso protecting their respective turfs.

But to this writer, Rosenow's work on the 1918-9 pandemic seemingly opened a new vista for exposure – a chance to show his genius through a prism un-fettered by the continuing controversy over the role of oral foci in causing or contributing to systemic diseases.

Rosenow's detailed "on the ground" examination of the 1918-9 pandemic was conducted with the full support of the Mayo Foundation and in cooperation with the finest researchers of the time. This work is a "must-read-thoroughly" for modern researchers who wish to understand the 1918-9 pandemic in depth (as well as subsequent and possible future pandemics, and the influenza-pneumonia interface in general. Rosenow's pandemic studies built on his prior work on pneumonia dating from 1903, including early reports on immunization (*JAMA* 59:795-796, 1912, and Science Mag., 1908) and treatment with autolysed pneumococci (*JAMA* 59:2203-2240, 1913, with L. Hektoen). Prior to 1919, he had already published over 30 articles in the medical literature with titles referring to "pneumonia" and/or "pneumococci".

- Rosenow's pandemic vaccine was also effective against influenza. Rosenow's results are supportive of and in concert with the idea, widely considered at the time, that both pandemic influenza and the associated distinctly-characteristic type of pneumonia may be caused by different phases of the same "pleomorphic" organism.

- But isn't influenza caused by a virus, and pneumonia by bacteria? Yes, but the virus associated with pandemic influenza and the bacteria associated with pandemic influenzal pneumonia are apparently related -- different and reversible phases of the same microbe, depending on environment.

Historically, the term "virus" fundamentally has denoted a small, filtrable size. The ability of an organism to pass through a filter of a given determinable size served as the dividing line between viral and bacterial forms. Notwithstanding the "modern" common misconception that the fundamental difference, the ability of some, if not all, microbes to change size and shape under varying environmental influences, or "pleomorphism", has been studied for well over a century (e.g., for early history, see Philip Hadley, *Jour. Infect. Dis.*1927, 1-312; and subsequent related articles, now available through Amazon.com as *Microbic Dissociation I-III,*). Specifically in the case of pandemic influenza, Olitsky [better known for work on polio with Sabin] and Gates (*J Exp Med.* 10/31/22) were among the first to show how the filtrable (viral) agent can be made to grow larger, to bacterial size, and revert to original smaller form, on appropriate culture media.

Rosenow: Over the years Rosenow conducted extensive tests demonstrating the relation between implicated pneumonia (bacterial/ streptococcal) and influenza (viral) microbes, as characterized in a 1953 article: **"The Streptococcus appears to be the toxicogenic, antigenic phase, and the virus the relatively non-toxicogenic, nonantigenic, but highly invasive phase."** (from *A.M.A. Arch. Otolaryng. 58:* 609 622, Nov. 1953)

- *Rosenow's pandemic vaccine was successfully used against influenza for several years afterwards*, having been preserved in glycerine-salt solution. The late C.F. Williamson, Bacteriologist and Dean of the College of Arts and Sciences, U. of Miami, Oxford Ohio, had worked directly with Rosenow and was the last to have produced Rosenow's vaccines. According to Dean Williamson, "for many years I supplied those to physicians who would give those prior to the season arriving, and with very good results." (Quote at 7:00 in a 1999 telephone interview with this writer; audio is posted at: https://www.youtube.com/watch?v=zqesi_Q88ok)

- *Great quantities of vaccine can be produced quickly*, i.e., within 48 hours. The U.S. Department of Health and Human Services has already committed more than a billion dollars to efforts to speed up the process of producing influenza vaccine, which currently takes months Rosenow's vaccine, which works against influenza as well as pneumonia, takes a mere couple of days to produce huge batches, and is available now. Rosenow's methodology is posted at instituteofscience.com/Ro-recdi.html, as described in *Am. Practitioner and Digest of Treatment*, 9(5), May1958, p. 755-761 and numerous prior articles (see also *Reference Manual Rosenow Et Al*, 1998, by S. H. Shakman available through *Amazon.com*.)

- *The Rosenow vaccine methodology does not involve chicken eggs*, thus avoiding the problem of egg allergies that afflicts many persons.

- *An oral version of Rosenow's vaccine yielded "striking results"* in preliminary tests in laboratory animals. "With its high concentration of hygroscopic sugars, bacteria are dehydrated, contaminants cannot grow, it does not require refrigeration, and dosage can be adujsted." (*Am. J. Clin. Path.* 8: 17-27, Jan. 1938, with FR Heilman)

- *Rosenow addressed the cause of epidemics and seasonality of respiratory infections* including influenza, as well as encephalitis and polio; he demonstrated how variations in the implicated causative organisms, directly attributable to variations in radiant energy, are the probable cause of seasonality. (*Postgrad. Med.* 7: 117-123, Feb. 1950; 8: 290-292, Oct. 1950.)

- *So why did some suffer severe consequences in the 1918-9 pandemic, and others did not?* This was the big take-away surprise of this research effort, i.e., as relates to Rosenow's pandemic work. As indicated above, Rosenow's foundational work on pneumonia and pneumonia vaccines preceeded, and was seemingly independent of, his well-known body of works implicating oral foci in a range of disease conditions. Thus it was hoped that the tremendous success of his pneumonia-related works could help shed fresh light on his monumental works overall.

Nonetheless, it was of great interest that, as research into Rosenow's pandemic vaccines progressed, it became increasingly clear that the organism responsible may well have been a virulent phase of a streptococcus (Streptococcus viridans) commonly found in the mouth, albeit usually in a relatively non-virulent form. This organism was apparently implicated first by Mathers and confirmed in depth by Rosenow and others (e.g., Tunnicliff, Schotmuller, Billings, etc). The distinctive age of victims, i.e., adults in their prime, versus the age of victims of common forms of influenza (generally the very young or very old) is further suggestive that pre-existing oral infections may have contributed to the severity of the pandemic in some persons.

- Weston Price's documentation of the correlation between dental infections and severity of pandemic complications: Adding evidence to this hypothesis is a study published by Weston Price in his 1923 book, *"Oral Infections and Systemic Disease"* (Volume I, Chapter xxi, p. 266-7), which reported:

"A study of two hundred sixty influenza patients in five different hospitals ... disclosed that when the patients were divided into two groups – those with, and those without clearly demonstrable dental infections – the percentage of individuals developing serious complications (in which we included pneumonia, empyema, carditis, severe neuritis, and severe rheumatism, was found to be in the group without dental infections 32 percent, and in the group with serious dental infections 72 percent."

Price noted that this contrast was likely much understated because "many cases of dental infection were undoubtedly overlooked" because "patients involved were frequently too ill to be questioned with sufficient care", "it was not possible to make roentgenographic studies", and "only those were included which were sufficiently gross to be determined definitely by oral examination, palpitation, etc."

Not proof positive, but certainly suggestive! (see Table 1)

Table 1 – from Weston Price, Oral Infections and Systemic Disease I, p. 267

ORAL INFECTIONS AND INFLUENZA COMPLICATIONS

Hospital	Date	No. of Flu Cases Studied	Flu Only	Flu with Various Complications	Flu with Pneumonia	With Oral Infection			Without Oral Infection		
						Total	Flu Only	Flu with Complications	Total	Flu Only	Flu with Complications
1 Lakeside, Cleveland Men's Ward	Nov. 30	20	13–65%	7–35%	7–35%	8–40%	2–25%	6–75%	12–60%	10–83%	2–17%
2 Lakeside, Cleveland Women's Ward	Dec. 1	6	1–17%	5–83%	5–83%	5–83%	1–20%	4–80%	1–17%	0	1–17%
3 St. Francis Columbus	Dec. 4-5	23	5–21%	18–78%	9–48%	18–22%	3–17%	15–83%	5–78%	2–40%	3–60%
4 Grant, Columbus Nurses	Dec. 5	50	41–82%	9–18%	2–4%	0	Held certificates from dentists		50–100%	41–82%	9–18%
5 Grant, Columbus Private Patients	Dec. 5	51	38–74%	13–26%	8–16%	0	None known		51–100%	38–74%	13–26%
6 City Hospital Cleveland	Dec. 7	26	· 8–31%	18–69%	15–51%	23–88%	7–30%	16–70%	3–12%	1–33%	2–67%
7 Mt. Sinai Cleveland	Dec. 19	31	14–45%	17–54%	10–32%	21–68%	8–38%	13–62%	10–32%	6–60%	4–40%
8 Mt. Sinai Cleveland Nurses	Dec. 16	53	38–72%	15–28%	13–24%	0	Clean mouths		53–100%	38–72%	15–28%
Eight Sources		260	158–61%	102–39%	69–26%	75–29%	21–28%	54–72%	185–71%	136–68%	49–32%
Private Practice Patients		37	14–38%	23–62%	14–23%	37–100%	14–38%	23–62%	0		

-The state of medicine prior to the pandemic of 1918-9: There were two particularly-relevant medical histories coming into the 1918 pandemic:

(a) The "influenza bacillus" or "Pfeiffer's bacillus" hypothesis, carried over from the Pandemic of 1889-92; and

(b) A more distinctly separate pneumonia vaccine experience, in the early 1900s, following on the prior works of Sir Almroth Wright, Leishmann, Rosenow and others.

(a) *The "influenza bacillus", or "Pfeiffer's bacillus", hypothesis*, carried over from the Pandemic of 1889-92, was the widely-considered but never-confirmed claim by Pfeiffer to have found the cause of the pandemic in the so called "Influenza Bacillus" (aka *Hemophilus influenzae*). Despite considerable and widespread doubt concerning the role of Pfeiffer's bacillus by the time the 1918-1919 pandemic struck, the lack of a proven alternative kept Pfeiffer's bacillus prominently in consideration. Thus it became somewhat of a requisite for inclusion in initially-proposed vaccines by various entities, particularly public entities such as the New York Department of Public Health and the Public Health Service.

And even today, nearly a century later, given the continued apparent lack of even consideration that the cause of pandemic influenza may have indeed already been well-established by the likes of Rosenow and others, it is nonetheless (to this writer at least) sadly surprising that some portion of the general medical population is still subject to this apparently-commonly-persisting wrongful impression, i.e., that Pfeiffer's bacillus (aka *Hemophilus influenzae*) caused the pandemic. Inertia is a tough nut.

This became particularly clear through a chance encounter with a USC internal medicine (obstetrics) visiting professor, in October 2011. As the writer was describing his Pandemic-related studies, the gentleman shared his conviction that the cause of the pandemic was established as "*Hemophilus influenzae*". In a follow-on email exchange, the professor kindly acknowledged receipt of and appreciation for the contrary and correct information and documentation as provided herein (specific references are available upon request).

(b) *The pneumonia vaccine experience*: Meanwhile, a distinct other body of work addressing the pandemic was coming from the pneumonia vaccine background, following on the prior works of Sir Almroth Wright, Lister, Leishmann, Rosenow and others. These were widely used during the pandemic, e.g., by Rosenow and the Mayo Foundation, by U.S. and British armed forces and many others. They made a lot of sense, because it was generally agreed that the cause of, and means of vaccinating against, pandemic influenza had not been established, but indeed there was a successful record of immunization against pneumonia. These vaccines used strains of the organisms isolated from victims.

While some of these pandemic pneumonia-directed vaccine efforts included some portion of "Influenza Bacillus", this seemingly was in reality a requisite "prevailing wisdom" inclusion – "insurance" of a sort. Indeed even Rosenow, as well as prominent British authorities under Leishmann who were doubtful about Pfeiffer's bacillus, were compelled to include it in their initial mix of vaccine microbes.

Some, such as Rosenow, dropped it out later in the course of improving the vaccine being used.

- What is the current thinking regarding Rosenow, pneumonia and pandemic vaccines? Notably, as evident from a review of the modern literature, Rosenow's pneumonia work continues to be prominently cited:

A 2004 article by Morton N. Swartz reprinted and lavishly praised Rosenow's 1904 study of pneumonia and pneumococcus, stating that "The large body of evidence presented in a logical sequence, the use of appropriate controls, and the clear and thorough explication of results in this article published a century ago in the first issue of the Journal set a suitable standard for future investigators." (Swartz, M.N., *J Infect Dis*, 2004: 189, 1, 128-164, *"Commentary: Rosenow EC. Studies in Pneumonia and Pneumococcus Infection. J Infect Dis 1904; 1:280-312"*).

And Chien 2010 (in this same journal) illustrates the continuing importance of Rosenow's pandemic (anti-pneumonia) vaccines. While not directly stated, most (~80%) of the total of all vaccines assessed by Chien 2010 (Appendix A) had been provided by Rosenow – i.e., his own plus ¾ of Cadham's civilian total [see Table 2].

Table 2 provides the raw data presented in Chien 2010 for "VACCINATED" and "NON-VACCINATED" persons, "Military" and "Civilian" categories, for all studies listed that provided totals of persons, influenza, pneumonia, and deaths. As shown in Table 2, vaccinated persons exhibited a huge advantage in terms of deaths.

Focusing on the last column in Table 2, Incidence Ratios for "per Totals – Died", with the glaring exception of the McCoy article, the incidence of death for unvaccinated was several times as high as for the vaccinated – i.e., it was 4.08 to 17.6 times more likely that the unvaccinated would die as compared to vaccinated!

Table 2. Data in Chien et al 2010 & Incidence Ratios

DATA AS PUBLISHED IN CHIEN TABLE 3, FIGURES 2 & 3								Incidence Ratios		
	VACCINATED				**NON-VACCINATED**				per Totals		
Source	Total	Influ	Pneu	Died	Total	Influ	Pneu	Died	Influ	Pneu	Died
Civilian - vaccines with pneumococci											
Watters	1638	89	13	8	1599	471	88	40	5.42	6.93	5.12
Rosenow	143760	13666	745	276	345133	97253	7534	2951	2.96	4.21	4.45
Cadham/Civilian	52999	5203	300	85	85941	21285	1869	563	2.52	3.84	4.08
McCoy	390	119	23	10	390	103	17	7	0.87	0.74	0.7
Military - vaccines with pneumococci											
Cadham /Military	4842	282	17	5	2758	238	41	17	1.48	4.23	5.97
Leishman	15624	221	26	2	43520	2059	583	98	3.34	8.05	17.6
TOTALS	219253	19580	1124	386	479341	121409	10132	3676	2.84	4.12	4.36

Table 2 Key:
Incidence ratios (IR) are calculated as IR = ARU/ARV. where
ARU = unvaccinated attack rate, and ARV = vaccinated attack rate.

An Essential Clarification of the Chien Data:
Chien 2010 states: "We identified and retrieved full texts of 485 publications for assessment. ... 13

studies were included in the final analysis". However, Chien specifically excluded five of these from their assessment results – four (Hinton-Kane, Wadsworth, Duval-Harris, Barnes) which involved "influenza bacillis" only, and one (Ely) involving only streptococci.

Of the remaining eight studies, one (Minaker) did not provide pneumonia data and two (Cherry, and Eyre) did not provide total inoculation data, therefore precluding determination of incidence of pneumonia and death as called for in the title/scope.

For the remaining five studies (including Cadham which included both civilian and military components), incidence data provided by Chien 2010 have been duly verified by the original texts – in terms of numbers of subjects and incidence of influenza, pneumonia and deaths.

These five studies involve a total of **219,253** inoculations, including 143,760 in Rosenow's Mayo reports; plus 39,749 (¾ of Cadham's civilian total 52,999) prepared from bacteria from Rosenow; plus 390 McCoy (Rosenow vaccines from Chicago, inappropriately used in California). Thus, **183,899 of the total (84 %)** were in fact Rosenow vaccines.

Further, all of the Cadham 52999 civilian and 4842 military vaccines adhered to protocols observed by Rosenow. Adding these and McCoy's 390 to Rosenow's 143,760 vaccines, some **201,991 of the total 219,253 inoculations, i.e., 92% of the total assessed by Chien, were Rosenow vaccines or otherwise in accord with Rosenow protocols** – a decidedly positive endorsement.

Given the choice, one might hope that Rosenow's influenza vaccine would be given serious consideration, if not preferred, as an alternate to products being proffered by contemporary pharmaceutical companies. Its attributes:

-- one vaccine for both influenza and pneumonia;
-- proven viability of epidemic vaccine strains over periods of years;
-- huge quantities produced within 48 hours after isolation, pandemic or not;
-- consequential huge cost savings in research and production;
-- avoiding the complication of allergies to chicken-egg vaccines.
-- availability of an already-developed oral vaccine method;
-- addresses the cause of epidemics and seasonality of respiratory infections;
-- explains why only some suffered severe consequences in the 1918-9 pandemic.

So please PHS, please NIH, why do we not have that choice? At this point we must be satisfied that we might, if only Rosenow's work were properly considered, and point to a couple of clues as to why we don't.

One clue jumps out from a brief scan of the last column in Table 2 (above). With the single glaring exception of the McCoy listing, the incidence of death for unvaccinated persons was several times as high as for the vaccinated – i.e., it was from 4.08 to 17.6 times more likely that the unvaccinated would die as compared to the vaccinated! The single exception, McCoy with 0.7, is so far out of line one with others that one might assume it was an error. However, surprisingly, the McCoy item is actually favored by Chien 2010 authors Chien, Klugman and Morens.

While the McCoy 1918 data is clearly an outlier relative to data listed for the other works assessed by Chien 2010, it must be noted that George McCoy occupies a unique place in the history of medicine. At the time of the pandemic, as noted above, McCoy was serving as director of the Hygienic Laboratory of the Public Health Service, which was renamed the National Institute of Health in 1930. McCoy served in this (combined) position for more than 21 years, more twice as long any other director in the history of the NIH. Accordingly he gained lasting historical recognition, notwithstanding the critical presentations made within this volume. Moreover, as noted on the NIH ALMANAC website, McCoy was, during his lifetime, the Nation's greatest authority on leprosy.

Beyond this, a central underlying historical issue can be traced back even earlier, to the 1880s and immunology giant Robert Koch, whose "dogma of the absolute constancy of specific bacterial types" [quote from Philip Hadley 1927, *Microbial Dissociation*] became strongly entrenched in predominant medical theory. This was despite the strong opposition, and evidence of variability, by Louis Pasteur and arguably a preponderance of others at that time and since. Nonetheless, the prominence of the Koch "monomorphist" dogma has prevailed even up to the present, and thus has served as a persistent thorn in the side of Rosenow's legacy and his decades of documentation of variability – e.g., between and within a range of bacterial and viral species.

The lingering effects in modern times of this 19th Century "dogma" are clearly evident in Chien 2010. While the Chien 2010 authors correctly report full data from a number of studies from 1918-1919, as listed in their Table 2, their assessment of this data is horrendously skewed. The original purpose of the 1918-9 (anti-pneumonia) vaccines, the very core reason they had been employed during the pandemic by their originators, was specifically based on their intention to combat pandemic pneumonia and associated death. This is clearly evidenced by the original authors and their articles. But when these pneumonia vaccines were employed during the pandemic against influenzal pneumonia, it was found that they were effective against the pandemic influenza as well.

Chien 2010 rejected consideration of this finding because it was "not consistent with our understanding of influenza etiology". Rather they ignored the extent that the pneumonia vaccination had already reduced the incidence of influenza by considering only persons with influenza in their assessments of the effects of anti-pneumonia vaccines on pneumonia and death. For example, in the case of data for Watters in Table 2 above, the incidence ratio of influenza was 5.42 times higher, and the incidence ratio of pneumonia was 6.93 times higher, in unvaccinated persons than in vaccinated persons,. This same pertains to the data shown in Table 2 for Rosenow, Cadham and Leishman. By discounting the effects that the vaccine had already had on the incidence of influenza [e.g. by the moving the demoninator in the equation], Chien 2010 appreciably under-valued the true effects of the vaccine on pneumonia and death. Nonetheless, the raw data listed by Chien 2010 serves as a comprehensive confirmation of the unassailable body of work by Rosenow on the pandemic; by extension, his follow-up work in subsequent decades; and exciting implications for future utilization.

Thus, Chien 2010 necessarily comprises the central, eye-opening, focus of this in-depth historical review. An overview/ summary of this review is provided herein as Chapter 2. More detailed critical reviews of Chien 2010 and Eyler 2009/2010 articles comprise Chapters 3 and 4 resp.; reviews/notes on a number of the actual historical articles comprise Chapter 5; a brief survey of additional modern articles comprise Chapter 6; and reviews/notes on significant theoretical works comprise Chapter 7.

Appendices A-L provide copies of the original historical articles, including particularly those articles assessed by Chien 2010. Hopefully these will enable the reader to independently confirm that we have been, and continue to be, badly misinformed as regards the substance of those historical articles, and thereby that we are being misinformed, by those most trusted resources on which we unfortunately rely, as regards the cause and prospective therapy – for pandemic-associated influenzal-pneumonia as well as as influenza and pneumonia in general.

Chapter 2. Perversion of the Legacy of Koch, Ehrlich and Rosenow
– A Necessary Reassessment of Chien 2010 and Implications

As noted above, one of the co-authors of Chien et. al 2010, David M. Morens, is Senior Scientific Advisor to Anthony Fauci of the NIH's National Institute of Allergy and Infectious Diseases (NIAID); and another co-author, Keith P. Klugman, heads up pneumonia research for the Bill and Melinda Gates Foundation. Thus, until superceded or disavowed by the powers that be at the National Institutes of Health, etc., this article may well continue to comprise the latest authoritative chapter/ continuation/ perpetuation of a misguided legacy implanted nearly a century ago by George McCoy within the bowels of the Public Health Service and NIH. (see Chien 2010 – Appendix A)

- How might the Chien 2010 article best be characterized?

Grossly misleading. Chien 2010 expresses an overall slightly positive view of efficacy of Rosenow's and the other anti-pneumonia vaccines; however, this work is hopelessly compromised due to a pervasive bias: Chien 2010's approach considers pneumonia and death among only persons influenza, not among the total numbers of persons in the given population sample – vaccinated or not. In this regard, Chien 2010 is dishonest from the start, even in its very title. They claim to assess the "Efficacy of Whole-Cell Killed Bacterial Vaccines in Preventing Pneumonia and Death... " – without further qualification. However, the article is indeed repeatedly highly qualified throughout as involving pneumonia and death only among "patients with influenza". Within the body of the article itself, there are 24 "patients with influenza" qualifiers and ten "influenza-associated" qualifiers that repeatedly emphasize this point. By "moving the denominator" in all of their considerations, from "total patients" to only "patients with influenza", Chien 2010 dramatically distorted the actual results of the very studies it was purporting to assess.

Rosenow and others had indicated that their anti-pneumonia vaccines had reduced the incidence of pneumonia and death as indended, and surprisingly had also reduced the incidence of influenza. Chien 2010 blatantly dismissed these results, citing as justification that this is "not consistent with our understanding of influenza etiology".

Detailed analyses of Chien 2010 and Eyler 2009/2010 reveals gross manipulation and misrepresentation perpetrated by them (as discussed in detail in Chapters 2 & 3), as well as by George W. McCoy (as discussed in greater detail in Chapter 4). In 1930, McCoy's PHS Hygienic Lab., of which he served as Director, was renamed as the "National Institute of Health". As the de facto first Director of NIH (although the NIH archival records retroactively give the title to 3 earlier Hygienic Lab Directors), McCoy's pandemic perspective is now an integral part of the NIH historical record, abetted and even further twisted by Eyler 2009/ 2010 and Chien 2010.

- Why is Chien 2010's approach inappropriate for Rosenow and Cadham, etc.?

Rosenow's vaccine specifically sought to prevent pneumonia and death --and **not** to diminish influenza (which coincidentally it did).

As Rosenow stated [*JAMA* . Jan. 4, 1919, **72**, p. 31], "In considering prophylactic inoculations in this epidemic of influenza, we put aside the debated question as to the cause of the initial symptoms and considered primarily the possibility of immunizing persons against the bacteria, pneumonia, streptococci, influenza bacillus and staphylococci, which are conceded by all to be the common causes of death in this disease."

And in a followup summary article in 1929 [*Minnesota Medicine,* June 1929, 366-368], Rosenow stated "The incidence of influenza was from three to six times as great and on the average was four times as great in the unvaccinated control groups as in the vaccinated groups. This observation was not anticipated since the vaccine was used only in the hope that the complicating pneumonia and the death rate might be lowered".

Rosenow's and the other pneumonia vaccines were based on prior successful results of Wright and Lister, 1912 to 1917, Cecil and Austin, 1918, Rosenow's own work on pneumonia from 1903 and immunizations from 1912, and others.

- But didn't Chien 2010 conclude that the pneumonia vaccine was advantageous?

Slightly, but the Chien article is far worse than merely too conservative: For example, if a given pneumonia vaccine reduced incidence of influenza and death equally, and if only persons with influenza are used as basis for comparison, those vaccinated would exhibit no added advantage in terms of whether they would die.

For specific example, in the Watters study (see Table 2 in the Introduction above and Table 2b below), unvaccinated persons were 5.4 times as likely to get influenza and 5.1 times as likely to die, compared with vaccinated persons. If one incorrectly assumed that the vaccine had had no effect on influenza, as the Chien article did, then the Watters vaccination would appear *disadvantageous* in terms of death.

- Chien 2010 (erroneously) claimed Rosenow and the others were biased,

Chien stated *"most vaccinations were given during the declining phase of the pandemic ...[and] usually compared with the same outcomes in unvaccinated individuals from the beginning of the epidemic ... This approach should diminish the bias caused by unequal observation periods."* This is absolutely not correct:

- Rosenow: "Vaccinations were begun soon after the onset of the epidemic.

1. Wright, A. E.; Morgan, W. P., et al.: "Observations on Prophylactic Inoculation Against Pneumococcus Infections and on the Results Which Have Been Achieved by It", *Lancet* **X**: 1-10 (Jan. 3) 1914..

2. Lister, F. S.: "Prophylactic Inoculation of Man Against Pneumococcal Infections and More Particularly Against Lobar Pneumonia; Including a Report on the Results of the Experimental Inoculation with a Specific Group Vaccine, of the Native Mine Laborers Employed on the Premier (Diamond) Mine and the Crown (Gold) Mines in the Transvaal and the de Beers (Diamond) Mines at Kimberley" — Covering the Period from Nov. 1, 1916, to Oct. 31, 1917, *Publications of South African Institute for Medical Research, Johannesburg, So Africa,* W. E. Horton and Company, Ltd., 1917, pp. 1-30.

3. Cecil, R. L., and Austin, J. H.: "Prophylactic Inoculation Against Pneumococcus", *J. Exper. M.* **28**: 19-41 (July 18) 1918.

Table 2b -- Data in Chien 2010 + Augmentations and Historical

Reassessment of Vaccine Efficacy: Influenza-Pneumonia Data in Chien et al. 2010, plus Augmentations and Historical Data

	DATA AS PUBLISHED IN CHIEN TABLES 3 & 4, FIGURES 2 & 3								EFFICACY		INCIDENCE RATIOS				
	VACCINATED				NON-VACCINATED				per Influenza		per Influenza		per Totals		
Source	Total	Influ	Pneu	Died	Total	Influ	Pneu	Died	Pneu	Died	Pneu	Died	Influ	Pneu	Died
Civilian - vaccines with pneumococci															
Watters	1638	89	13	8	1599	471	88	40	10%	13%	1.279	0.94	5.42	6.93	5.12
Cadham/Civil	52999	5203	300	85	85941	21285	1869	563	27%	25%	1.523	1.62	2.52	3.84	4.08
Rosenow	143760	13666	745	276	345133	97253	7534	2951	29%	26%	1.421	1.5	2.96	4.21	4.45
Minaker	6400	111		2	1233782	43671		3716		5%		4.72	2.04		9.64
Cherry		1148	180	36		2002	676	213	26%	22%	2.154	3.39			
McCoy	390	119	23	10	390	103	17	7	9%	9%	0.854	0.81	0.87	0.74	0.7
Chien's "pooled" results - Civilian									34	42					
Averages of straight calculations											1.45	2.17	2.3	3.14	4
Averages ... excluding McCoy											1.59	2.44	2.6	3.76	4.66
Military - vaccines with pneumococci															
EyreHosB T5	1817	25			492	18			Chien -% wt				2.66		
EyreHosB T6		92	9	0		96	17	8	10%						
Cadham /Mili	4842	282	17	5	2758	238	41	17	28%	32%	2.858	4.03	1.48	4.23	5.97
Leishman	15624	221	26	2	43520	2059	583	98	65%	33%	2.407	5.26	3.34	8.05	17.6
McCoy Non-existent	1008			38		130		11		34%		2.24			
Chien's "pooled" results - Military									59	70					
Averages of straight calculations											2.63	3.83	3.8	6.15	11.8+
Ely-StrepOnly	4212	144	0		8486	1409		96					4.86		96/0
Pfeiffer bacillus only -- in Chien data but not calcalations; acknowledged as NOT cause of pandemic influenza/pneumonia															
Hinton-Kane	461	163		28	518	178	na	24							
Wadsworth	44	12		1	102	27	na	0							
Duval -Harris	981	27	0		338	130	41								
Barnes	152	25			113	23	na								
AUGMENTATIONS: Cadham-Civilian & Rosenow: Benefits of 1-3 versus one vaccination; & Rosenow Table 9 Controlled Study															
Cad.C-1+2:0	52999	5203	300	85	85941	21285	1869	563					2.52	3.84	4.08
Cad.C-1x : 0	28,815	2843	177	61	85941	21285	1869	563					2.51	3.54	3.09
Cad.C-2x : 0	24184	2360	123	24	85941	21285	1869	563					2.54	4.28	6.6
Ros.1+2+3:0	143760	13666	745	276	345133	97253	7534	2951					2.96	4.21	4.45
Ros. - 1x : 0	26936	3184	242	81	345133	97253	7534	2951					2.38	2.43	2.84
Ros. - 2x : 0	23348	2265	75	61	345133	97253	7534	2951					2.9	6.8	3.27
Ros. - 3x : 0	93476	8217	428	134	345133	97253	7534	2951					3.21	4.77	5.96
Ros. Table 9	8306	257	8	4	9388	1878	113	52					6.47	12.5	11.5
HISTORICAL															
Cecil Austin	12519		17	2	19481		173	48						6.54	15.4
Cecil Vaughn	13460		363	79	3415		327	73						3.55	3.64
CV-ex 1st wk	13460		155	19	3415		327	73						8.32	15.1
Sherman-	19913	561		15	1687	588		42					12.4		33.1

Explanation of calculations in Table 2b:

A. DATA AS PUBLISHED IN CHIEN 2010

Table 2b provides the raw data presented in Chien 2010, for a number of 1918-9 studies involving killed mixed-pneumococci vaccines, plus one using streptococci and four with Pfeiffer bacillus. Available data for each study indicating numbers of persons "vaccinated" versus "non-vaccinated" are presented, although only the vaccines with pneumococci are being assessed.

B. VACCINE EFFICACY (VE) Calculations

In Table 2b, under "Vaccine Efficacy/ Efficiency", the vertical section labeled "Chien", lists percentage weights and "pooled results" directly as in Chien.

Under vertical sections labeled "Calcs. per Yule15,Orenstein85", calculations use the formula:
VE = (ARU - ARV)/ARU (x 100), where
ARU = unvaccinated attack rate and ARV = vaccinated attack rate. Thus for Cadham / Military the VE for "per Influenza","Pneumonia" is:
$((41/238 - 17/282)/(41/238))(x100) = 65$
The remaining "Vaccine Efficacy" values in the "Vaccine Efficacy/ Efficiency" section are calculated in this manner.

C. INCIDENCE RATIOS (IR) Calculations

Incidence ratios (IR) are calculated as
IR = ARU/ARV. Thus for Cadham /Military, the IR for "Pneumonia", "per Influenza" is:
$(41/238) / (17/282) = 2.858$.

Focusing on the last column in Table 2b, Incidence Ratios for "per Totals – Died", with the single glaring exception of the McCoy "study", the incidence of death for the unvaccinated was universally several times as high as for the vaccinated – i.e., it was from 4.08 to 17.6 times more likely that the unvaccinated would die as compared to the vaccinated!

D. Miscellaneous Notes re Data:

"Cadham/Military" – died (vaccinated and non; cols. F and J) are mislabled as "Eyre" in Chien's Fig. 3. These items are shown correctly here.

"EyreHosB T5" – Eyre Military Hospital B Table 5 as shown in Chien Table 3. These are not used in Chien's assessment.

"EyreHosB T6" – Eyre Military Hospital B Table 6 as used in Chien'a Fig.2. Data shown for totals of vaccinated receiving 1+2 inoculations

"McCoy Non-existent" – This data does not exist anywhere in Chien article except Chien Figure 3. This appears to be mangled (inconsistent) data from Duval and Harris. See discussion on p. 27, Ch. 3.

E. AUGMENTATIONS

– Particularly notable details and other data listed in Table 2b that had not been discussed or listed in Chien 2010.

For a number of studies, the odds of survival increased when a more complete series of vaccines was administered:

For Rosenow, incidence of death in the unvaccinated (last column) was 5.96 times higher than in those receiving a full series of 3 vaccinations, 3.27 times higher than in those receiving 2 vaccinations, and 2.84 times higher than those receiving one vaccination – for an average of 4.46 for those receiving 1-3 doses. And in one relatively more "controlled" study of Rosenow's (Table 9), incidence of death for unvaccinated was 11.5 times greater than for the vaccinated.

Similarly for Cadham/Civilian, incidence of death in unvaccinated was 6.6 times that in those receiving 2 vaccinations, and 3.09 times that in those receiving one vaccination – for an average of 4.08 for those receiving 1-2 doses.

F. HISTORICAL

Also included in Table 2b is pneumonia-only vaccine data from Cecil and Austin (*J.Exp. Med.* July 1, 1918) [see discussions pages 63-5 below] and Cecil and Vaughn (February 15 1919 *J Exp Med,* 457-83) [see discussions pages 88-90 below]; and influenza-only data of Sherman (in *JAMA* 71, Dec. 21, 1918) [see table/discussion on page 82 below]. Also shown for Cecil and Vaughn is edited data excluding cases in first week after vaccination versus no vaccine [as discussed on page 89-90].

- Cadham: "The majority of these inoculations were given in the earlier stages of the epidemic."
- Watters, Minaker and Leishmann indicated most of their vaccinations came early in the epidemic, and involved equal observation periods.
[See Appendices H, D, G, K, E, resp.]

- How might this Chien 2010 error be explained?
Chien 2010 cited U.Minn. historian J.M. Eyler (Appendix C – *J. Hist. Med. Allied Sci., 2009*). Eyler, referring to Rosenow and the other pneumococcus vaccines, had erroneously stated: "*Such vaccines were used more often later in the epidemic*", citing McCoy *(JAMA* **73**, p.402, 1919*)*. But Eyler was absolutely incorrect regarding Rosenow's etc. vaccines (see above); and had clearly misread McCoy. In fact, **McCoy had clearly been referring to "a vaccine made from the influenza [Pfeiffer's] bacillus alone"**! Eyler wrongfully referred to this as involving vaccines other than Pfeiffers, and Chien 2010 adopted Eyler's (erroneous) perspective, apparently without checking either the original McCoy 1918 article [Appendix L] nor Eyler 2009 [Appendix B]. Thus might Chien 2010's statement that: " ... *the scientific quality of 1918 vaccine studies was low by today's standards ...*" be

properly challenged, both from perspective of the expemplary quality of most of the historical pandemic articles (Appendices A-L), particularly so in the face of the extenuating circumstances of the pandemic, and the decidably-unscientific quality of Chien 2010 itself.

- Chien 2010's dilemma – methodology versus ethics:

Regarding the Chien 2010 charge that the reviewed pandemic articles suffered from "such methodological flaws as lack of subject randomization", it must be further noted that the "absolute" theoretical standards advocated by Chien 2010 were (and still are to an extent) in fact absurdly impossible, particularly given the exigencies of the pandemic – and, moreover, innately unethical. In attempts purportedly to discredit Rosenow and others, who actually did succeed in developing and using effective vaccines, McCoy sought to exclude from consideration any vaccines developed after an epidemic had started; therefore the two worlds could never meet. And in their defense of McCoy's legacy, Eyler and Chien enthusiastically rallied in support. Indeed, even modern standards are more, and necessarily so, flexible on this point.

Insofar as locally-produced pneumonia vaccines had already been shown to be effective by Cecil and Austin (and in prior studies by Wright, Lister, Rosenow and others), Rosenow and the others could not morally blanketly employ a random sample that purposely denied this methodology from a particular population. Indeed, once a vaccine methodology had been proven, to purposely withhold it from a "control group" that was not receiving vaccine, then as now, would have clearly been unethical. [e.g., for modern discussions of "field efficacy", please see Chapter 7, Theoretical Considerations, and source articles: A Weinberg & PG Szilagyi, *JID* 2010:201 (1 June), 1607; WA Orenstein, RH Bernier, AR Hinman, *Epidemiol Rev* 1988; 10:212–241; WA Orenstein, RH Bernier, TJ Dondero, Chien 2010, *Bull World Health Organ* 1985; 63:1055–1068.]

> Historical Side-bar: As per Neuhauser etal., 2008, as of the time of Cecil's death in 1965, his Textbook of Medicine had made him "the best known American physician in the world". Neuhauser praised Cecil for his "clear … methodological awareness" of the role of controlled trials throughout his career. His pioneering and contributions to the history of controlled trials began soon after joining the U.S. Army in 1917, when he was asked by the Surgeon General to study pneumonia, and "carried out two very large trials to assess the value of vaccination." [i.e., the Cecil-Austin and Cecil-Vaughn studies]. Cecil was noted as "creative in conducting his vaccine trials in circumstances largely outside his control", i.e., the 1918 pandemic, given the impossibility of a "textbook" controlled trial under such circumstances.

- Chien 2010's flaws don't stop there. As if the above fatal flaws were not already cause for retraction of the Chien 2010, the "buck" cannot simply be passed off to Eyler and McCoy.

For example, of a total of four final results of their assessment [see Table 2b – "pooled results" under "Vaccine Efficacy"], Chien 2010 refers to the "military/fatality" category as the **"most accurate"**, which is pretty sad, in that it is anything but accurate. The source of one of three data sets used in this "most accurate" result simply does not exist (the listed McCoy "military" study), and the data Chien lists for it are not to be found in any of the assessed studies. A second of these three data sets is mislabeled, "Eyre" instead of Cadham – a less serious error, but raising further questions about the Chien 2010 work overall. Thus aside from the blind acceptance of the Eyler polemics as gospel, Chien 2010 itself is highly suspect on its own.

- *"Historian" Eyler plays it loose with history.* Referring to "vaccines made up of organisms ... that had been isolated ... during the outbreak", Eyler stated: *"Such vaccines were used more often later in the epidemic when confidence in the causal role of the Pfeiffer's bacillus waned. Such vaccines were usually defended as measures to prevent the bacterial pneumonias that so often kill influenza's victims."* [John M. Eyler; see Appendix B]
- *This statement is grossly incorrect on multiple counts*:
   1. Confidence in the supposed causal role of Pfeiffer's was clearly lacking even before, and certainly by early in, the pandemic.
      a. October 14, 1918, in England: At a conference at the UK War Office on Oct. 14, 1918 chaired by Sir William Leishman, the committee concluded "the majority of those present were agreed that there was considerable doubt as to the primary etiological significance of the Bacillus influenzae of Pfeiffer ..." [The Lancet, October 26, 1918, p. 565]
      b. Dec. 8-11, 1918, in the U.S.: At the APHA Annual Meeting held in Chicago Dec. 8-11, 1918, report in "Society Proceedings", Col. Victor Vaughn stated: "We have used influenza vaccine in great quantities, all they could make in the Army laboratory, and have used all that Dr. McCoy could spare, and also have used that which Dr. Park has furnished us from the New York laboratory, and I do not hesitate to say that it has not done one bit of good. Speaking on this point with the evidence of the Pfeiffer bacillus not being the cause of influenza, I can agree with those who have spoken." [JAMA 71, Dec. 21, 1918]
   2. As documented above, the locally isolated vaccines (anti-pneumonia) were in use from the very start of the pandemic and indeed to some extent had been proven effective against pneumonia for years prior.
   3. And these anti-pneumonia vaccines were **specifically intended**, not **"defended"**, as measures to prevent the bacterial pneumonias.

- *Eyler's penchant for polemics:* Eyler keeps the Pfeiffer's bacillus hypothesis on life support by dedicating half of his 2009 article to discussions of it, playing up the (failed!) Park and Leary Pfeiffer's-bacillus vaccines, and slamming the *"other vaccines and other producers, most of whom were less cautious than these two ... [and who] added ... other organisms to concoct witches' brews of injectable fluids"*. [i.e. including Rosenow and the other legitimate investigators! – see Eyler, p. 404-5].

- *Eyler - omitting relevant data to accentuate the negative - a few examples:*
   Eyler offers a rejection of efforts on Puget Sound (Ely, Lloyd and Hitchcock) based on the circumstance that none of the units under observation could be deliberately divided into experimental and control groups and *"It was possible to*

observe vaccinated and the unvaccinated men simultaneously in only two of these units."

Eyler neglects to mention that in these two units, of 2931 vaccinated there were 94 cases (81 of these before vaccination completed) and no deaths; compared to 4327 unvaccinated with 596 cases overall and 63 deaths. In the entire camp, among 4212 vaccinated, there were 144 cases (112 before vaccination completed) with no deaths; compared to 8486 unvaccinated with 1409 cases and 96 deaths. [p. 411]
Likewise regarding Minaker and Irvine's work at the Naval Training Station in San Francisco, Eyler rejects the validity of the study based on the circumstance that "they were unable to divide naval units into vaccinated and unvaccinated groups". [Eyler p.412] No mention is made of the actual results reported by Minaker and Irvine, i.e., of 6400 vaccinated, 111 came down with influenza and 2 died (0.031 %); whereas among 1,233,782 unvaccinated, 43,671 with influenza and 3716 died (0.301 %), or 9.6 times more deaths among unvaccinated on a percentage basis.

Indeed, had Eyler or Chien 2010 merely mentioned Cecil's well-documented successes with pneumona vaccines, their attack on the anti-pneumonia vaccines (based on their supposed lack of controls) would have been substantially undermined.

Referring to Rosenow's work as *"Among the largest and most ambitious of these early vaccine trials"* [clearly inconsistent with Eyler's own false assertion that these studies occurred late in the pandemic], Eyler criticizes Rosenow for his insistence that the vaccine be comprised of the organisms from the epidemic itself, and seeks to reject Rosenow's method because it did not begin before the epidemic [which of course was not possible if organisms from the epidemic were to comprise the vaccine].

Further seeking to dismiss Rosenow's results as "disappointing", Eyler states that *"Although ... over 140,000 individuals had received his vaccine, he received reports from only 530 physicians which were complete enough to use in compiling his results"*. Whereas, as detailed in Rosenow's published data [JAMA 73 (1918) p. 398], sufficiently complete reports were indeed received from 530 physicians reporting on a total of 488,893 persons, which were in fact comprised of 143,760 vaccinated persons, 13,666 (9.5%) of whom got influenza, with 276 (0.19%) deaths, compared with reports received of 345,133 not vaccinated of whom 97,252 (28.2%) got influenza and 2951 (0.85%). [Eyler 412-13]

Eyler 2009's polemics and misrepresentations continue, as exemplified in his transition from slamming Rosenow to his pandering characterization of the George McCoy "study": *"More definitive and provocative was the article of a single-column's length in JAMA by George McCoy ... The team tested Rosenow's vaccine, the influenza vaccine with the greatest scientific pretensions. ... McCoy and associates concluded that Rosenow's vaccine offered no protection whatever. ..."* (Eyler referring here to GW McCoy, *JAMA 71, p. 1997, 1918*; see Appendix L.)

- *Speaking of pretensions:* Insofar as McCoy 1918 had claimed he was using, and had disproved, "Rosenow's vaccine", several curious aspects are noted:

1. Critical details in McCoy's one column JAMA article are missing or even misleading, e.g., notably the location. Insofar as McCoy stated the vaccine was obtained from F. O. Tonney of the Chicago Dept. of Health [known to have complied with the Rosenow methodology], a reader might logically assume [as had this writer] that the test took place in Illinois.

2. Indeed, as Rosenow had emphasized (*JAMA 72, p. 34, 1919)*: "The vaccine should contain freshly isolated strains ... [and] conform as nearly as practicable to the respective flora of the disease in the communities in which the vaccine is to be used."

3. However, the location, while not disclosed in this *JAMA* item, was disclosed elsewhere as a mental institution in California (see p. 27, below). So the McCoy vaccines were neither freshly isolated nor strains in circulation within the McCoy study area.

4. Whereas, when this vaccine was properly used locally in Chicago by F. O. Tonney: "The ratio of influenza patients developing pneumonia in the unvaccinated of industrial groups studied was 1 in 21, while in the vaccinated it was 1 in 184. The ratio of influenza cases terminating fatally in the unvaccinated of the industrial groups in Chicago was 1 in 48, and in the completely vaccinated there were none in the 1201 cases reported. The influenza in vaccinated individuals occurred almost exclusively in those who had received one vaccination." [*JAMA* 71, Dec. 21, 1918, p. 2098]

Table 3: EC Rosenow (& BF Sturvidant) 1918-1919 vaccine results:

			Incidence in Each 1,000 Persons		
	Groups	Persons	Influenza	Pneumonia	Deaths
Nineteen counties in Minnesota	Vaccinated	17,532	102.8	4.2	0.8
	Unvaccinated	36,100	373.5	20.4	6.35
Olmsted County, Minnesota	Vaccinated	9,300	41.0	3.0	0.64
	Unvaccinated	8,700	248.0	13.1	4.00
Institutions	Vaccinated	8,306	31.0	1.0	0.5
	Unvaccinated	9,388	200.0	12.0	5.9
Hospitals	Vaccinated	57		21.0	5.0
	Unvaccinated	609		57.0	22.0
Results from questionnaires	Vaccinated	93,476	87.0	4.4	1.43
	Unvaccinated	345,133	281.0	21.0	8.55
Influenza complicating pregnancy	Vaccinated	997	109.0	27.0	14.0
	Unvaccinated	3,656	294.0	80.0	59.9

[Data from Rosenow's Tables 6-11 in *JAMA* 1919, 73, 396-401; E.C. Rosenow and B.F. Sturdivant, as summarized in E.C.Rosenow, *Minnesota Medicine*, June 1929]

- How does the McCoy civilian study compare with the other items listed in Chien?
Noting particularly the last column in Table 2b, incidence of death in unvaccinated versus vaccinated, the results of the McCoy civilian study stick out like a sore thumb as compared to all of the other studies listed. Calculated from the data for the other

six studies for which death data is listed within the Chien 2010 report, the incidence of death for the unvaccinated is from 4.08 to 17.6 times greater than that for the vaccinated, versus 0.7 for McCoy.

- How was McCoy's work viewed by his contemporaries?   On August 16 1919, Dr. Will Walter, in J.R. Herrick's concluding article in JAMA's 8-part 1919 Symposium on Influenza, stated: "Dr. McCoy's records, so far as they relate to preventive inoculation, show a violation of the fundamental principles laid down by Wright, who always was very emphatic and still insists on the postulate that if you are going to do preventive inoculation in the presence of an epidemic you must use very small doses – infinitesimal doses. In the cases I have seen reported by Dr. McCoy as failing to show results, enormous doses were given [2-3 times larger than Rosenow], and not only that, but they were repeated on the third and again on the fifth day [versus 7 days per Rosenow]. This would be the very method to bring about a negative phase and therefore to increase the susceptibility of the patients to the organisms against which we are inoculating. It must not be forgotten that this is done not to prevent influenza, the cause of which is unknown, but to immunize, as Dr. Rosenow says, against the known organisms which kill."

Chapter 3. A Critical Review of Chien 2010 (Appendix A) – Raw Notes

http://jid.oxfordjournals.org/content/202/11/1639.full and
http://www.ncbi.nlm.nih.gov/pubmed/21028954
Yu-Wen Chien, **Keith P. Klugman** and **David M. Morens**, *Journal of Infectious Diseases*, December 2010 Volume <u>202</u>, Issue <u>11</u>, Pp. 1639-1643, "Efficacy of Whole-Cell Killed Bacterial Vaccines in Preventing Pneumonia and Death during the 1918 Influenza Pandemic"

Most of these (bacterial) vaccines did in fact reduce pneumonia and death; however, they also substantially reduced the incidence of influenza, often in nearly the same or even greater proportions. By obscuring this fact, by "moving the goalposts", this study is worse than worthless. Given the prominence of its authors within the ruling hierarchy of NIH, this study is indeed extremely harmful to the prospects of conducting an honest and legitimate discussion of the 1918-9 pandemic, and beyond this it is damaging to our basic understanding of pandemics, influenza and pneumonia overall.

Chien 2010 incorporates discussions of two distinct types of vaccine efforts – one based on the already-largely-discredited idea of Pfeiffer's 1892 so called "influenzae bacillum", and the other based on historical work on pneumonia vaccines of Wright and Lister, from 1912, and by others, e.g., Rosenow.
Rosenow had been publishing on pneumonia and the pneumococcus from 1903, with 33 articles listed in the Index Medicus prior to the pandemic including 13 in *JID* from 1904, and 8 in *JAMA* from 1905. For example, see Rosenow, E.C., "Immunization in pneumococcus infections", *JAMA* 59:795-796, 1912, and *Science Magazine*, 1908; treatment of pneumonia with autolysed pneumococci, based on research dating from 1910, *JAMA* 59:2203-2240, 1913 (with L. Hektoen); *JAMA* 67:1929-1930, 1916 (with F. H. Falls.); and "Results in two hundred cases." *JAMA* 70:759-763, 1918.
Given the general uncertainty regarding the cause of influenza at the time of the start of the pandemic, Rosenow specifically emphasized that his work was directed not at influenza but rather at reducing pneumonia and pneumonia death. The attempt by Chien 2010 to filter it through influenza incidence is absolutely inappropriate, and impossibly biased against objectively assessing the possible relation between the cause of so-called pandemic influenza and the cause of the so-called pneumonia that is commonly associated with it. Such a possibility is not merely ignored; it is rejected out of hand by Chien 2010 as being "not consistent with our understanding of influenza etiology". It is noted that even McCoy had addressed, and not totally dismissed, this possibility.
Chien 2010 is highly qualified throughout as limited to comparisons among patients that had contracted influenza, i.e., not between totals of all persons. For example, on the first page are two qualifying references to "*patients with influenza*" and two additional "*influenza-associated*" qualifiers; on the second page, six of the former and one of the latter, asserting this approach was supposedly "*addressing methodological flaws*" of the studies. Notwithstanding its assertions of "*significant*

methodological problems" and "*systematic biases in these studies*" being considered, the restriction of consideration to only those persons with influenza in fact introduced a gross methodological problem and bias relative to the studies being considered, grossly misrepresenting their intentions and results.

The alleged fundamental bias Chien 2010 sought to address is the claim that the original pandemic articles involved unequal observation periods.   Yet when the individual original historical articles are reviewed, one is impressed by the efforts taken by each to provide some measure of respectable valid control and consistency, exemplary efforts indeed given the emergency circumstance.

And Chien 2010 repeatedly dismisses the competency of these early 20th century articles while playing up a very short McCoy 1918 article (Appendix L) as the best quality study. On the contrary, McCoy 1918 was grossly deficient, e.g., for reasons of small-sample size, and using a vaccine in California that had been specifically designed for Illinois (and arguably trying to obscure its geographic impropriety). In comparison, the other original historical items [Appendices D-H, K are for the most part thoughtful and detailed presentations of decent scientific investigations, which are clearly worth far more consideration that given by (and deserving of) Chien 2010.

p. 1639 From the outset, the Chien 2010 authors posit a number of assumptions that underly their study, which on examination tend to irreparably render their entire article problematic, even beyond its improper framework, e.g.

"*Many contemporaneous investigators erroneously believed that bacteria, in particular Bacillus influenzae [Pfeiffer's bacillus, aka "Haemophilus influenzae"] was the cause of influenza [6]. ...*

[NO, by this time, most did not, as discussed in more detail below!]

"*It was also generally believed, however, that most 1918 pandemic influenza deaths resulted from secondary bacterial pneumonia following primary influenza infections of whatever cause [2]. ...*

[No, a substantial portion believed there was one cause of both, even discussed as a possibility by McCoy; and de facto in essence documented in reduced influenza incidence in vaccinated individuals!]

"*In attempts to prevent the primary disease of influenza, to reduce pneumonia and mortality, and to investigate the etiology of influenza, many bacterial vaccines were produced, tested, and administered during the 1918 pandemic. ...*

[No. most of the bacterial vaccines were specifically directed at the pneumonia/ streptococcal cause. They were NOT intended to prevent influenza, but in fact did!]

"*Here we review studies of whole-cell bacterial vaccines administered to healthy subjects during the 1918 pandemic to examine their efficacy in preventing influenza-associated pneumonia and mortality ...*

[Here the Chien 2010 authors appear to contradict their basic (albeit-faulty) methodology involving "influenza-infected" versus "healthy" subjects, nonetheless here using weasel-worded justification for filtering results through influenza cases in any case.

"An important concern about such a review is that the scientific quality of 1918 vaccine studies was low by today's standards, owing to such methodological flaws as lack of subject randomization. ...

[None seemingly were as deficient as Chien 2010 from an objective scientific perspective, as further documented below]

"Moreover, whereas most vaccinations were given during the declining phase of the pandemic (fall–winter 1918–1919), the incidences of influenza, influenza-associated pneumonia, and deaths in vaccinated individuals were compared with the same outcomes in unvaccinated individuals from the beginning of the epidemic [6, 7], introducing unequal observation periods more favorable to vaccinated individuals."

[NO ... WRONG -- this is not true; most were used early! McCoy, Chien's ref.7 (Appendix J), discussed this possible problem as relates to vaccines employing **Pfeiffer's bacillus only**!; Eyler wrongfully referred this to the vaccines other than the Pfeiffers vaccines, and Chien took it all further from reality!. [see also Chapter 4 (Eyler), Chapter 5 (History) & McCoy, August 1919 (Appendix J)]

CHIEN 2010 resumes:

"In addition, vaccinated individuals might come from select populations with reduced exposure or susceptibility to influenza because they had not had influenza between the appearance of the pandemic and the start of vaccination. Not fully appreciating such potential design flaws, investigators studying bacterial vaccines often believed that they had demonstrated a reduction in the incidence of influenza, which is not consistent with our understanding of influenza etiology. We reasoned that any true effect of bacterial vaccines on influenza disease might more plausibly result from reduced attack rates of secondary bacterial pneumonias and consequent reduced case fatality rates among patients with influenza. To examine this possibility while addressing methodological flaws of the original studies, we reanalyzed published data, asking whether vaccinated patients who developed influenza had lower attack rates of pneumonia or lower case fatality rates than unvaccinated patients with influenza. This approach should diminish bias caused by unequal observation periods, because these measures were less likely to be influenced by changing influenza incidence during the progress of the pandemic. In addition, the attack rate of pneumonia and case fatality rates among patients with influenza seems to be higher in the later phase of influenza epidemics [8–10]. Therefore, this approach may result in more conservative estimates of vaccine efficacy (VE), because the vaccinated individuals were more likely to be from the later phase of the 1918 pandemic."

There is a lot packed in here, some of which arguably may be wrong: e.g., that the pneumonia was secondary, rather than an extension of the inciting disease, that the bacterial vaccines did not reduce influenza "which is not consistent with our understanding of influenza etiology", and the charge of "unequal observation periods". In particular Rosenow's work had explicitly "put aside the debated question as to the cause of the initial symptoms and considered primarily the possibility of immunizing persons against ... the common causes of death in this disease." And since most (3/4) of Cadham's civilian vaccines were also provided by

Rosenow [see Appendix D – Cadham, p. 886], some 80% of the total vaccines in the studies considered by Chien 2010 involved vaccines primarily directed at the pneumonia and deaths – but did in fact reduce influenza substantially in any case. The Ely streptococcal vaccine, which specifically was directly targeting influenza, did likewise reduce influenza as well deaths.

It is noted that Rosenow also provided a more highly qualified set of controlled data, whose results were even more positive than his larger total report. Further, death-ratios of unvaccinated to vaccinated for three of the remaining five civilian studies in Chien were closely on the order of the Rosenow larger report (Watters 5.12, Minaker 9.63, Cadham 5.97, Rosenow 4.45). Thus the overall results seem to buttress the validity of the Rosenow larger report results. The Leishmann/Military ratio of 17.59 admittedly might be partly attributed to the small sample size, e.g., at least small number of deaths among the inoculated.

Regarding the McCoy 1918 "study", Chien again states " ... *the best-quality study [by McCoy] with a small sample size suggested no vaccine effect ... .*" Aside from the fundamental disqualifying nature of the McCoy "work", i.e., involving non-local and non-current organism(s), the small sample size itself undermines the suggestion that it is the "best" quality study or even of sufficient quality to be considered.

Discussion: Chien 2010 correctly note that Rosenow had included B. influenza in an earlier vaccine, as per Rosenow's preliminary report from 6 months prior to the Rosenow report that was included in the Chien study. However, Rosenow had deleted it from subsequent vaccines, and emphasized the (polymorphic) green-producing diplococcus-streptococcus-pneumococcus strain as the predominant and seemingly most important strain in his studies, as did several other studies. Granted that many studies were undecided as to a predominant strain, but of those that indicated a suspect predominant strain, the green-producing streptococcus (S. viridans), as the overwhelming choice.

Insofar as McCoy claimed he was using and had disproved "Rosenow's vaccine", several curious aspects are noted:

1. Critical details in McCoy's one column JAMA article are missing or even misleading, e.g., notably the location. Insofar as McCoy stated the vaccine was obtained from the Chicago Dept. of Health [which is known to have worked with Rosenow on its vaccines], a reader of the JAMA item might logically assume [as had this writer] that the test took place in Illinois.

2. Indeed, and as noted in the Chien article as per above, it was well known that Rosenow had emphasized the need for freshly isolated strains composed of strains in circulation.

3. However, the location, while not disclosed in this JAMA item, was disclosed elsewhere (by Kellog, July 1919, *California State Journal of Medicine*, **17** p. 230) as a mental institution in California. So beyond the above-referred issue of use of strains other than those being used in the study under comparison, even if the McCoy vaccines were of the same composition, they were neither freshly isolated nor strains in circulation within the McCoy study area.

4. But most damning of McCoy was criticism of McCoy's vaccine efforts as misguided and doomed to have failed, as particularly discussed by Will Walter above.   As is shown in the Chien article, McCoy used much larger doses of respective comparable strains (2-3 times larger) and at far more frequent intervals (48 hours versus 7 days per Rosenow). See comments by Dr. Will Walter, page 22-23 above [from *JAMA* August 16 1919: James R. Herrick, p. 486].

It may also be noted that data presented in Chien is not consistent; e.g.:
- Minaker is excluded from Chien's Figure 2, but included in Figure 3. This exclusion is necessary, as Minaker does not include pneumonia data, which raises the question as to why Minaker was included in Chien 2010 study in the first case.
- Data given for Eyre and Lowe in Chien's both Table 1 and Figure 2 are from Eyre and Lowe's data for Military Hospital B only, from Eyre and Lowe's Tables 5 and 6 resp. This data is far below Eyre and Lowe's totals otherwise presented. Moreover the totals of influenza cases in these two instances are not consistent; the former gives figures of 25 and 18 for vaccinated versus not, resp., whereas the latter gives figures of 92 and 96, resp.
- In Figure 3 data given for Eyre and Lowe is clearly from Cadham, as seen in corresponding denominators for Cadham in Figure 2 and numerators for Cadham in Table 3.
-   Also in Chien's Figure 3, data given in Military studies section for presumed McCoy article is a total mystery, having no relation to the minimal data McCoy otherwise cited, and rather might speculatively be suggested to be somewhat mangled data from Duval and Harris; at least that seems to be the only data from the cited sources that sort of fits the numbers of Chien: Data presented in Duval and Harris's Tables 1 and 2 for groups A and B is indeed consistent with that in Chien's Table 3, i.e., influenza incidence of 27/981 vaccinated versus 130/338 unvaccinated; however, the numbers Chien presents for McCoy/military in his Figure 3 of (a) 1008, which happens to equal the sum of numerator and denominator of $27 + 981$, makes no sense at all; and (b) 130, happens to equal Duval's number of influenza cases among unvaccinated, a combination of coincidences albeit nonsensical. Duval and Harris do not offer mortality data at all, and there is no clue as to where the number 11 came from; but another coincidence is that the above cited number 27 plus the mystery 11 equals 38, the other number given by Chien in his Figure 3 for the nonexistent McCoy military study. And since this unexplained and arguably bogus data set is given 34% weight in Chien's Figure 3, i.e., the largest weight value in this key presentation in his study's so-called meta-analysis, i.e., the component relating to fatality rates, and is clearly worthless, on this alone the entire Chien article fails.

Chapter 4. A Review of the Fabrications of John Eyler 2009-2010

John M. Eyler: The significance of Eyler's work cannot be overstated; his is the primary historical reference work. As documented herein, Eyler was heavily relied upon by Chien 2010, and thereby a key underpinning of current assessments of the actions to be taken relative to the possibility of a future pandemic, etc.

Eyler's work is beyond merely sloppy and unprofessional in its unsupported presumptions and lack of proper scholarship.   It is blatantly misleading and seemingly purposely so, and absolutely incorrect in a number of areas.

Eyler 2009

John M. Eyler, "The Fog of Research: Influenza Vaccine Trials during the 1918-9 Pandemic", *Journal of the History of Medicine*, **Volume 64**, October 2009, 401-428.
 ["Research funding was provided by ... the Burroughs-Wellcome Fund" (Burroughs-Wellcome is a division of Glaxo Smith Klein)]

p. 401 - Abstract [*annotated by shs*]

"ABSTRACT. Bacterial vaccines of various sorts were widely used for both preventive and therapeutic purposes during the great influenza pandemic of 1918–19. Some were derived exclusively from the Pfeiffer's bacillus, the presumed cause of influenza, while others contained one or more other organisms found in the lungs of victims. Although initially most reports of the use of these vaccines claimed that they prevented influenza or pneumonia, the results were inconsistent and sometimes contradictory ...
[Whereas, some early vaccines were exclusively from Pfeiffers, by this time there was already a general consensus that Pfeiffer's was no longer "the presumed cause" of pandemic influenza, and in fact most of the others did not claim to prevent influenza.   Rather most of the others were specifically not intended to prevent influenza and were directed against pneumonia and pneumonia death, were effective in doing so, were internally consistent, and in the main not contradictory among themselves.   In fact, there is an impressive consistency among the various and generally successful vaccine attempts, as shown in Tables 2 and 2b herein, and Appendices D-H,K].
"... During the course of the debates over the efficacy of these vaccines, it became clear that the medical profession had no consensus on what constituted a proper vaccine trial. Even among those who asserted that clinical impression was not enough, there was no agreement on how a trial ought to be conducted. The American Public Health Association, through its Working Program on Influenza, sought to establish standards for the profession. The standards the APHA set in December 1918 guided American vaccine trials for a quarter century."
 "KEYWORDS: influenza vaccines, vaccine trials, clinical trials, American Public Health Association, William Park, George McCoy."

Eyler presents the situation as an indeterminate mish-mosh, into which are inserted early public health officials Park and McCoy. Insodoing, Eyler changes the subject from what did and did not work in the pandemic to an academic approach of how to conduct vaccine trials under ideal circumstances.

Eyler here is essentially rejecting the overwhelmingly positive clinical results in the same fashion that Park and McCoy, whom he cites below, had attempted to do so in 1918-9, in the very midst of the great pandemic. The pandemic was underway, and Park and McCoy sought to impose an impossible standard, under the circumstances, somewhat retrospectively and arbitrarily. In essence they were attempting to change the rules in the middle of the game, with apparent success, and in-so-doing sought to discredit or at least subjugate proven methods of assessment of vaccine effectiveness, e.g., including agglutination tests, animal experiments, antibody tests ("opsonins), etc., as well as considerable and well documented efforts to compare vaccinated and non-vaccinated (controls) involving thousands of persons in a number of studies conducted under particularly-difficult conditions.]

[Neither Park nor McCoy was successful in developing a vaccine, as discussed further in this paper; as to why McCoy in particular sought to discredit the works of others who were successful is not clear. However, as a result of his close relationship with the editor of the Journal of the American Medical Association as well as his position on JAMA's all-powerful committee on chemistry and pharmacy, in conjunction with his position at PHS, his unsupported and unsupportable assertions have taken on an aura of credibility up to and including the present time.]

Excerpts and commentary:

Eyler 2009 is replete with misinformation and prejudicial innuendo. Following are some examples:

pp. 402-4, Eyler discusses attempts by Park and Leary to vaccinate with Pfeiffer's bacillus, notwithstanding that by this time its role had been generally discredited. No mention was made of Park's results; however, at the APHA Annual Meeting held in Chicago Dec. 8-11, 1918, as per a *JAMA* 71, Dec. 21, 1918, report in "Society Proceedings", Col. Victor Vaughn stated: "We have used influenza vaccine in great quantities, all they could make in the Army laboratory, and have used all that Dr. McCoy could spare, and also have used that which Dr. Park has furnished us from the New York laboratory, and I do not hesitate to say that it has not done one bit of good."

As reported by Watters, neither he nor Leary were at first able to isolate the Pfeiffer bacillus. Later, when Leary was able to do so, he decided to attempt a vaccine using only that organism. And Barnes, using Leary's vaccine, concluded "The morbidity was only slightly lower among the vaccinated, and the mortality among those who developed influenza was practically the same whether vaccinated or not."

p. 404 Eyler notes that in addition to the Park and Leary Pfeiffer vaccines, *"there were other vaccines and other producers, most of whom were less cautious than these two."* This slam is totally unsupported and unsupportable, seemingly intended to discredit the many very thorough and cautious attempts at vaccines at this critical time. Eyler's use of the word "most" in this sentence is beyond rude.

In opening his discussion of mixed vaccines, Eyler states:

"Other vaccines were also in use during the great pandemic. These were most often mixed vaccines made up of organisms, known and newly discovered, that had been isolated in wards and death houses during the outbreak. Such vaccines were used more often later in the epidemic when confidence in the causal role of the Pfeiffer's bacillus waned. Such vaccines were usually defended as measures to prevent the bacterial pneumonias that so often kill influenza's victims."

The term "defended" is grossly misleading; in fact the vast majority of these vaccines were specifically "intended" to prevent pneumonia and pneumonia death; and as noted elsewhere in this paper, were actually used early in the epidemic.

p. 404-5. Mentioning the mixed vaccine produced by the Naval medical officers in San Francisco (Minaker and Irvine) which contained pneumococci and streptococci, in addition to Pfeiffer's bacillus, Eyler states: *"Other vaccine producers added staphylococci and several other organisms to concoct witches' brews of injectable fluids"*

[Here Eyler also cites the credible works of Watters, Stone, and Kolmer (Watters who was a close associate of Leary, who otherwise was praised above by Eyler, as discussed elsewhere in this paper) as a prelude to discussing Rosenow's work. In fact virtually any and all organisms included in the mixed vaccines that Eyler refers to, were derived and cultured from Influenzal and Influenzal Pneumonia victims (with the possible exception of some cases wherein stock Pfeiffer's bacillus from Rockefeller were included). Eyler's snarky "witches' brew slam was indeed nothing other than his prejudicial polemics — and utter nonsense.]

p. 405, proceeding to discuss Rosenow's work, Eyler acknowledges that Rosenow's avowed target was the pneumonia, albeit mischaracterizing it as "secondary" infections. Whereas Rosenow's work arguably demonstrated that these were not actually secondary, but rather directly related to the cause of the primary influenzal infection (see particularly E.C. Rosenow, *Studies in Influenza and Pneumonia*, Amazon.com etc.).. Eyler correctly acknowledges the "green producing diplostreptococcus" that Rosenow indicated was of primary importance, but neglected to acknowledge that this organism had been previously and subsequently implicated by several investigators, notably, seemingly initially, by Mathers.

p. 406, Eyler notes: *"Rosenow developed his vaccine **during the early phases** of the outbreak in Minnesota and administered it to doctors and nurses in his own institution, and, when he was convinced that it was safe and effective, the Mayo Foundation distributed it to physicians throughout the upper mid-west."*

Whereas the criticism that vaccines were started in the later phases of the pandemic, as per Eyler's own introduction, is hereby contradicted by …. Eyler!

Eyler further notes Mayo and Rosenow received questionnaires reporting on more than 150,000 vaccinated persons, neglecting to mention that the returned questionnaires involved about a half million persons in all, including those not vaccinated. Rather Eyler seemingly sought to diminish these results with the statement that '*The number of people who received the vaccine distributed by the Mayo Foundation is unknown … .*"

Eyler then states that Rosenow's vaccine was adopted by the Chicago Health Department, for the city and "for distribution throughout Illinois".
[Thus it is acknowledged these were not intended for use in California, by McCoy or anyone else.]

At this point, mid-p. 406, Eyler breaks off from discussion of Rosenow's vaccine, morphing into a reference to pandemic vaccines in general and then a discussion of the ineffective stock vaccines by drug companies, which while totally unrelated and contraindicated by Rosenow's work, were in a sense being lumped with it.

Furthering an intended slam by association, Eyler then states "*Proprietary hucksterism was not limited to the drug industry*" here launching into an attack on Exner and his claimed successful use of vaccines developed 6 years earlier by Ellis Bonime. Eyler notes Bonime was "*a partisan of the oposium theory of immune response and of the therapeutic use of vaccines*".

By "oposium", Eyler undoubtedly was referring to "opsonins", relating to antibody assessment, as originated and employed by Sir Almroth Wright (mentor of Andrew Fleming and originator of autogenous vaccines). Indeed, even Rosenow's and all autogenous vaccines to the present day owe a debt to Wright.

[Specifically regarding the anti-pneumonia vaccine studies assessed by Chien 2010, we find citation of the prior works of Wright and/or his associate Lister (along with Cecil and Austin) in Eyre and Lowe 1918, Minaker, and Rosenow and Sturdevant; and indirect reliance on these original sources in Cadham (via Rosenow) and Leishman (via Eyre and Lowe). This further substantiates that the vaccines listed and assessed in Chien 2010 were in fact directed at pneumonia, not influenza; thus Chien's attempt to measure or filter their effectiveness as against only those patients with influenza is doubly totally bogus.]

Eyler is apparently attempting to write off the great works and legacy of Sir Almroth Wright and his followers as "hucksterism". (Indeed, autogenous vaccines are currently all the rage in medical science as of 2017, even more heavily so in the case of cancer.) Eyler continues trashing Exner for 2/3 of page 407, characterizing Exner's efforts to gain wider use of his vaccine as "boosterism". But Eyler offers no supporting details for his negativity other than the (positive) circumstance that no one who received all three doses of Exner's vaccine contracted influenza, and the only death was among those refusing a second and third injections!

Eyler then again proceeds to merge reference to the perils of stock vaccine with slams on vaccines in general, clearly and improperly implicating Exner's as among them, as without "public or professional constraints". Then Eyler again injects his charge of "hucksterism" against the stock vaccines (which, again, had absolutely nothing to do with Wright and his followers, e.g. Exner), citing pronouncements by the AMA in general against stock vaccines, conflating this improperly with Exner's etc.

P. 408 And in mid-paragraph comes an even more blatant, prime example, of the deplorable manner of Eyler's general rude manner, as he interjects and misrepresents a discussion in the AJPH about vaccines. Here Eyler implies that the AJPH was discussing these same stock vaccines, which is absolutely not the case.

Firstly, quoting Eyler, "*The American Journal of Public Health editorialized that, although it might be better to err on the side of using a useless vaccine rather than to risk preventable influenza deaths, the early experience with these vaccines were contradictory; therefore the public should be warned that they were experimental, so that should these vaccines prove ineffective, public confidence in other vaccines would not be shaken.*"

In fact the *AJPH* article was discussing specific vaccines being used by the state of Massachusetts, with apparent success, i.e., summarily providing details for (1) 44 nurses at Boston City Hospital – 32 vaccinated with no influenza, 8 partly vaccinated with all with mild influenza, and 4 refusing vaccination 2 of which died; and 169 persons at Wretham (Mass.) State School – 66 vaccinated 6 of which had mild influenza, one partly vaccinated died, and of 58 not vaccinated, 33 were sickened and 1 died.

In contrast to Eyler's characterization, here we quote the *AJPH* editorial in entirety (*American Journal of Public Health*, Vol 8 # 10 Oct 1 1918, p. 788): "*The results which are available are interesting and suggestive, but not conclusive; for they all have the weakness that vaccination was not begun until influenza had developed in the institution, and had taken down a number, possibly the most susceptible, who might have taken the disease even if vaccinated. But while we wait for more conclusive statistics, the epidemic rages; any community is, therefore, justified in employing the vaccine, for it is safer to gamble with the cost of preparing and administering the vaccine than with the lives endangered. It will be well to emphasize to the public that the vaccination is experimental, and is not compulsory; otherwise, in the event of its ultimate failure, the whole system of vaccination may be discredited by the public, including that against smallpox, typhoid, etc.*"

Clearly, the *AJPH* editorial did not indicate in any way that the results were "contradictory", only that they were "not conclusive", but nonetheless "suggestive". Within the context of the actual text of this editorial, Eyler here is purposefully being misleading, seeking to use the editorial against vaccines in general. Unfortunately, his comments are neither appropriate to nor anywhere-nearly reflective of the text in the editorial. Of course, all those who are relying on Eyler 2009's failed analyses would do well to take notice of this deficiency, and adjust their derivative work accordingly (i.e., including the likes of Chien, 2010) i.e., supposedly authorative PHS/NIH information relative to the Pandemic of 1918-9.

Still on p, 408: Eyler states "*W.H. Watters, the pathologist at the Massachusetts Homeopathic Hospital, placed heavy reliance on the reports of community physicians who used his vaccine. Most reported that as far as they knew, no patient they vaccinated developed influenza.*" [For the record, Watters reported 8 deaths among 1638 vaccinated persons, versus 40 deaths among 1599 unvaccinated, i.e., a death rate of 5.12 times greater for unvaccinated persons.]

On page 411, Eyler offers a critical rejection of efforts on Puget Sound (Ely, Lloyd and Hitchcock) based on the assertion that adequate separate vaccinated and control groups were not observed. *"Nonetheless, they concluded that their vaccine prevented many illnesses and mitigated the severity of the illnesses in other cases."*

Whereas Ely et al. acknowledged that "It is fair to say that no unit was divided into two parts for the purpose of running experimental subjects and controls side by side. Circumstances were such that this could not well be done. It is also fair to say that in our largest unit (Seamen's Barracks) many cases had already occurred before vaccination could be done; we do not know how many. ... The period of observation was from Sept. 17 to Oct. 21, 1918."

Eyler neglects to mention that among the small sample in the Philadelphia Unit, with 131 vaccinated, there were no deaths, whereas among the 855 unvaccinated there were 21 deaths, or 12.5% deaths; and among the 2800 vaccinated at the Seaman's Barracks, there were also no deaths, compared with the 3472 unvaccinated with 42 deaths, or 9.8 % deaths. And overall, in the entire camp, among a total 4212 vaccinated, there was a total of 144 cases with no deaths; compared to 8486 unvaccinated with 1409 cases and 96 deaths.

Clearly, Eyler's characterization was anything but objective. Actual Ely data:

	Vaccinated					Not Vaccinated				
	Total	Cases	%	Deaths	%	Total	Cases	%	Deaths	%
Philadelphia Unit	131	37*	28.2	0	0	855	168	19.6	21	12.5
Seaman's barracks	2800	57*	2.03	0	0	3472	428	12.3	42	9.8
Subtotals	[2931]	[94]	[3.2]	[0]	[0]	[4327]	[596]		[63]	
Seattle Training Camp 1	---	---	---	---	---	4159	813	19.5	33	4.1
Seattle Training Camp 2	662	11	1.60	0	0					
Marines, Yard & Depot	425	5	1.2	0	0					
Filipino Unit	111	2	1.8	0	0					
Aviation Unit	83	32*	38.5	0	0					
Subtotals	[1281]	[50]		[0]		[4159]	[813]		[33]	
Totals	4212	144*		0		8486	1409		96	

Eyler, on page 412, turns to the Naval Training Station in San Francisco (clearly referring here to Minaker), again giving no details of results, but rather rejecting the validity of the study based on lack of proper control groups, in essence parroting the rejection of all legitimate studies by McCoy, in 1918-9 on this (admitted by many as impossible) standard, which at the time was just being developed by McCoy.

However, in the actual article Minaker makes a point of correlating periods of unvaccinated with vaccinated; "Inoculations of the 1080 of the civilian population were completed by October 16, twenty four days after the start of the pandemic in San Francisco, and the incidence and mortality figures for the city represent the period of time, beginning with the inoculation and running until December 1, when the original epidemic subsided."

Minaker, referring to Mare Island Marines and Mare Island personnel, "The low incidence of the disease in the inoculated persons can only be appreciated when we compare with it the morbidity and mortality of the large population with whom they associated at the same period. We also ask attention to the low incidence of disease of our inoculated hospital corpsmen detailed in military and civilian hospitals in San Francisco, in comparison with the nonvaccinated civilian nurses exposed to the infection under identical conditions. The 3100 men from the San Pedro Naval Camp were inoculated about November 15, at which time the epidemic was in its recrudescence in Los Angeles and vicinity, and the figures given represent only the cases reported in Los Angeles during the period of twenty four days following the inoculation of the men."

In any case, the actual results reported by Minaker and Irvine were certainly worthy of mention, i.e., of 6400 vaccinated, 111 came down with influenza and 2 died (0.031 %); versus among 1233782 unvaccinated, 43,671 with influenza and 3716 died (0.301 %), or 9.6 times more deaths among unvaccinated on a percentage basis. This data was omitted by Eyler, who stated: "None of these difficulties kept the authors from concluding that their vaccine provided a 'noteworthy degree of protection against influenza and its complications'." Indeed, 9.6 times the incidence of death among the unvaccinated, if not noteworthy, what is?

And on page 412, Eyler returns to Rosenow's work. Leading in with the somewhat loaded "Among the largest and most ambitious of these early vaccine trials was that of Edward Rosenow at the Mayo Clinic." Eyler immediately criticizes Rosenow for his insistence that the vaccine be comprised of the organisms isolated from the epidemic itself, and then seeks to reject the Rosenow method because it did not begin before the epidemic.

On page 413, Eyler notes *"the Mayo Foundation distributed the vaccine gratis to physicians and hospitals who requested it and agreed to provide a record of results. The returns, however, were disappointing. Although Rosenow knew that over 140,000 individuals had received his vaccine, he received reports from only 530 physicians"*.

Whereas, as detailed in Rosenow's published data, reports were, indeed, received of 143,760 vaccinated persons, 13,666 of whom got influenza, with 276 deaths (0.192%), compared with reports he received of 345,133 not vaccinated of whom 97,252 got influenza and 2951 died (0.855%). Undoubtedly the number of returns had to be negatively affected by the fact of the pandemic; however, reports were in fact returned involving about a half-million total persons, including more than 140,000 vaccinated individuals.

Eyler 2009 in large measure is easily characterized as a "hatchet job" on Rosenow in particular, throwing the various other 1919 studies "under the bus" at the same time. The actual results of these many studies were blanketly rejected by Eyler 2009 as not complying with the theoretical and generally recognized impossible standards being set mid-pandemic by McCoy. More later.

P. 413: Eyler states *"He [Rosenow] also published tables for two sets of institutionalized patients who were said to be under closer observation. One gave the rates for some 17,000 inmates of unidentified institutions, distinguishing those receiving three injections from the unvaccinated. The other gave incidence rates for influenza and pneumonia, and deaths from pneumonia, among those vaccinated one, two, or three times, and among the unvaccinated in the hospitals of Rochester. In neither instance did Rosenow provide detail on how the vaccinations were conducted or the trial arranged."*

Regarding the "17,000 inmates of unidentified institutions", Eyler clearly intended to refer to data presented in Rosenow's Table 9, JAMA 73, page 400; however, they were NOT inmates – they were factory workers, hospital personnel and office workers.

    Rosenow, E.C., Studies in influenza and pneumonia. IV. Further results of prophylactic inoculation. *Jour. Am. Med. Assn.* 73:396-401, 1919. (With B. F. Sturdivant.)

As per Rosenow: "The results obtained in institutions in which the conditions among the vaccinated and the unvaccinated [Rosenow, p. 400] were comparable are summarized and given in Table 9 in order still further to check the figures. The number of persons in most of the institutions included (fifty- three in all) was small. The opportunity for accurate observation was, therefore, favorable. The institutions included factories, personnel of hospitals, schools, and offices. The proportion of the vaccinated and unvaccinated varied between wide limits. The period of observation in the two groups was the same. The incidence of disease and the number of deaths in almost all instances were lower in the vaccinated than in the unvaccinated group. The total average, as given in Table 9, compares favorably with that of the others. The death rate among the vaccinated is decidedly lower than among the unvaccinated."

Following is the data from Rosenow's Table 9 for these 17,688 persons:

| | Total # | Incidence per 1000 persons | | |
		Influenza	Pneumonia	Death
Vaccinated 3 times	8300	31	1.0	0.5
Not Vaccinated	9388	200	12.0	5.9

As shown in this Table, the persons not vaccinated suffered pneumonia at 12 times the rate of the vaccinated, and died also at a rate equal to 12 times that of the vaccinated.

    The second table to which Eyler referred was totally unrelated to Eyler's above discussion relating to Table 9, but rather a Table 10 and discussion of the relation between vaccination and pregnancy complications. After this came a Table 11 discussing the Rochester hospital results to which Eyler had referred.

    In this latter case Rosenow did not claim that these were comparable groups of vaccinated and unvaccinated. Indeed, immediately prior to Table 11 Rosenow stated, concerning the inability to provide comparisons in Rochester: "A reliable morbidity and mortality rate for each thousand of the vaccinated and unvaccinated could not be determined because such a large percentage of patients remained in Rochester for too short a time. "It was thought that a study of the cases of influenza admitted to the hospitals might, however, be worthwhile."

    This data did not in any way provide comparisons between incidence of influenza in vaccinated versus non-vaccinated; rather All of the persons reported in Table 11 were influenza patients. Although the incidence of death was considerably smaller in the vaccinated persons, Rosenow himself had acknowledged that "The mortality figure in the unvaccinated is abnormally high because only the patients with relatively severe attacks were admitted to the hospitals."

p. 414   provides another example of Eyler finding an aspect of Rosenow to criticize, and ignoring the overwhelming positive data:

In his Table 7, Rosenow provides data from reports from 19 Minnesota counties exclusive of the Mayo Foundation. As per Rosenow's reports received, there were 0.8 deaths per 1000 among 17,532 vaccinated (3 inoculations) versus 6.35 per 1000 among the 36,100 unvaccinated; thus per capita there was an eight times incidence of death among unvaccinated compared with fully vaccinated. For further comparison, Rosenow noted: "Through the cooperation of the Board of Health of Minnesota we were able to check the results as reported to us with the morbidity and mortality figures as reported to them." This data reported 3.2 deaths per 1000 among a population of 472,584 (the death incidence was exclusive of deaths which occurred prior to the use of the vaccine and exclusive of the Mayo Clinic cases, all of which were subtracted from the raw State data; indeed, the raw State data had reported 4.2 deaths per thousand prior to the adjustment downward by analysis), or four times the incidence of death compared to Rosenow's fully-vaccinated in reports. The State Board also provided a total for reported influenza incidence, which was low relative to the State reported death rate, at least in comparison to Rosenow's data. Accordingly, insofar as "Mortality figures … may be considered as fairly accurate", Rosenow suggested "The figures in the table indicating the cases and the deaths as reported to us are believed to be more accurate."

Eyler ignored all of this data, made no mention of death rates which was the substance and purpose of Rosenow's inclusion of this data, focused instead only on the incidence of reported influenza cases in Rosenow's data versus that in the State reports, and mischaracterized the entire table and associated very detailed study as an "attempt [by Rosenow] to determine the incidence rate for influenza in the general population". Thus Eyler sought to dismiss the significance of all of Rosenow's results on that basis alone.

Recapping, Eyler was off base on several counts:

(1) he totally ignored the central importance of the death rate comparisons; the influenza rates were incidental to the central importance of death rates, and in any case shown to be too low relative to the death rates;

(2) Rosenow's detailed data set for 19 counties had all come from the same, very detailed and comprehensive reports from a uniform set of respondents, whereas the State influenza incidence data was from two distinct sources
(a) actual influenza cases serious enough to be reported to the State, compared with
(b) total population; and

(3) Rosenow had clearly stated that given the uncertainty over the cause of influenza, his efforts were directed at lowering the death rate from pneumonia, thus rejecting his work on the basis of influenza incidence is irrelevant and arguably-intentionally ignorant.

p. 414 As he transitioned out of attacking Rosenow in his concluding sentence, Eyler attempts to diminish the significance of the data in Rosenow's Table 7 with an improper inference that it based on Rosenow's opinion rather than fact; and them morphs into his next paragraph with a slam on vaccine effectiveness in general, with an inescapably clear inference of inclusion of Rosenow. **This treatment by Eyler is so typical of his characteristic approach / attack, so inherently perjorative, that it is quoted here in entirety:**

"… Based on this evidence, Rosenow concluded that individuals who received three doses of his vaccine experienced one-third the incidence and one-quarter the mortality from influenza as the unvaccinated.

"Regardless of the vaccine they tested or the approach they used, most researchers who published the results of influenza vaccine trials in 1918 concluded that their vaccine was effective. …"

This is a bit tricky, insofar as Rosenow's vaccine was a pneumonia vaccine and not an influenza vaccine, nonetheless was implicated by association. However, Eyler proceeds here to discuss "influenza vaccines" specifically, i.e., vaccines that employed the influenza bacillus; notably, most of these were recognized as NOT having been effective, contrary to Eyler's assertion; Eyler mentions efforts of Barnes and Wadsworth, the latter modeled on a Park vaccine, and both of whom themselves had indicated failure with the influenza bacillus.

[Of course a conspiracy theorist might speculate some connection between Klugman's (of Chien 2010.) having received funding from GlaxoSmithKline and Eyler's article having been funded by the Burroughs-Wellcome Fund (Burroughs-Wellcome merged into GlaxoSmithKline (1995, 2000)]

P. 415 Here we arrive at Eyler's pandering characterization of the "work" of George McCoy: *"More definitive and provocative was the article of a single-column's length in JAMA by George McCoy et al. 1918 (see Appendix L). The team tested Rosenow's vaccine, the influenza vaccine with the greatest scientific pretensions."*

The terms "definitive" and "provocative" are worthy of clarification, as well as the "loaded" reference to Rosenow's "pretensions". The McCoy column was anything but definitive (and certainly not objective), providing no details of the location of this "trial" or other specifics; and indeed "provocative" in that it actually occurred in California and not in Illinois (for which the Chicago Health Department vaccines were intended). Indeed Eyler acknowledges that the vaccine had been produced "for use in Illinois", and goes on to say McCoy "conducted the trial in a single institution, an unnamed state insane asylum." One would naturally assume the state was Illinois; it was not.

Aside from the circumstance of admonition from Rosenow and others that a vaccine be produced locally, other issues enabling the proper characterization of McCoy's "article" as a total sham include (1) the competence of McCoy in the area of vaccines, i.e., using improper technique doomed to failure (see comments page 22-3), (2) the failure of McCoy to state in his 1918 single column article that his "test" was conducted in a state other than Illiniois (for which the vaccine was intended), and (3) his cozy relationship with the editor of JAMA on the all-powerful committee on Pharmacy and Chemistry that enabled such a meagre article to be published in any case (holding sway over disposition of drug claimants and advertisers), and (4) a seemingly disqualifying small sample size. Rather, it serves as further evidence of Eyler's total capitulation, falsification and pandering to the powers that be at the Public Health Service, and, indeed, McCoy's negative impact on health and life, as reflected in his continuing impact on PHS policy.

Eyler accepts as gospel that "McCoy and associates concluded that Rosenow's vaccine offered no protection whatever. ... [and that] the closer a study was to equalizing risk and to obtaining complete information, the more likely it was to conclude that the influenza vaccines of 1918-19 were useless. The contrast between McCoy's study and many of those that concluded that a vaccine was effective serves to illustrate the point."

Indeed, McCoy's study was a total joke, so that the contrast between that and any and all of the many other, reputable studies conducted in 1918-19 illustrates clearly and fully how Eyler's entire article, aka hatchet job, is totally shameful.

It is very difficult to read what is in effect an editorial supporting the shameful Pandemic record of George McCoy, who was recognized separately as an expert on Leprosy. McCoy's work on the Pandemic area unfortunably may come to be best viewed as simply dishonest, insofar has his long-standing tenure at PHS and NIH seemingly argues against a lack of competency. But Eyler does not disappoint with a correspondingly worthy degree both of dishonesty and incompetence.

P. 416 Eyler referring to vaccines used in 1918-9, states "What deserves notice ... is how little concern the authors of these reports of 1918 showed for the design of their trials or for the circumstances in which the vaccinations took place ... ".

Whereas, a review of the many contemporary articles on the subject, including particularly the several mixed or streptococcal vaccines included in the Chien 2010 "assessment", clearly shows the great concern and great efforts the several authors actually did take to attempt to properly measure the efficacy of their vaccines. One wonders if Eyler even looked at the actual papers. Certainly he did not read or understand them!

Eyler continues, stating *"Even more significant is the willingness of editors of some of the nation's leading medical journals to publish these studies ..."*; whereas, the clearly-worst offender in this area is indeed the McCoy column, which would never have seen the light of day were it not for the special relationship between McCoy and the editor of JAMA, George Simmons.

At the bottom of this page, Eyler notes that McCoy and Park had both attempted to make a useful Pfeiffer's vaccine, without success:

"By late 1918, they were convinced that there was no evidence that any influenza vaccine worked, and [p. 417] that no such evidence would be forthcoming unless certain basic standards were met in testing it. Both men explained the fallacy of beginning a vaccine trial during an outbreak, when disease might already have claimed the most susceptible and have selected a more resistant population for vaccination who might have escaped infection even without the vaccine. They also stressed the necessity of large vaccinated and unvaccinated control groups matched by age, sex, and exposure."

Thus we find Eyler rationalizing if not excusing the failures of McCoy and Park, and thereby to some extent rationalizing the failure of Pfeiffer's vaccines overall, by asserting the problem was in methodology.

Eyler goes on to refer to: *"use of Leary's vaccine in twelve institutions in Massachusetts as reported in April 1919 by William Hinton and Edna Kane, both of the Massachusetts State Department of Health. The trial was conducted in ways similar to those we have seen take place in multiple institutions during the 1918–19 epidemic. But in this case, the authors concluded retrospectively that the evidence from all but one of the institutions was unreliable either because vaccinations had begun as the outbreak had reached its peak, because there were too few cases in the institution, or because the vaccinated and the control groups were incomparable. In only one institution, an institution for epileptics, did the authors believe they had reliable data. In the Monsol State Hospital, alternate inmates in each cottage were vaccinated, and the vaccination began just as the first cases appeared. Hinton and Kane concluded that Leary's vaccine caused no harm, but it did not prevent influenza, moderate its course, or lessen its complications."*

Thus did McCoy, and now Eyler, reject in essence (in advance!) the proven works of many competent scientists during the period, who clearly demonstrated that the vaccine needed to be produced from the organism that caused the problem. Through McCoy and Park's esteemed and inept leadership, the Public Health Association in January 1919 [quoting Eyler] *"declared ... that the cause of influenza was unknown. Since that was the case, there was no 'scientific basis' for a vaccine against the disease itself. There was a logical basis for a vaccine against secondary infection, but no evidence had yet come to light proving that such a vaccine was effective."*

Thus McCoy, and now Eyler, ignores all of the information produced prior and subsequent to January 1919 bearing on this issue (i.e., evidence that showed a pneumonia vaccine was effective), and clearly demonstrating that McCoy, and now Eyler, are absolutely wrong.

p. 418 Eyler refers to a report in JAMA discussing the APHA annual meeting in December 1918: "In the discussion at that meeting following his paper, Rosenow found himself on the defensive. The discussion began inauspiciously for Rosenow by McCoy's directing the audience's attention to his own recent paper demonstrating that Rosenow's vaccine was worthless."

It is noted that McCoy said nothing, except for the citation of his single column item: "See the article on 'The Failure of a Bacterial Vaccine as a Prophylactic Against Influenza." JAMA Dec. 14, 1918, p. 1997. That's it! That is all McCoy said in this meeting, according to this JAMA report!! So once again, Eyler exposes himself as a propagandist.

Eyler continued his misinformation campaign against Rosenow in a 2010 article, with reference to this PHS meeting in JAMA, , using the same lead, i.e., "Rosenow found himself on the defensive" (see further discussions of/ references to McCoy 1918 on pp. 27-8, 39, 43, 46, 54, 83-84, 101, 111).

p. 418-9 Eyler refers to "both of" Rosenow's articles on the pandemic published in JAMA (actually there were four, plus an additional seven in the Journal of Infectious Diseases, for a total of eleven in this series). Eyler then refers to a "critical editorial" as having "explicitly suggested that Rosenow was more receptive to favorable than to unfavorable evidence and that his study was vague and lacking in critical details."

Eyler would again refer to this editorial in his 2010 article as "anonymous"; whereas it was published by *JAMA* Editor George Simmons, a close associate of McCoy, and it may have well written by McCoy. Certainly, had Eyler actually read what Rosenow said, rather than the out of context excerpt quoted in the editorial, he would have readily seen how the writer of the editorial, and thus Eyler himself, totally missed the point and mischaracterized this quotation.

The editorial stated "It may be questioned, perhaps, whether the greater receptivity for positive rather than negative results shown in the phrase, 'because, after all, the results from prophylactic inoculation must be sufficiently favorable to be apparent under the conditions included in this report,' is justified in an inquiry demanding such a rigorously critical attitude as the one in hand."

Yet when the actual statement of Rosenow is viewed in entirety, it is clear that the quoted phrase absolutely did not reflect a bias for the positive over the negative in any way, but rather that the results must stand on their own notwithstanding constraints on conducting control comparisons. Rosenow had stated, with specific reference to controls (thus e.g., directly contradicting the misleading assertion of Eyler that 1918-9 investigators were not interested in controls: "The total incidence and death rate in the uninoculated controls are well within the average, as they occur during the present epidemic and hence serve as a fair basis for comparison. Experiments in which alternate control persons were inoculated were not done because of difficulty to obtain consent, and because, after all, the results from prophylactic inoculation must be sufficiently favorable to be apparent under the conditions included in this report."

The editorial did call for additional details that had not been provided in this "Preliminary Report" by Rosenow, which details were provided in the subsequent 10 parts of this series of eleven articles, spanning well over a hundred pages in JAMA and the Journal of Infectious Diseases, a circumstance totally ignored by Eyler 2009 his 2010 continuation.

The third main point raised in the editorial was the circumstance that the Rosenow pneumonia vaccine was clearly intended to reduce pneumonia and death, but then was found to also reduce incidence of influenza. The editorial criticized Rosenow for this as being an inconsistency; whereas, it actually indicated that there was a relation between the causative organism in influenza and that which caused the pneumonia and death, a circumstance supported by the studies of many of the other pandemic/pneumonia investigators, as discussed elsewhere in this current work.

p. 419 Eyler cites Kellog, in the Cal. State Journal of Medicine, as indicative of a supposed "changing opinion" against Rosenow, and concluding that McCoy's bogus anti-Rosenow position, purportedly as characterized by Kellog, "*definitely disposes of vaccine as a preventive measure worthy of consideration.*"

Going to the actual Kellog article, it is here we learn that the McCoy 1918 charade (Appendix L) was conducted not in Illinois, for which the Chicago-generated vaccine was intended, but in a California mental institution. It is thus arguably-significant that McCoy 1918 made no mention of this circumstance, which itself rendered McCoy 1918worthless by definition. Further, in Kellog's 2-1/2 page, 40 column inch article, he includes only a brief 3-inch paragraph on vaccines, citing only McCoy 1918 (in California) and a prior McCoy study involving the Pfeiffer bacillus, as the basis for his statement that "vaccines have definitely proven to be of no value as a preventive measure …".

A couple other points: Kellog incorrectly referred to the McCoy 1918 California vaccine as involving a "Rosenau-type" vaccine. Milton Rosenau was a close associate of McCoy at the Public Health Service, and a predecessor as head of the Hygienic Laboratory (which later became the National Institute of Health). Of course this was an understandable error, confusing the spelling of Milton Rosenau's last name with that of E.C. Rosenow. Further, it is noted that Kellog was Executive Officer of his state's board of health, thus arguably not fully objective relative to the national Public Health Service as represented by McCoy.

p. 419 Eyler, as a general observation, seems intent on ignoring all bacterial and other evidence in support of vaccination against pneumonia, and rather rejects vaccination categorically, based on standards regarding controlled studies in an ideal situation (which were only at that time being devised by McCoy). In this context he refers to a study by Jordan and Sharp that was favorable on this point, but "did not demonstrate any protection against influenza; Jordan and Sharp could not rule out the possibility that the vaccine offered some protection against pneumonia, although they cautioned that the number of cases in their study was too small to be certain."

A few points:

1. Eyler ignores all of the efforts at control comparisons in the many other articles involving mixed vaccines. Moreover, the arguably most important articles worthy of mention in this context, the two articles co-authored by Cecil that reported vaccine results against pneumonia, were totally ignored by Eyler and Chien as well.

2. Regarding sample size, an important consideration in control group comparison methodology in general, it is noted that the sample size of the Jordan and Sharp study, acknowledged as too small, was in fact much larger than that in the Jan. 1919 McCoy piece; The Jordan and Sharp study involved 2873 vaccinated versus 3193 unvaccinated; whereas the Jan. 1919 McCoy piece involved reportedly 390 vaccinated versus 390 unvaccinated, a much smaller sample.

3. Jordan and Sharp in any case state: "Both the influenza and pneumonia attack rates are hence somewhat lower among the vaccinated, but the difference is not great. Pneumonia, not associated with influenza, was also less frequent among the vaccinated, only 6 of 19 pneumonia patients having been vaccinated. The small numbers hardly warrant, although they suggest, a favorable conclusion regarding some slight prophylactic value for pneumonia."

It is a minor point, but nonetheless illustrative of the negative slant of Eyler, that the Eyler characterization is that "Jordan and Sharp could not rule out the possibility that the vaccine offered some protection against pneumonia …"; while the Jordan and Sharp characterization allowed/stated that the results "suggest a favorable conclusion regarding some slight prophylactic value …".

4. Rosenow, in a subsequent article, referred back to the Jordan and Sharp study as having involved a non-local organism, thus doomed to failure, or at least a less

successful conclusion.   Rosenow, E.C., Minnesota Medicine, June 1929, p. 367, "Observations on the Cause and Prevention of Influenza and Influenzal Pneumonia" (Appendix A in Studies in Influenza and Pneumonia) commenting on this Jordan and Sharp article:

"The largely negative results of Jordan and Sharp obtained in 1920 should not be interpreted as nullifying the positive results which I have obtained. In their work no particular care was exercised to incorporate freshly isolated strains, especially of the green-producing and hemolytic streptococci, which were so predominatingly present. I used freshly isolated strains. They worked at a time when the bacteria found, as well as the clinical manifestations, were far more heterogeneous and the disease less virulent. The amount of streptococcus viridans, the peculiar green-producing streptococcus in their vaccine, was approximately a half of the amount which was present in my vaccine. A sixth of their vaccine consisted of *Bacillus influenza,* against which, as is well known, it is more difficult to immunize than against pneumococci or streptococci. My vaccine contained at first a smaller proportion of influenza bacilli than theirs and later no influenza bacilli, but staphylococci instead. Their organisms were killed by heat; mine were killed by cresol. Moreover, in their series, as in mine, most of the patients declared that they had received definite protection against colds. Differences in epidemics and in the vaccines used may readily explain the discrepancies in the results obtained."

From mid-page 420 through p. 422, Eyler discusses the history of criteria of an adequate vaccine trial and his own research on influenza vaccines relating to it, applauding again McCoy and associates, and Jordan and Sharp for their contributions in this area; and ignoring the pivotal and successful prophylactic pneumonia vaccine work of an acknowedged master of controlled trials, Cecil, with Austin and then with Vaughn.

At the end of page 422 into page 423, comes the acknowledgement that McCoy's associate Park had been involved in human experimentation, with diphtheria, with child patients at Willard Parker Hospital and "inmates at an orphanage". Eyler justifies this exploitation of children in experimentation as having contributed to the Schick test as a measure of immunity in diphtheria. [Whatever the value of these tests, we are reminded of the great sophistication of skin tests, diagnostic cutaneous reactions, developed by Rosenow in the decades following the 1918-9 pandemnc, i.e., tests for specific antibody and/or antigen in the blood.]

p. 423   Eyler notes that after the war, in 1922, Park and colleagues obtained parental permission to Shick-test and immunize in public schools, with the result that diphtheria incidence in unimmunized persons was four times that in the experimental group, with 90,000 in each group. But because failure to assure equal susceptibility, Eyler offers that Park's cannot be considered *"the clear model for the new standard for vaccine trials [and] that we need to look elsewhere for the intellectual origins of these new standards."*

On p. 424 Eyler states *"None of the documents I have located refers to previous discussions of vaccine testing or trial design or cites earlier authoritative works on such subjects. ..."*

[In others words, Eyler seems to be saying that even by 1922 there was no clear model of proper vaccine trials. Thus Eyler is rejecting all of the work during the pandemic as it did not comply with a proper vaccine trial model, which model did not yet exist as of 1922! Of course this would have been impossible, in that the time machine had not been developed prior to 1922, except in H.G. Wells' mind.]

"... subjects ... American discussions in these years are remarkable for the absence of theory or statistical principles. It is difficult to believe, however, that the authors of the APHA Working Program, especially George McCoy and William Park, were unaware of the literature that would seem to be the most relevant to the issue they faced—the controversy over the value of Almoth [correcting here the spelling "Almroth"] Wright's typhoid vaccine ignited by its use during the Boer War ... "

Eyler then reviews the history of discussions of these subjects, going back to Wright's vaccines in 1899; however, incredibly, no reference was made to Wright and Leishman's work with pneumonia, a necessary fore-runner for most of the pandemic pneumonia vaccines!

Eyler gives particular attention to Greenwood and Yule's theoretical work of 1914-5 (see THEORETICAL CONSIDERATIONS below). It is in Greenwood and Yule that we find expression of the position that "the use of a vaccine during an epidemic skews the statistical results by ensuring that the vaccinated and the unvaccinated are exposed to risk for unequal periods." It is this concept, adopted to the extreme by McCoy and accepted by Eyler, that closes off consideration of Rosenow's and virtually all of the successful vaccines used during the Pandemic. It is a classic, complete and inescapable "catch 22".

As Rosenow and many others maintained and demonstrated, one must use the specific organism associated as the cause of the particular pandemic and from that organism produce the vaccine against the pandemic disease, or you have nothing. McCoy and Eyler reject the possible validity of a vaccine developed after the pandemic starts insofar as a "proper" control mechanism is by then impossible. The two approaches cannot meet.

From p. 425 to the bottom of p. 427, Eyler continues discussion of history of standards of control trials, recounting thought experiments of Greenwood and Yule, and McCoy, on which their views were based. Beyond the work of Park, rejected as a model for a proper trial, no subsequent model was provided. Rather, the only foundation for the minimum acceptable standards of McCoy and Eyler are based on the thought experiments of Greenwood and Yule. So it's thought experiments and ideals of wishful thinking, versus bacteriology and satisfaction of Koch's postulates by Rosenow et al; and according to Eyler, the thought experiments and McCoy's bogus "perfect" "trial" win.

p. 425: *"McCoy ... in August 1919 ... provides a similar [to Greenwood and Yule's] but not identical explanation of the statistical fallacy of vaccinating during an epidemic and of including as illnesses among the controls all illnesses that occurred among the unvaccinated during the course of the epidemic.81 Both the British and American authors pose a thought experiment to the reader in which half a population of 1000 is inoculated with a useless substance after the beginning of an epidemic and subjected to equal risk of illness thereafter. "*

Bottom of page 427, Eyler sums up use of a large number of vaccines during the pandemic: *"Some of these vaccines, especially those developed by Park, Leary and Rosenow, were very widely used."*   Again, please note the gross impropriety of lumping these three together, insofar as the Park and Leary vaccines used Pfeiffer's bacillus, which by the turn of the year 1918-1919 was universally rejected as the cause of the pandemic; and Rosenow's was a mixed vaccine made up from organisms isolated locally and currently.

p. 427 *"We have thus seen that during the influenza pandemic of 1918–19, American health workers developed a large number of influenza vaccines. Some of these vaccines, especially those developed by Park, Leary, and Rosenow, were very widely used. The medical literature during the pandemic contained frequent reports of the use of these vaccines claiming to prove their efficacy. Readers of the medical literature in those months faced the remarkable circumstance that all these vaccines, regardless of their composition or mode of administration, were proven to prevent influenza."*

NOT TRUE ON SEVERAL COUNTS: THE LEARY AND PARK VACCINES USED PFEIFFER'S BACILLUS ONLY, WERE NOTED TO BE FAILURES AND WERE NOT WIDELY USED.   IT IS WHOLLY INAPPROPRIATE IF NOT EXTREMELY DISHONEST TO LUMP LEARY AND PARK'S EFFORTS WITH ROSENOW'S!!

More lies in Eyler's concluding comments: *"A turning point was clearly the trial of Rosenow's vaccine conducted by George McCoy in a California mental institution. Using stricter standards to guard against selection bias and to ensure the equal exposure of the experimental and control arms, McCoy showed that Rosenow's vaccine offered no protection at all ..."*

Again, as stated elsewhere, among the several problems with the McCoy hoax were (1) use in California of a vaccine developed for use in Illinois; (2) too large doses at too frequent intervals as discussed in APS meeting (see HISTORY file); (3) smaller sample that that rejected by McCoy himself (see McCoy article in Ch. 2).

Thus, while acknowledging that the McCoy experiment was conducted in California, not in Illinois where the vaccine was to be properly used, this alone wholly nullifying McCoy, Eyler proceeds to accept this as totally negating Rosenow's vaccine.

Eyler adds a concluding couple of sentences promoting the memory of McCoy and Park, and thus the PHS, to which he is a dedicated ... apologist. Shame Shame.

Eyler resumes his lying report on the 1918 APHA meeting, as reported in JAMA in his 2010 article.

Eyler 2010

This article, entitled "The State of Science, Microbiology, and Vaccines Circa 1918" deserves a more appropriate title:
"The Sorry State of the PHS's Contrived History of Medicine" or
"Medical History – Making It Up As you Go Along"

Featured in Eyler's synopsis and occupying half of 8 pages of text, is the wholly discredited Pfeiffer's bacillus, aka the influenza bacillus. This article is a total sham.

p. 27 Eyler, in the Synopsis, states:

"Pfeiffer's bacillus (Bacillus influenzae) was a major focus of attention and some controversy between 1892 and 1920. The role this organism or these organisms played in influenza dominated [NOT REALLY!] medical discussion during the great pandemic.

"Many vaccines were developed and used during the 1918–1919 pandemic. The medical literature was full of contradictory claims of their success; there was apparently no consensus on how to judge the reported results of these vaccine trials. The result of the vaccine controversy was both a further waning of confidence in Pfeiffer's bacillus as the agent of influenza and the emergence of an early set of criteria for valid vaccine trials."

Whereas:

1. The possible role of Pfeiffer's bacillus was generally discredited by the end of 1918, and it did not dominate discussion during the pandemic, although it was a consideration.

2. There was a general consensus that the severe consequences of the pandemic were due to a streptococcus, and not Pfeiffer's bacillus.

3. Albeit constraints on ideal controls for comparison, there was a consensus on the failure of Pfeiffer's bacillus vaccines, and success of mixed vaccines containing current strains of organisms, particularly streptococcal, diplostreptococcal and pneumococcal.

4. There was absent a basis for rejection of the several successful vaccine efforts, other than the set of criteria retrospectively/ on-the-fly applied by George McCoy (via his bogus attempted refutation of Rosenow's vaccine) and his cronies. It is not clear to what extent collusion with JAMA Editor George Simmons, and revenues from the drug and stock vaccine companies solicited by Simmons via the committee on Pharmacy and Chemistry (on which George McCoy served for a couple of decades) may have been a factor.

Of particular note is that Eyler, with his above-attempted summary dismissal, writes off all of the important and constructive efforts conducted during the pandemic, which efforts if properly utilized could have saved, and could continue to save, untold thousands of lives and untold billions of dollars over the years.

Of course, while an apologist and cover-up propagandist for the PHS is of course entitled to his own opinions, however ill-formed and fallacious, he is not entitled to his own facts.

p. 29 Eyler states *"Pfeiffer was never able to find an animal model for influenza, although he innoculated mice, rats, guinea pigs, rabbits, pigs, cats, dogs, and monkeys. ... The failure to satisfy Koch's Postulates by producing an experimental disease in animals by the inoculation of pure culture was not in itself damning."*

YES IT IS!   IT MEANS YOU DON'T HAVE THE CORRECT CAUSATIVE ORGANISM!

At the outset, it must be noted that Rosenow, by the time of the second article in his series of eleven, did in fact satisfy the most important of Koch's criteria of replication in laboratory animals. The existence of this part of Rosenow's work is cited by the likes of Morens and Fauci, as per their detailed bibliography, but nowhere discussed by them or the likes of Chien 2010: "Rosenow EC. Studies in influenza and pneumonia. II. The experimental production of symptoms and lesions simulating those of influenza with streptococci isolated during the present epidemic. Journal of the American Medical Association 1919;72(22; 31 May):1604-1609."

p. 30   Eyler: *"By 1918, the successful use of some vaccines, especially those against rabies, typhoid fever, and diphtheria, as well as the use of diphtheria anti-toxin, had raised high expectations for a vaccine against influenza.[12]"*

Actually it was the successful use of vaccines for pneumonia, particularly the work of Cecil and Austin in 1918, that spurred the wave of constructive and successful vaccines during the pandemic. These vaccines were directed not against influenza but rather against pneumonia. The circumstance that they were also beneficial relative to influenza was demonstrated by a number of investigators, and explained as due to a common cause, i.e., different phases of the same organism. The pivotal and unassailable work in this area was that of Olitsky, who was not only the first to show that influenza was caused by a filterable organism, but also among the first to show that this organism was variable in size, ranging from a filterable size, commonly considered a virus, to a larger size commonly considered bacterial.

p. 30 Eyler refers to 1918-9 new laboratory techniques, albeit widespread as exemplified in U.S. Army active participation, as *"rudimentary by 21st century standards. ... filterable viruses were known to exist, but very little was known about them, and there were very few techniques for working with them."*

Eyler notes that *"Drug manufacturers aggressively promoted their stock vaccines for colds, grippe, and flu. ..."* Arguably these may have been the same drug purveyors that were advertising in JAMA, courtesy of Editor Simmons and his crony George McCoy.

As in his 2009 hatchet job on Rosenow and all bacteriological efforts during the pandemic, Eyler again morphs, within the same paragraph, from *"stock vaccines ... of undisclosed composition ... price-gouging and kickbacks"* [as approved by Simmons and McCoy] to *"Preexisting vaccines of undisclosed composition ... endorsed by physicians such as M.J. Exner ... developed some six years earlier by his colleague, Ellis Bonime ... an adherent of the opsonin theory of immune response ... ."*

Thus again does Eyler reject the monumental epochal works of Sir Almroth Wright, originator of the opsonin antibody work, pioneer in vaccine and vaccine-therapy, and advocate of developing vaccines from the directly attributable causative organism. Again Eyler seeks to denigrate Exner's effort as "boosterism"; yet, no reference is made to results, be they success or failure; thus we clearly have her an unsubstantiated attack on any and all vaccine attempts during the pandemic, in accord with Eyler's PHS and drug company sponsors. And, in keeping with the pattern of Eyler having ignored any and all favorable information that contravened his negative vendetta against the pandemic vaccines, it may be confidently offered that the Exner efforts were indeed successful; had they failed one could be certain this would have been noted by Eyler!

As for the methodology of Bonime, the major work is available in print form via Amazon.com and on-line digitally (free) at:
http://books.google.com/books?id=PRqrSTqYGBMC&pg=PA166&lpg=PA166&dq
=bonime+vaccine&source=bl&ots=cHCTjzO9NB&sig=QxuPu9-
ntFPt_eq3jUkSRYKkDAc&hl=en&sa=X&ei=KD0DT_LTK4XGtgff6YHQBg&sqi=
2&ved=0CDkQ6AEwAQ#v=onepage&q=bonime%20vaccine&f=false
e.g. 191 clearly indicates that *these, indeed, were not "vaccines of undisclosed composition"*:

TABLE OF DOSAGE

	Beginning Dose	Increase
Streptococcus	50 million	20 million
M. Catarrhalis	25 million	5 to 10 million
B. Friedlander	25 million	5 to 10 million
M. Paratetrogenus	50 million	10 to 20 million
Pneumococcus	25 million	5 to 10 million
B. Influenza	25 million	5 to 10 million
Staphylococcus { Albus / Aureus }	200 million	25 to 50 million

P. 30 bottom of page, Eyler exposes his clear bias towards the Pfeiffers bacillus, actually moribund for a century: *"Early in the pandemic, more highly respected [relative to Exner and Bonime] and well-placed authorities developed vaccines based explicitly on Pfeiffer's bacillus"*, citing (p. 31) W.H. Park, Leary, Holman/ Pittsburgh, Duval, and others.

Seemingly defending this bogus direction, *"It was not only heads of [the very few, cited] bacteriological laboratories who acted on the assumption that Pfeiffer's bacillus was the cause of influenza and developed vaccines on that assumption. Some private physicians did the same."*
IN FACT, MOST DID NOT; THEY RELIED ON THE ABLE SERVICES OF THE LIKES OF THE MAYO FOUNDATION I.E. ROSENOW, ETC.

p. 31 Eyler discusses Pfeiffer's bacillus vaccine, referring in text to Park, Leary, U. of Pittsburgh (Holman), Duval and Harris, Horace Greeley, and including citations also to Hinton and Kane, Barnes, Hawes and Wallace, and stating *"Almost without exception, those reporting on the use of these Pfeiffer's bacillus vaccines reported that they were effective in preventing influena."*

THIS IS NOT CORRECT; INDEED, THE absolute OPPOSITE IS MORE ACCURATE.

On closer review of a number of the actual articles cited or referenced by Eyler, it is noted, regarding FACTUAL ERRORS:

1. Park: As per Col. Victor Vaughn (JAMA 71, Dec. 21, 1918, report in "Society Proceedings", on APHA Annual Meeting held in Chicago Dec. 8-11, 1918:): "We have used influenza vaccine in great quantities ... [including] that which Dr. Park has furnished us from the New York laboratory, and I do not hesitate to say that it has not done one bit of good. Speaking on this point with the evidence of the Pfeiffer bacillus not being the cause of influenza, I can agree with those who have spoken."

2. Leary:

   a. (American Journal of Public Health, Vol 8 # 10 Oct 1 1918): "Dr. E. R. Kelley appointed two committees to study the value of an influenza vaccine prepared by Dr. Timothy Leary of Tufts Medical School. The Board of Scientific Investigation ... concluded ... The evidence at hand affords no trustworthy basis for regarding prophylactic vaccination against influenza as of value in preventing the spread of the disease, or of reducing its severity.

   b. Barnes, using Leary vaccine, concluded "The morbidity was only slightly lower among the vaccinated, and the mortality among those who developed influenza was practically the same whether vaccinated or not."

3. University of Pittsburgh: p. 112, concludes: "it is apparent that there is very little to indicate that an immunity to epidemic influenza is conferred by the use of a prophylactic vaccine composed of inert Pfeiffer bacilli alone."

4. Duval and Harris reported 2-3 months prophylactic protection in the 2nd part of the epidemic (influenza incidence of 27/981 vaccinated versus 130/338 unvaccinated); however, they offer no mortality data. Indeed, this seems to be the only study that reported a clear advantage to the use of Pfeiffer's bacillus.

5. Greeley: no comment; did not access this item as it was not cited by Chien, or significantly elsewhere.

6. Hinton and Kane: As summarized in Chien 2010, influenza incidence reported was about the same for vaccinated (163/461 or 35.4%) versus unvaccinated (178/518 or 34.4%)

7. Barnes

   a. using Leary vaccine, Barnes concluded "The morbidity was only slightly lower among the vaccinated, and the mortality among those who developed influenza was practically the same whether vaccinated or not."

   b. As summarized in Chien, influenza incidence reported was about the same for vaccinated (25/152 or 16.4%) versus unvaccinated (23/113 or 20.4%). Subtracting out the children, who were quarantined, and two wards with one case each that were promptly isolated, as per Barnes preference p. 1899, this leaves 24/90 or 26.7% vaccinated, versus 22/64 or 34.4% unvaccinated.

   c. Barnes also provides limited mortality data, i.e., 4 of 25 vaccinated versus 9 of 57 unvaccinated; it is not clear where the 57 came from, except it does not correlate with anything else in the article. Perhaps it is an error; or there is data left out of the article.

8. Hawes, Wallace: not accessed.

9. Wadsworth 1919 (included in the Chien article) reported "on use of influenza vaccine in New York state comprising scattered reports from different physicians and health officers, general reports from all the state institutions, and reports of special selected institutions. ... it is evident that the vaccines ... failed to give reliable protection against influenza or influenzal pneumonia."

From this brief summary, it is clear that the assertion by Eyler, that *"almost without exception"* proponents of the Pfeiffer vaccine reported they were effective, is absolutely false.

p. *32 "By early 1919, evidence was running more strongly against Pfeiffer's bacillus"*: BACK UP TO 1918!

True to form, Eyler, machinates for another half-page-plus over the dying corpse of the Pfeiffers' hypothesis, allowing "Park and His associates" the final shovel on it's grave, notwithstanding it had been dead all along. Then Eyler goes to a subchapter entitled "Alternative Etiologies, other vaccines", as if to say "the king is dead, but who are the pretenders ...".

Eyler starts off here rejecting the most potent phase of the actual causative organism, i.e., so-called "Mathers streptococcus:

"Other candidates had been proposed as the cause of influenza during the pandemic, but these were disposed of rather quickly. An Army medical officer, Captain George Mathers, who died of influenza during his investigation, isolated and characterized a streptococcus that produced a green color on blood agar plates. ... The Mathers streptococcus attracted some attention during the early months of the pandemic. Jordan, for example, systematically looked for it in his study but found no evidence that made it seem a more probable cause than B. influenzae. [ABSOLUTELY WRONG!] Then ..."

TIME OUT !! [We'll pick this up a bit later, noting that: HERE, IN MID-PARAGRAPH, AS IS HIS CUSTOM IF THIS ARTICLE IS USED TO JUDGE, EYLER CHANGES THE SUBJECT; PICKING THIS UP BELOW, FOLLOWING THIS CLEAR EXPOSURE OF A "BLATANT LIE"; OK, FACTUAL ERROR]:

IN FACT, Jordan reported a closer association of the Mathers streptococcus with pneumonia, as compared with B. influenzae: "The Mathers coccus was found about as frequently and abundantly as the Pfeiffer bacillus, although its occurrence was quite independent of that of the latter. Its association with the pneumonia cases seemed to be closer than that of the Pfeiffer bacillus, but it was also found in all the later cases of simple influenza. ... Practically pure cultures of the Mathers coccus were obtained from the nasopharynx of some patients."

Indeed, the October group, of 8 cases of Influenza-Pneumonia, all 8 yielded the Mathers cocci, compared to 3 that yielded the Pfeiffer bacteria.

Jordan also notes: "This is apparently very similar to, if not identical with, the organism described by Zingher (JAMA, 1919, 72, p. 1020)."

It is also the same as that isolated by Rosenow, Olitsky, and many others.

BACK TO EYLER; IN MID-PARAGRAPH HE CHANGES THE SUBJECT TO THE QUESTION AS TO THE CAUSE OF INFLUENZA:

... Then, in both Europe and America, investigators considered the possibility that influenza might be caused by a filterable virus. ... "

p. 32-3 Eyler refers to *"the disputed finding that influenza could be caused in humans with inoculation of material from the noses or throats of influenza patients that had been passed through a bacterial filter. French and Japanese investigators had reported succeeding in transferring influenza by this method. American researchers failed to confirm these findings. ... These negative findings were also confirmed by extensive human experiments with influenza sponsored by the U.S. Navy and the U.S. Public Health Service."*

Notably, Eyler abstains from naming names; however, from the literature of the day, McCoy and his associate in the PHS, Milton Rosenau were prominent in these human experiments. (JAMA 73, 5, August 2, 1919, p. 311-3, by Milton J.Rosenau, refers to experiments "by a group of officers ... from the US Navy and the US Public Health Service, consisting of Dr. G.W. McCoy ...). Thus is disclosed McCoy's perfect record – an inability to vaccinate against influenza and an inability to cause influenza with experiments on volunteer humans.

However, it was indeed an American, Olitsky, who seems to have been the first to pass the viral organism to rabbits, thus demonstrating the suspected role of the virus in the cause of pandemic influenza. As reviewed by Charles H. Calisher (Croat Med J. 2009 August; 50(4): 412–415., **"Swine Flu"**:

"In 1921, ... Peter Olitsky and Frederick Gates of the Rockefeller Foundation published their filtration results, which demonstrated that nasal secretions from patients infected with the 1918 influenza virus (influenza A H1N1, *vide infra*), and passed it through a filter that excluded bacteria, still caused pneumonia in rabbits (4,5). Olitsky and Gates had isolated the etiologic agent of this disease but did not recognize that."

[As discussed elsewhere herein, Olitsky was also among the first to show that the organism was polymorphic, i.e., that it morphed between smaller (filterable, viral) size to larger (bacterial) size.]

p. 33 In the sentence and paragraph immediately following his [August 2, 1919] discussion of Milton Rosenau and George McCoy's failed human experiments, Eyler states:

"As confidence in the role of Pfeiffer's bacillus in influenza waned, the strategy of prevention by vaccine changed. Vaccines developed later in the pandemic – almost all developed in the middle of the country and on the West Coast -- were composed of other organisms either singly or in mixtures. Increasingly vaccines were justified as preventing the pneumonias that accompanied influenza."

A couple of points to be raised here:

1. From the outset of the pandemic, vaccines of other organisms were developed, insofar as a pandemic-role for Pfeiffers was in question, long before the Milton Rosenau/McCoy August 1919 human experiments.

2. From the outset, the emphasis of many of these vaccines, including but not limited to E.C. Rosenow's, was preventing pneumonias and death from them. This was the **intention**, not a second-hand "justification" as stated/insinuated by Eyler. Indeed, Eyler's citation #43 refers to Ely and Lloyd, JAMA 1919, vol. 72, p. 24-8, i.e., work published in January 1919 which necessarily was referring to work with mixed vaccines accomplished during 1918, i.e., earlier rather than "later in the pandemic" as suggested by Eyler.

p. 33 Eyler turns here to discussing Rosenow, noting that "Rosenow argued that the exact composition of a vaccine intended to prevent pneumonia had to match the distribution of the lung-infecting microbes then in circulation." Eyler notes that Rosenow's vaccine including the "green-producing streptococcus", which Rosenow and others recognized as one and the same as Mathers, but Eyler makes no mention of this. Eyler acknowledges that the Mayo Clinic received returns for 143,000 persons who had received from one to three injections, and that more than 500,000 doses were produced by the Chicago department of health. "Some of it was distributed to Chicago physicians and the rest was turned over to the state health department *for use throughout Illinois*." Indeed the Mayo Foundation received returns from doctors reporting on a total of half-million patients, 143,000 of whom had received vaccines and the remainder not.

Moreover, here Eyler has acknowledged (1) that Rosenow prescribed that the pneumonia vaccine was to be made from the locally obtained organisms, and (2) the doses produced by the Chicago department of health were intended for use in Illinois. Hereby Eyler indirectly is acknowledging that McCoy's attempt to use this vaccine in a California institution was ill-fated from the outset [aside from methodology errors (see comments by Dr. Will Walter, above pp. 22-23, and associated discussions elsewhere in this work) which would have doomed McCoy's efforts even if he was using a proper organism].

And of course, immediately following this discussion [i.e., the sentence and paragraph immediately following "for use throughout Illinois", separated by a heading "Vaccine Controversy and Standards for vaccine Trials", Eyler attempts to degrade/ distract from Rosenow's work with:

"As was the case with Pfeiffer's bacillus vaccines, most of the early reports on the use of these mixed vaccines indicated they were effective. ... all vaccines, regardless of their composition ... were held to prevent influenza or influenzal pneumonia. [Again, this was ABSOLUTELY not true, particularly in the case of the Pfeiffer's bacillus vaccines which for the most part were found to be not effective. Continuing with Eyler --] *Something was clearly wrong. The medical profession had at the time no consensus on what constituted a valid vaccine trial, and it could not determine whether these vaccines did any good at all."*

Thus did Eyler again abruptly change the subject, i.e. changing the focus to theoretical considerations ("what constituted a valid vaccine trial"), and insodoing insinuate that Rosenow's and the others' vaccines were not effective. And of course he injected PHS-associated luminaries Park and McCoy as saviors of the process of developing standards for trials.

Eyler repeats the McCoy challenge that the pandemic-associated-vaccine "trials" were not valid in that *"Most trials began after the first cases of influenza had appeared, often after the epidemic peak had passed ... "*, without giving any specific references. Eyler criticizes these studies, charging: *"little effort was usually made to minimize selection bias ... and too many trials operated with poor observation and imperfect data collection."*

Eyler then focuses on the bogus vaccine 'trial/study' that McCoy had used to ignore all of the constructive work by many investigators. To top it all off, Eyler then acknowledges McCoy's bogus "trial/study" occurred in California, with a vaccine intended for use in Illinois, as having demonstrated that "Rosenow's vaccine offered no protection whatsoever."

p. 34 We now are treated with additional blatant fabrication and misrepresentation by Eyler. Middle of first column, page 34:

"By the beginning of 1919, Rosenow, the most vocal defender of vaccines, found himself on the defensive. ... " Here, with use of the term "defender", Eyler attempts to characterize Rosenow's work as subjective, which it was not; the facts of his scientific work spoke volumes, which Eyler again seeks to ignore. Eyler continues] *"... defensive. During the discussion of his paper at APHA's annual meeting, he faced hostile comments from both McCoy and Victor Vaughan."*

In fact, McCoy did not comment at all, except to say "See the article on 'The Failure of a Bacterial Vaccine as a Prophylactic Against Influenza." JAMA Dec. 14, 1918, p. 1997. McCoy did not even mention Rosenow's name, or say anything else at all, so we can easily categorize this as "fib" or "white lie" at best.

As for *"hostile comments from ... Victor Vaughan"*, THIS IS AN ABSOLUTE LIE. On the contrary:

(1) While Victor Vaughan was indeed very negative, it was not regarding Rosenow, but rather regarding McCoy! At the APHA Annual Meeting held in Chicago Dec. 8-11, 1918, as per a *JAMA* 71, Dec. 21, 1918, report in "Society Proceedings", Col. Victor Vaughan stated: "We have used influenza vaccine in great quantities, all they could make in the Army laboratory, and have used all that Dr. McCoy could spare, and also have used that which Dr. Park has furnished us from the New York laboratory, and I do not hesitate to say that it has not done one bit of good."

(2) Regarding Rosenow specifically, Col. Victor Vaughan makes absolutely no mention of or reference to Rosenow or his vaccines. Vaughan, whose comments comprised about 80% of the text in the discussion section, refers to "vaccines for influenza", rejecting the efforts of McCoy and Park as per (1) above, concluding with "Speaking on this point with the evidence of the Pfeiffer bacillus not being the cause of influenza, I can agree with those who have spoken."

However, regarding vaccines for pneumonia, again, although Vaughan makes no specific reference to Rosenow, he notes "encouraging results" in this area, implicitly and clearly favorably endorsing Rosenow's efforts. Further, summarizing Cecil and Austin's work at Camp Upton, updated to a latest report within the prior day or two, Col. Victor Vaughan notes the same number of cases of pneumonia among the 20% of unvaccinated cases as among the 80% unvaccinated; in other words, Victor Vaughan acknowledges a four-times greater incidence of pneumonia per person among the unvaccinated compared to the vaccinated.

Eyler continues: "The next month, *JAMA* ran an anonymous critical editorial on the use of his [Rosenow's] vaccine."

The JAMA editorial of January 1919, which Eyler refers to as "anonymous", would presumably have been written by the editor George Simmons, a close associate of McCoy, and may well have been influenced if not written by McCoy. It asserts that data on prophylactic inoculation "are simply too inadequate to permit a competent judgment." Specifically regarding the immediately preceding report of Rosenow, the editorial asks for details regarding communities, population, incidence, mortality, and numbers, location and results of vaccines (all items which Rosenow responded to in detail in subsequent articles); and two paragraphs down, reduntantly calls for "dates, places, ages and population inoculated and uninoculated ..." etc.

Particularly exemplary of the intrinsically negative perspective of this Simmons / (sic McCoy) piece are comments relative to the effect of Rosenow's vaccines on initial attacks of influenza. As Rosenow had stated at the outset, his intention was to reduce the severe effects of pneumonia and death, rather than the initial influenza. However as Rosenow reported, somewhat to his surprise, the vaccines did in fact seem to reduce the incidence of influenza as well. The editorial adopts the position that this reflected an inconsistency in Rosenow's position.

Again, Eyler switches back [sic diverts] to the issue of "professional standards ... in trial design and analysis", citing the work of Park et al., and Jordan and Sharp with a single mixed vaccine in 1920, "which concluded the vaccines used were ineffective". On the contrary, and indeed, Rosenow had specifically commented, in 1929, on the Jordan and Sharp article [see page 52 and further discussion of Eyler 2009].

At the same time, Eyler here contradicts his own 2009 article, where he had acknowledged (p. 419): "Jordan and Sharp could not rule out the possibility that the vaccine offered some protection against pneumonia, although they cautioned that the number of cases in their study was too small to be certain." [It is noted again that the Jordan and Sharp study involved more than 7 times the unvaccinated and 8 times the unvaccinated numbers as compared with the brief McCoy 1918 article (Appendix L).

p. 35 On this last page of text in Eyler 2009, he devotes about half of his text to human experiments of Milton Rosenau and McCoy, although he does not name McCoy in the text itself. [McCoy is mentioned by Milton Rosenau in his primary *JAMA* article, and McCoy is also listed as author on a follow-on PHS piece.] Milton Rosenau concluded, regarding influenza, "we are not quite sure what we know about the disease." And Eyler summed up these failed efforts: *"It seemed that what was acknowledged to be one of the most contagious of communicable diseases could not be transferred under experimental conditions."*

Eyler and McCoy et al had to know from the very title of the second in E.C. Rosenow's series of eleven articles, that Rosenow had succeeded in transferring the disease to laboratory animals, e.g.:

(1)   Rosenow EC. Studies in influenza and pneumonia. II. The experimental production of symptoms and lesions simulating those of influenza with streptococci isolated during the present epidemic. *JAMA*; **72** (22; 31 May 1919):1604-1609; and other published works, of which McCoy was, and Eyler would advisably be, aware:

(2)   *American Journal of Diseases of Children*, **23**, p. 275 (January 1922), By American Medical Association: Rosenow: "Through a painstaking study of the infecting powers of the streptococcus in influenza and influenzal pneumonia throughout several epidemic waves, it has been possible to reproduce in animals by various methods of injection, but particularly by intratracheal injection, the picture of influenza as seen in man. The symptoms both of influenza and influenzal pneumonia have been grossly simulated in these animals as far as possible. Likewise the gross and microscopic changes which have come to be regarded as quite characteristic of influenzal infection have been reproduced. The same varied picture that often supervenes in the later stages of influenzal pneumonia in man such as leukocytosis as evidence of pleural involvement and pleural infection, becomes manifest and the varied pathologic picture in the lung of patients who died late has been noted in guinea-pigs injected intratracheally with these strains. The tendency to involvement of the female generative organs with a high mortality in pregnancy and a high incidence of abortion, of lesions of the heart, abscess in the rectus muscle, and interstitial emphysema, have been noted in the experimental animal quite as they occur in man."

(3)   *JAMA* August 16, 1919, p. 482: In discussion following James R. Herrick, "Treatment of Influenza by Means Other than Vaccines and Serums", in which McCoy was likely in attendance: Dr. E.C. Rosenow:

"The vaccine which we used was made to contain as soon after isolation as possible the bacteria isolated in influenza and the accompanying pneumonia together with type pneumococci. It contained, as we found months later, a high percentage of strains of green-producing streptococci which, according to their serologic reactions, appear to bear etiologic relation to this disease and with which the picture of **influenza has been closely simulated in animals**. ... The difficulties in evaluating the results, as pointed out by Dr. McCoy, have been considered and the sources of error eliminated. ... Averaging all the results obtained, it appears that the incidence of influenza was about three times as common and the death rate five times as high among the uninoculated as among the vaccinated persons".

In a sweeping statement that seeks to reject all science up to that point, Eyler proclaims: *"If anything, the experience of 1918-1919 served to deconstruct existing biomedical knowledge."* If anything, Eyler's many fabrications, distortions, yes LIES, totally deconstruct any claims to validity.

In his concluding comments, Eyler fully discloses how fully his head is buried in the sand of "ignoration", asserting that the agent of influenza was "still unknown" as of 1927, and that the three decades following the pandemic of 1897 *"had seen remarkably little addition to the fund of basic scientific knowledge of influenza, in spite of concerted efforts by researchers employing the best available research tools."*

Wrong. What a disgrace.

Chapter 5 – A Chronological Review of Historical Pandemic Articles

"The only thing new in the world is the history you don't know"
Harry Truman
(As quoted in *Plain Speaking...* 1974, by Merle Miller)

This is a file of notes and commentary on historical articles accessed in the process of compiling and writing an introductory Foreword to the eleven part series written in 1919-1920 by E.C. Rosenow reporting on the 1918-1919 pandemic. [That work is currently available on Amazon.com and Kindle books as *Studies in Influenza and Pneumonia* by E. C. Rosenow.]

Particular attention is given here to those articles specifically cited in, and included in assessments and discussion by, Chien 2010 (Appendix A).

However, beyond brief mention, those Chien 2010 items involving *only* the use of "Pfeiffer's bacillus" (aka the so-called and previously suspected "influenza bacillus" or "hemophilus influenzae") are not discussed here (1) insofar as the alleged role of "Pfeiffer bacillus" in causing the 1918-9 pandemic had already been generally rejected relatively early in, if not prior to, the 1918-9 pandemic; and moreover, (2) substantive assessments of these items are excluded by Chien 2010.

Also included in this Chapter are numerous historical items not cited in Chien 2010 nor Eyler 2009/2010, perhaps due to their falling outside the specific pandemic time frame imposed by Chien 2010 (1918-1920). Some of these articles particularly referred to a **"purulent bronchitis"**, e.g., a measles epidemic of 1917 and presumed 1918 epidemics of mastoiditis and catarrhal infections, which were characterized as associated with particularly deadly episodes of "purulent bronchitis". As such, these seemingly may have been a precursor, or otherwise related, to the deadly "influenzal pneumonia" of 1918-1919. Thus it may be noted that the pneumonia vaccine work of Cecil and Austin, decidedly an essential factor in development of pandemic anti-pneumonia vaccines discussed herein and in Chien 2010, had been referred to by Cecil and Austin as a catarrhal epidemic associated with "purulent bronchitis". Similarly, Lathrop had referred to an epidemic of mastoiditis as involving "purulent bronchitis".

Detailed discussions of most of Rosenow's series of eleven pandemic articles are excluded from this chapter, insofar as these articles are incorporated in entirety in as *Studies in Influenza and Pneumonia* by E. C. Rosenow. However, it must be noted that Rosenow had been addressing the issue of pneumonia and associated therapy for several years prior to the pandemic, e.g., "The Blood in Lobar Pneumonia, with remarks concerning treatment, JAMA 44:871-873, (March 18) 1905, 871-3.

In Sept. 1912, Rosenow discussed successful immunization of pneumococcus infections using autolysed pneumococci. [*JAMA* **LIX**, no. 10, Sept 7 1912 p. 795 Immunization in Pneumococcus Infections, p. 796]: "For the treatment of lobar pneumonia, so far chiefly the autolyzed pneumococci have been used. ... A study by the statistical method during the past two years at the Cook County Hospital has shown a definite reduction in the mortality of the 130 treated cases. The number of patients treated, however, is too small to allow definite conclusions to be drawn; but when we consider that the patients treated in this way belong to the most unfavorable group, it looks as if this antigen really was of definite value."

Cecil and Austin, as well as Rosenow as well as others cited below, place particular emphasis on Sir Almroth Wright's work with pneumonia vaccines in South Africa, from 1912, and the follow-on additional detailed studies of his assistant Lister published in 1917, as immediate forebears of the bulk of the pandemic anti-pneumonia bacterial vaccines discussed herein.

In retrospect, it is noted that while a purported causal role for Pfeiffer's (influenza) bacillus had been generally discredited even prior to the pandemic, also even prior to the pandemic attention had been directed to the possible role of a **green** streptococcus, or **streptococcus viridans**. Indeed as we review the various accounts of possible culpability in article at the time, this organism and its various incarnations seem to have been far more dominant than any other entity – along with discussions of pleomorphism and other possibly related forms e.g., diplococci and hemolytic streptococci.   These terms are accordingly scattered throughout this chapter as encountered.

Some early citations: Rosenow (*JAMA* **63,** 1914,   906) in an article on bacteriology, found **S viridans** in 16 of 25 stomach ulcer cases; and in 14 of 25 cystic ovaries cases. And Billings, (*JAMA* **63,** 1914, 900), "Focal Infection", got pure cultures from deep in tonsils of rheumatism patient.

Frank Billings MD –*Focal Infection* 1916 (Lane Lectures); his "finest hour":
Page v., "the etiologic relation of focal infection to systemic disease has been a subject of study in the clinical material of Rush Medical College, in affiliation with the U. of Chicago and the Presbyterian Hospital for the past 12 or more years."
p. 26   Billings cites his own work and that of Rosenow as confirming "the report of Schottmüller [*Münch. Med. Wchnschr.* 1903, L, 845] in the isolation from the blood during life of the patient of a pure culture of **streptococcus viridans**. Schottmuller isolated a streptococcus from patients with chronic infectious endocarditis, which grew fine colonies on blood agar plates, was non-hemolyzing, but produced a greenish halo around the colonies. In consequence it was named S. viridans and because of its low virulence for animals it was also called streptococcus mitior."

Frank Billings MD. in *JAMA* Sept. 16, 1916 **67** (12):847-850, "The Principles Involved In Focal Infection As Related To Systemic Disease", p. 848:
"Schottmueller classified streptococci pathogenic for man, by growing them in solid blood agar medium, into S hemolysans longus S mucosus and S viridans Mitior We have learned that any one of these types may change in general and special pathogenicity and the degree of virulence S viridans so named because of the green colored halo produced by the colonies on blood agar is usually of very mild pathogenicity for man It is a very common surface parasite of the mucous membrane

of the mouth and tonsil Apparently this type of streptococcus may acquire special pathogenicity for the endocardium and especially for old valvular scars and cause enormous vegetations and thrombus formation on the heart valves A person so affected suffers from a constant viridans streptococcemia In other instances a green producing streptococcus of less virulence than the foregoing may be isolated from the infected tissues of the patients suffering from myositis arthritis and other chronic diseases Evidently the property of green color production on the blood agar plates only affords a name but does not signify the pathogenic character or virulence The type may even lose the property of green color production on culture media."

- - - - - - -

Rosenow Towne and Wheeler, *JAMA* **67** Oct 21, 1916 p. 1204, discussed the relation of poliomyelitis to to S viridians.

- - - - - - -

JAMA 67, Nov. 4, 1916, Isaac Arthur ABT, MD, and A. Levinson MD, Chicago, "A Study of Two Hundred and Twenty-Six Cases of Chorea", p. 1343

"G. F. Still goes to the extreme of regarding chorea as much an evidence of rheumatism as gumma is of syphilis. Attempts have been made to establish the relationship of the two diseases bacteriologically. Poynton and Paine, who cultivated the *Micrococcus rheumaticus* in cases of articular rheumatism also found the organisms in the brains in cases of chorea associated with rheumatism. Richards reported two cases of chorea in which a *Streptococcus viridans* was found in the blood. He found the organism to be culturally identical with the description of **the green-producing streptococcus of Schottmueller** and probably not different from the description of the *Micrococcus rheumaticus* of Poynton and Paine. *JAMA* Jan 10 1914, p. 110 (Note: This writer can't find the Richards article ?)].

- - - - - - -

The Mathers article seems the first to have conclusively identified the cause of the pandemic – a strain of S. viridian and its related forms.

GEORGE MATHERS, M.D., *JAMA* 1917 March 3, **68** (9):678-680 "Etiology of the Epidemic of Acute Respiratory Infections, Commonly Called Influenza", Chicago, From the Memorial Institute for Infectious Diseases.

p. 678 "Epidemics of acute respiratory infections have occurred at irregular intervals for centuries in various parts of the world, and their prevention has been one of the most formidable problems in preventive medicine. These infections, different from other epidemic diseases, seem least liable to modification by hygienic or geographic conditions, and at some time in its history almost every race of people has suffered from their ravages. During these visitations, recorded in centuries of medical history, the general mortality is greatly increased; the etiologic agent, independent of its own virulence, may increase the death rate by combining with preexisting diseases, or by lowering the resisting power of the individual to such an extent that other more formidable infections gain a foothold and cannot be overcome. Furthermore, it is very striking that, notwithstanding the wide diversity of conditions under which these great epidemics have occurred, the clinical manifestations of the disease have always been the same. ..."

" .... Whether or not Pfeiffer's bacillus was the causative factor in the great pandemic of 1890, there has been little evidence brought forward in recent years to support the view that it is of any great importance in the etiology of the disease.

"During the winter of 1915-1916, the United States was visited by a severe epidemic of acute respiratory infections which resembled in every detail the great epidemic of 1890. This outbreak was apparently first noticed in the middle western states, and it spread rapidly over the entire country, taking a heavy toll of human life. December and January were the months in which these infections were most prevalent, and the epidemic had almost completely lost its impetus by March, 1916. During the height of this epidemic in Chicago, sixty-one cases of the disease were studied bacteriologically, and the results form the basis of this paper.

"In all the cases the nasal discharge and sputum were examined, and in a few instances blood cultures were made. In forty-six instances, hemolytic streptococci [p. 679] were found in predominating numbers, and in six of these cases these organisms were isolated from the nose and throat in pure culture. **Green-producing streptococci were found in thirty instances with one pure culture,** and pneumococci in thirty cases with four pure cultures. Staphylococci were isolated in fifty cases, *Micrococcus catarrhalis* in six, and Freidlander's bacillus in one case. **In only one instance was the influenza bacillus found, and then in small numbers.** Anaerobic cultures were also made in the majority of cases, but there were no findings of any great interest. The *Bacillus rhinitis,* which has been described by Tunnicliff in connection with acute rhinitis, was found in the nasal discharge in two cases, and fusiform bacilli were not uncommonly observed in these anaerobic cultures.

"The majority of the patients were studied early in the course of the disease, and, in the earliest of these, hemolytic streptococci were almost constantly found, especially in the throat. These different strains of streptococci grew on standard blood. agar plates as small round semitranslucent colonies of variable moisture surrounded by a clear zone of hemolysis from 2 to 3 mm. in diameter. They were gram-positive, arranged in pairs and short chains, medium sized and slightly oblong, and occasionally faintly staining capsules were visible. They were highly virulent for rabbits, doses of 1 c.c. of a twenty-four hour broth culture usually causing multiple arthritis and death in from five to ten days.

"The pneumococci isolated were usually in small numbers, and often presented the characteristics of the organism found in the mouths of normal persons which Cole and his associates call Group 4 or the atypical type of pneumococci. The green-producing streptococci were also usually found in small numbers, and were in the instances studied relatively avirulent. ...

"... bacteriologic studies of material from these cases, both antemortem and postmortem, revealed the presence in predominating numbers of hemolytic streptococci in most instances. **In no instance** in which postmortem material was examined **was the *Bacillus influenzae* found**."

- - - - - - -

HAMMOND *The Lancet*, July 14, 1917

Hammond   reports on a breakout of purulent bronchitis at a British base in northern France in the winter of 1916-7. Following early cases in December, it assumed epidemic proportions late January, abating later with the frost.

"Patients suffering from this unusually fatal disease present a symptom complex so distinctive as to constitute a definite clinical entity."

The results of bacteriological and post-mortem examinations

p.43 "In cases here shown the following organisms other than B. influenzae were found:

	Cases.
Pneumococcus	 13
M. tetragenus	 2
Streptococcus	5
A Gram-positive diplococcus	 1
A Gram-negative diplococcus resembling D. catarrhalis	 5
A large Gram-negative bacillus	 1
Staphylococcus	 3
B. tuberculosis	 1

In most of the cases in which B. Influenzae are present in large numbers the pneumococcus also occurred.

CONCLUSIONS.

1. We are here dealing with an epidemic of a variety of **purulent bronchitis**.

2. For the following reasons we consider the cause of the disease to be the influenza bacillus :

 (a) The almost constant **occurrence of this organism in the sputum** ;

 (b) its presence in the pus of the affected bronchioles;

 (c) in some typical cases it occurs apart from the presence of any other organism ;

 (d) the outbreak of the disease in epidemic form at the time of year when influenza epidemics are most common and whilst one was actually in progress;

 (e) the marked signs of toxic poisoning which are found during life and post mortem.

3. There are **well-marked clinical features** which distinguish these cases from ordinary cases of bronchitis. The most prominent are the **characteristic sputum, the extreme tachycardia, the cyanosis, the course of the temperature (notably the ante-mortem fall), and the extremely high mortality**. ... [evidence of septicemia]

4. Treatment has so far been unsatisfactory. The most encouraging results have been obtained by use of a steam tent. Vaccines have not yet had a trial, but it is unlikely, in view of the blocked condition of the bronchioles, that they would be of great benefit.

5. The morbid anatomy consists of **three groups of changes**.

(a) **The lung condition**: Marked purulent bronchitis, the smaller bronchi being filled with thick pus, from which air is notably absent. In some cases secondary broncho-pneumonia and edema, pleurisy, and emphysema are common.

(b) **Evidence of toxemia**: Especially seen in kidneys, spleen, liver, lymphatic glands, and heart muscle.

(c) **Signs of right side heart failure** and passive congestion. Some cases die of the toxemia and others of the cardiac failure.

6. The histological changes are those of an acute purulent bronchitis affecting the smaller bronchi with or without some surrounding catarrhal pneumonia. Degenerative changes are seen in other organs, notably in the kidneys, where the appearances of a toxic nephritis may be found.

- - - - - - -

Abrahams, Hallows, Eyre and French, *The Lancet*, Sept 8 1917
"PURULENT BRONCHITIS: ITS INFLUENZAL AND PNEUMOCOCCAL BACTERIOLOGY".

p. 377 "One point which has impressed all … in the Aldershot Command … is the occurrence of a considerable number of cases of a definite type, clinically recognisable almost at sight, yet different from anything we have been familiar with in men of military age in civil life. To this peculiar type of case we have applied the designation "purulent bronchitis" on account of the characteristic nature of the expectoration. [deserving] … special attention … two chief reasons. In the first place, the affection has a very high mortality-very much higher than that of lobar pneumonia ; secondly, there are features and circumstances which suggest an epidemic nature."

"A typical case of purulent bronchitis

"A typical case is as follows. The onset is usually acute ; the early symptoms are those of a "cold in the head." The temperature may be 101° or 102° F., but there are no features to distinguish the condition from acute coryza "or febricula, so that in the majority of cases the patient does not report sick for two or three days, by which time he is sent to hospital. At this stage two features attract particular attention.

"First, the character of the expectoration: this consists of thick pale yellow dollops of almost pure pus, not the frothy expectoration familiar in ordinary bronchitis; it has no particular odour and it becomes increasingly abundant until in a day or two it may amount to several ounces in the 24 hours.

"Secondly, the rapidity of the patient's breathing : this may be so evident that pneumonia suggests itself, yet on examining the chest the only physical signs consist of few or many rhonchi scattered widely, but most marked at the bases of the lungs behind, associated with wheezy vesicular murmur ; resonance everywhere is unimpaired and bronchial breathing is absent. The characters of the temperature, pulse-rate, and respiration rate are exemplified below.

"A little later a third point attracts notice : a peculiar dusky **heliotrope type of cyanosis of the face, lips, and ears**, so characteristic as to hall-mark the nature of the patient's malady even on superficial inspection. By this time dyspnoea is very pronounced ; respiration consists of short, shallow movements, which in bad cases amount almost to gasps, reminiscent of the effects of gas poisoning. Recovery at this stage may occur, but by the time the cyanosis has become at all pronounced the prognosis is extremely bad, though the number of days the patient may still live in spite of the severity of his distress is often surprising. One of the most striking features of these cases is the great respiratory distress and the peculiar **heliotrope cyanosis of the face** in the fatal cases.

"In a sequential series of 8 cases, 2 of which died: Sputum. ... The bacteria, although numerous, were in some instances limited apparently to two species- namely, (a) minute Gram-negative bacilli often exhibiting bipolar staining and so simulating **diplococci**, chiefly intracellular but also in extracellular bunches; and (b) extracellular Gram-positive lanceolate **diplococci.** ... in every instance the Gram- negative bacillus predominated. ...

"General Bacteriological Conclusions.

"It seems not unlikely that these patients suffer from a primary invasion of their lung tissues by the B. influenzae, and that pneumococci, present at the same time, are at first of low virulence. The earlier symptoms seem to be attributable to a B. influenzae toxaemia. Exaltation of the virulence of the pneumococci by symbiotic growth with B. influenzae would appear to follow, **a fatal termination being due to pneumococcal septicemia.** ... When a patient has become decidedly cyanosed no treatment that we have been able to devise appears to do any good."

- - - - - - -

Cecil and Austin, *J.Exp. Med.* July 1, 1918 (published); April 22, 1918 (received for publication)

p.34 "The vaccination of the troops began on February 4, 1918. The Division was transferred from Camp Upton about April 15, 1918. The following figures are based on the period extending from February 4 to April 15, about 10 weeks. The number of troops vaccinated was 12,519. The number of unvaccinated was approximately 19,481. The latter figure varied, of course, from day to day as new men came and others departed."

p. 19 – notes that pneumonia was responsible for probably 80 percent of the deaths in various training camps in this country ... " many caused by streptococcus but pneumococcus also played a prominent part. Notes that while prior work on pneumonia prophylaxis had been carried out by Wright in 1911 and 1912, these earlier works had not differentiated between types of streptococcus, rendering interpretation of results difficult."

Cecil/Austin show protection against pneumonia/deaths, but make no mention of Influenza except in relation to similar anti-typhoid shot symptoms. They used a mixed vaccine of Pneumococcus I, II and III.

"There were twenty-eight cases of streptococcus pneumonia among the unvaccinated half and only two cases of streptococcus pneumonia among the vaccinated half, yet these men were living in the same part of the camp and closely associated on drill-grounds, and in recreation and amusement halls. ... The incidence of pneumonias, pneumococcic and streptococcic, was approximately equally distributed in the two groups of organizations previous to the beginning of the vaccination."

p. 21-30 Preliminary experiments indicated protection in extensive mouse tests and volunteer disease tests in trials, serum tests, agglutination titer, mouse protection experiments (after Douchez)

p. 34 Vaccinations began Feb. 4, 1918, through April 15.

Before vaccinations, 30 % of pneumonias were streptococcal.

p. 37 Pneumonia death rate per 1000 – vaccinated

Table VI
Incidence of Pneumonia among Vaccinated Troops, February 4 to April 15, 1918.
Average strength of command, Feb. 4 to Apr. 15, 1918 32,000
No. of troops vaccinated against pneumonia . . . . 12,519 (40 per cent)
No. of unvaccinated men (average) . . . . 19,481 (60 per cent)

Incidence of pneumonia among the vaccinated troops, Feb. 4 to Apr. 15:
Total No. of pneumonias among the vaccinated troops 17

Table VII.
Incidence of Pneumonia among the Unvaccinated Troops, Feb. 4 to April 15 ,1918.
Total No. of pneumonias among the unvaccinated troops 173

TABLE VIII.
Mortality Rates. Feb. 4 – April 15, 1918
Type of pneumonia.   Deaths.

Among unvaccinated troops.

	(*Txt table vii*) Tot # pneu	#	%
Pneumococcus.			
Types I, II, and III .	26	7	27
Type IV	33	. 6	18
Streptococcus haemolyticus	72	26	36
" *viridans*	34	. 4	12
Type undetermined	7	5	
Totals	**172**	**48**	**28**

Annual pneumonia death rate per 1,000 for unvaccinated troops   12.8
[actual = 48/19481 = .002464]

Among vaccinated troops.   Table vi
Pneumococcus
Type 1   1   0
Type 4   9   0
Streptococcus h¢molyticus   6   2

"	viridans........	1	0	
Total.........		**17**	**2**	**11.8**

Annual pneumonia death rate per 1,000 for vaccinated troops 0.83
[Actual = 2/12519 = .000160]

Whether calculated on an "annual" or "actual basis, unvaccinated were 15 times as likely to die. A summary of the control shows that there were twenty-six cases of pneumococcus pneumonia of Type I, II, or III. There were thirty three Pneumococcus Type IV cases, making a total of fifty-nine pneumococcus pneumonias. There was a total of 106 streptococcus pneumonias, 72 of which were of the hemolytic type and 34 of the *viridans,* or non-hemolyzing type. Altogether there were 173 pneumonias among the unvaccinated troops.

p. 38 There were seven deaths among the Pneumococcus Type I, II, and III cases, or 27 per cent (Table VIII). There were six deaths among the Pneumococcus Type IV cases, or 18 per cent. Of the streptococcus cases, hemolytic type, twenty-six died, or 36 per cent. There were only four deaths, among the *viridans* cases, the mortality being 12 per cent.

- - - - - - -

Lathrope, August 10, 1918 JAMA 71 (6), p. 451-55,
    "Acute Mastoiditis as a Complication of Infectious Diseases"
Lathrope notes that during the prior winter the southern Army camps were invaded by streptococcus infection, with the highest mortality attributed to the Streptococcus hemolyticus. The epidemic at Camp Shelby was not of the severest type, with "only about 300 cases of pneumonia and 35 cases of empyema. ...[but] among the empyemas, the hemolytic streptococcus is not the prevailing agent ... by far the larger number ... are due to a streptococcus of the S. viridans group." The Camp Shelby experience also differed from the other bases in that "there is a large number who suffered invasion of the middle ear and mastoid. ... In all 123 soldiers developed acute mastoiditis of one or both sides... ."

Lathrope correlates the timing of the mastoid cases, from dec. 15 to Feb. 1, with a preceding measles epidemic, beginning in October, peaking in late November, and declining rapidly in Jamuary. Lathrope posits that measles was "responsible for 36 percent of the mastoid cases" and suggests "a greater number were due to respiratory infections" with "a definite history of it in only 28 percent of the cases. Lathrope notes a considerable number of such cases with complicating bronchitis, and several developing pneumonia.   A few cases developed so rapidly that it suggested hematogenous infection, despite the proximity of middle ear to the nasapharynx via the middle ear.

"Captain Zingher, in his report on the bacteriology of the empyema cases occurring at Camp Shelby, thus describes this organism:

"The streptococcus viridans isolated from a large number of the cases of empyema occurring in this camp produces on blood plates rather large, moist colonies, resembling somewhat those of the Streptococcus mucosus.   This appearance of the colonies is most marked at the end of 24 hours. At the end of 8 hours, these colonies become flat and dry. The size of these colonies is in striking contrast to the small pin point colonies usually produced by the ordinary Streptococcus viridans. The blood medium is turned slightly green, especially where colonies are numerous. There is no evidence of hemolysis. In broth cultures the organism produces a sediment, which consists of very long convoluted chains of cocci. The supernatant fluid is clear. The organism has no capsule and is not soluble in bile. It does not ferment inulin. The morphology of the organism is interesting. When grown on a solid medium the cocci are generally uniform in appearance; the organism shows, however, a tendency to polymorphism, many of the cocci appearing unusually large, oval or rod shaped."

" ... out of our 27 measles-streptococcus cases, only one showed a hemolyzing streptococcus. The proportion of deaths in this group was very high, three out of five."

Lathrope concludes that the mastoid infection epidemic is one expression of the general streptococcus incidence in the camp, and this in turn "but a sideshow in the very widespread wave of streptococcus disease throughout southern Army camps."

- - - - - - -

American Journal of Public Health, Vol 8 # 10 Oct 1 1918
George T Palmer, MD

"Boston, with a total population of less than 800,000, has had about 4000 deaths from the beginning of the disease in early September to October 19." Epidemic in Boston started around September 8, showing a peak in Boston around Sept. 30 1918.

		#pers	# influ	% influ	# died	% died
Boston City Hosp. Persons -	Vaccinated	46	0			
	Not Vacc	88	28		Not mentioned	
Boston City Hosp. Nurses -	Vacccinated	32	0		0	
	Part.Vacc	8	8 mild		0	
	Not Vacc	4	2		2	
Wretham State School	Vaccinated	66	6 mild		0	
	Part.Vacc	1	1			
	Not Vacc	58	33		1	
TOTALS	Vaccinated	144	6 mild		0	
	Partly vac.	9	9 (8 mild)		1	
	Not Vacc	150	63		3	(2.0%)
[Boston Total Population		800,000			4000	(0.5%)]

p. 788 "Among the curative measures [that] have been advocated: use of serum from convalescent patients, and again, anti-influenza vaccine. In the reduction of contact infection, the face mask, the stagger-hour system of transportation, the education of the public in personal hygiene, and the closing of schools, assemblies, etc., have probably helped somewhat. There seems to be little hope for controlling the epidemic along these lines, however, for the scourge is more communicable than measles."

"As for the vaccine [referring here to 'anti-influenza vaccine'; no specifics are given], the Massachusetts scientific and statistical commissions have concluded that it has no therapeutic effect,* that the prophylactic effect merits further investigation, and that no ill effects follow the use of the vaccine.

"The South Department of the Boston City Hospital reports 46 vaccinations, none of which were followed by influenza; on the other hand, of the remaining 88 attendants and patients, 28 contracted the disease-about a third.
"Another analysis from the same figures shows that of 32 vaccinated nurses none contracted influenza; 8, who had been incompletely vaccinated, contracted mild cases. The remaining 4 nurses refused to be vaccinated: of these, two developed influenza and died.

"At Wrentham (Mass.) State School, 66 vaccinations are said to have been followed by 6 mild cases, and no fatal cases. One incompletely vaccinated individual developed a fatal case. Of the remaining 58, who were not vaccinated, 33 sickened, and one died.
"**The results which are available are interesting and suggestive, but not conclusive**; for they all have "the weakness that vaccination was not begun until influenza had developed in the institution", and had taken down a number, possibly the most susceptible, who might have taken the disease even if vaccinated. But while we wait for more conclusive statistics, the epidemic rages; any community is, therefore, justified in employing the vaccine, for it is safer to gamble with the cost of preparing and administering the vaccine than with the lives endangered. It will be well to emphasize to the public that the vaccination is experimental, and is not compulsory; otherwise, in the event of its ultimate failure, the whole system of vaccination may be discredited by the public, including that against smallpox, typhoid, etc.
"Turning to therapeutic efforts, the serum described in this issue by McGuire and Redden seems promising and should by all means be tried. As with vaccine, however, it is too early to make definite statements.
"The open-air treatment of Brooks was found by the Massachusetts State Health Department to be the most valuable factor in reducing mortality. Apparently the fatality of hospital cases was reduced from 40 per cent to* about 13 per cent by the treatment. An invaluable incident to this treatment is the fact that in the open air, the immunity of the nurses and physicians is enormously increased, leaving them to carry out the great amount of work confronting them.

"What should health officers do in those communities where the disease has not yet struck? Shall they build fences to try to keep people from falling off the cliff or shall they invest in ambulances to take care of those who will have fallen?
"It must be confessed that to date the preventive measures have not averted the epidemic. It would seem advisable for the health officer first to organise his open-air hospitals and relief agencies as far in advance as possible; let him organize for efficiency the doctors, nurses, social workers, teachers, and volunteers. Money and assistance will be easy to get, for the public has been aroused. With one in two

hundred persons of the stricken populations dying, no community will criticise the health officer who may have prepared too thoroughly.

"The health officer should also put into effect with great vigor all of the preventive measures at his disposal. Let him not neglect, however, to plan for those who are sure to become sick-and as pointed out to the investigator in the first paragraph for those who will die. Regrettable and discouraging as it is, we must nevertheless admit that in this specific catastrophe, the ambulance possibly will help more than the fence. [* See the notes section of this issue, p. 802.]

p. 802 notes: Massachusetts. "-Influenza apparently first reached Boston about August 25, and by the middle of September had reached epidemic proportions. On October 4, the disease was made reportable over the state, and from 6,000 to 8,000 cases were reported daily. The fatality is very high-about 5 per cent. By October 12, influenza was on the decline in Boston, only about 120 deaths being reported daily from influenza and pneumonia, as opposed to 200 when the epidemic was at its height.

"However, the western part of the state, which was attacked later, was becoming more seriously involved about the middle of October.

"Dr. E. R. Kelley appointed two committees to study the value of an influenza vaccine prepared by Dr. Timothy Leary of Tufts Medical School. The Board of Scientific Investigation, consisting of Drs. M. J. Rosenau, G. W. McCoy and Frederick F. Gay, concluded as follows:

"1. The evidence at hand affords no trustworthy basis for regarding prophylactic vaccination against influenza as of value in preventing the spread of the disease, or of reducing its severity. The evidence from the present epidemic, though meagre, suggests that the incidence of the disease among the vaccinated is smaller than among the non-vaccinated. The Board, therefore, concludes that further experimental evidence should be collected.

"2. The evidence at hand convinces the Board that the vaccines we have considered have no specific value in the treatment of influenza.

"3. There is evidence that no unfavorable results have followed the use of the vaccines. The Board of Statistical Investigation reached substantially the same conclusions. It consisted of the following: Prof. G. C. Whipple, Dr. W. H. Davis, Dr. Frederick C. Crum. It was further pointed out that open air treatment and the use of face masks were effective in protecting exposed persons.

"It is recommended that the distribution of influenza **vaccine be encouraged for prophylactic use** in order to obtain further experimental evidence, but that the State neither furnish nor endorse the vaccine at present for therapeutic use."

- - - - - - -

Oct. 5, 1918 Jama editorial 71 14 p. 1101

"THE INFLUENZA OUTBREAK -- As set forth elsewhere in this issue[1], widespread outbreaks of acute respiratory infection have occurred at irregular intervals for many centuries. The general clinical manifestations and the complications have been always practically the same. Owing to conditions that are far from being adequately understood, such infection now and again spreads over the world with great rapidity and in a manner that was altogether mysterious and disconcerting until we learned that it never spreads faster than human travel. It seems as if in the course of evolutionary processes there suddenly is liberated a form of infectious agent against which large numbers of people offer little or no resistance and which is transmitted readily from person to person under the most diverse hygienic and geographic circumstances. That the peculiarly subtle nature of these outbreaks was recognized long before the bacteriologic era is indicated by the introduction of the name influenza, which means, literally, influence. The question as to the real nature of this "influence," it must be acknowledged, is not settled definitely. The discovery by Pfeiffer in 1890, at the time of the last pandemic, of the influenza bacillus *(B. influenzae)* in the sputum and respiratory tract of influenza patients seemed, it is true, to have settled the matter. At any rate, **Pfeiffer's claim** that he had discovered the cause of influenza secured fairly general acceptance except possibly in France.

"Since then, **however, the influenza bacillus has been found to be present in practically all cases of whooping cough and in a large percentage of the cases of measles and scarlet fever, as well as in tuberculosis and chronic bronchitis.** Minor epidemics of acute respiratory infection, clinically regarded as epidemics of influenza, have occurred in which the influenza bacillus was not present regularly in the sputum [2] or the respiratory tract. In such epidemics, as well as in the great pandemic of 1889-1890, streptococci and pneumococci occurred quite regularly in the respiratory tract; indeed, a large group of French and German investigators regarded the great pandemic as a streptococcus or mixed streptococcus and pneumococcus infection. We see that as a matter of fact the only evidence that influenza is caused by the influenza bacillus, up to the time of the present outbreak, is the demonstration by Pfeiffer and others of the presence of the bacillus among other bacteria in the respiratory tract of patients with influenza. The production of influenza in animals by injections of pure cultures of the bacillus has not given any decisive results. No distinctive immunologic reaction has been discovered, showing that the body reacts specifically to the influenza bacillus in the course of influenza. In truth, the evidence in favor of the influenza bacillus is not any stronger or different from that which can be urged in favor of the streptococcus, pneumococcus or other bacteria. And if we grant the possibility that the influenza bacillus may cause outbreaks of influenza, wherein lies the deep difference between such strains of the bacillus and the strains found in whooping cough, measles and other conditions?

"The "influence" in influenza is still veiled in mystery. It is also too early to consider in detail the outcome of the etiologic investigations of the present outbreak; already contradictory results have been recorded, and for the present we await further developments. We may anticipate, however, highly valuable and interesting contributions when the full observations on the outbreaks at the Great Lakes Naval Training Station and other military camps, as well as in civil groups, are published. The recent remarkable work on the spread and prevention by selective isolation of streptococcus bronchopneumonia in measles; and other conditions in our Army camps sets a fine example, which we believe will be duplicated in connection with influenza.

References:

1. Epidemic Influenza, Therapeutics Department, this issue, p. 1136.

2. Mathers, George: Etiology of the Epidemic Acute Respiratory Infections Commonly Called Influenza, Proc. Inst. Med. Chicago, 1916, 1, 84; Bacteriology of Acute Epidemic Respiratory Infections Commonly Called Influenza, Jour. Infect. Dis., 1917, 21, 1

- - - - - - -

Park Oct. 12, 1918, *NY Med J,* announces the testing of "a pure influenza [bacillus] vaccine made from a current strain of influenza bacilli, rather than one of a mixture of cocci and bacilli." The vaccine was saline, heat-killed, given in 3 injections at 2-day intervals, in quantities of one half billion, one billion and two billions; was being given to a limited number of persons in corporations, among troops in several camps, and was being furnished to New York City physicians who promise to provide information on results. The clinical aspects of 15 fatal cases are discussed, but no vaccine results are given, implying that they were not yet available.

- - - - - - -

JAMA Volume **71** part 2, p.1573 -- ABSTRACTS OF FOREIGN LITERATURE COMPILED BY BRITISH MEDICAL RESEARCH COMMITTEE

"[NOTE.—The following abstract on influenza is taken from the Medical Supplement compiled by the Medical Research Committee of Great Britain and issued by the General Staff under date of October 1. It apparently covers all the important recent literature on this subject, and especially German literature, which is not now available in this country.—ED.]

BRITISH EPIDEMIC OF 1915 -- " The Leipzig epidemic was not an isolated instance of a European influenzal disturbance. Shera early in 1917 gave an account of an influenzal epidemic of the spring of 1915 in London and the southern counties, in which he claimed to have occasionally isolated a bacillus similar to *B. influenzae,* but it is somewhat difficult to identify it from the scanty details given. Lenz drew attention to very frequent occurrence of pneumonias in 1915 in German prisoners' camps. Coincidently with both the epidemics observed by Stephan, catarrhs and bronchitic infections localized in the bronchioles appear to have been very prevalent in December, 1916, and January, 1917, in military hospitals in France and also at home. The *British Medical Journal* drew attention to their extent in a special article, stating generally that their bacteriologic character was rather undecided, though a coccal (mainly pneumococcal) nature was assumed. The infections were stated to have run an acute course. At about the same period, in the late winter of 1917, a "grippal" outbreak visited Vienna and lower Austria, but *B. influenzae* was not found, because **Economo** *(Medical Supplement,* 1918, 1, 220), in his account of encephalitis lethargica, insists in his differential diagnosis on this fact. Von Wiesner *(Medical Supplement,* ibid.), describing the **diplococcus which, he claimed, had caused the epidemic of encephalitis,** emphasized the frequent findings on postmortem examinations of that period of lesions indicative of hemorrhagic diathesis, produced, in his opinion, by the **"diplococcus of encephalitis." It may be noted that this organism was held to behave variably toward gram-staining, to have been pleomorphic, and insoluble in bile. The pleomorphic diplococcus discovered and described by Rosenow and his collaborators in America at the time of the 1916 and 1917 epidemics of poliomyelitis falls undoubtedly into the same group of organisms.** Incidentally it may be added that bronchopneumonias were often found to have been the determining cause of death in both the Viennese and the American outbreaks of poliencephalomyelitis."

...

INFECTIVE ENCEPHALITIS -- "The late winter and spring of this year witnessed the epidemic of infective encephalitis in this country, while isolated outbreaks of virulent pneumonias seem also to have been observed. At one of the London hospitals (unpublished observation) a **diplococcus identical with that of Rosenow** was obtained in several cases of encephalitis and frequently found in the routine examination of throat swabs. "During the first week of May of this year an acute febrile disease with symptoms resembling those of influenza invaded three factories and one industrial home for boys in Glasgow," to quote MacLean. "The bacillus of influenza was invariably absent. ... A gram-negative **diplococcus resembling the pneumococcus** has frequently been obtained from the nose, throat, lungs and membranes of the brain." A few months ago Rosenow found streptococci in an outbreak of "grip" in Chicago.

Thus it is clear that in the three years 1915 to 1917 diplococci were the predominating organisms associated with influenza-like infections, although it is difficult to pronounce as to the identity of the several strains described.

...

BRITISH LITERATURE

-- "Little, Garofalo and Williams flatly deny that the pandemic is a true influenza. For, first, no relapses or complications were observed by them in France; secondly, in the twenty cases examined by them, there was very slight leukocytosis with a proportional lymphocytosis of a small mononuclear variety, and lastly, **as in all the twenty cases, a very small gram-positive diplococcus was of "universal predominance."** It was absent from the two blood cultures that were undertaken. It was recovered from nasopharyngeal and throat swabs and from the sputum. Morphologically it was flattened out on apposing sides. **It appeared sometimes in pure culture. Grown on legumin-serum agar, it developed in small transparent granular streptococcal-like colonies.** It showed a slight tendency to anaerobic growth, fermented no sugars and was nonpathogenic to animals.

Gotch and Whittingham examined carefully fifty cases. Leukopenia with a neutrophilia at the height of fever, accompanied by a slow pulse, were pathologic features observed. In 8 per cent, of the throat swabs and sputums, *B. influenzae* was found. In the remaining cases there was constantly present a gram-negative **diplococcus** not unlike *M. catarrhalis,* while in 10 per cent, of cases there was also a coccus similar to the meningococcus. The fairly large predominant **diplococcus** was also recovered from the blood, and its cultures proved pathogenic to man in the two instances in which the disease was experimentally transmitted by means of its cultures. The organism, if properly investigated, might be found related to the larger group of cocci previously dealt with.

......

-- "Averill, Young and Griffiths had under their care 1,439 patients, of whom sixteen developed lobar pneumonias with seven fatal issues. No account is given of postmortem examinations. Forty-three cases were examined bacteriologically. *B. influenzae* was not detected in the nasopharynx, a grampositive **diplococcus** being predominant. The sputum of forty-one patients showed in thirty-two cases the presence of the same diplococcus associated with a gram-negative bacillus often in clumps. In nine other instances the diplococcus retained the field to itself.

...

-- " Simmonds maintains that the only difference as against the 1890 pandemic consists in the more frequent occurrence of secondary streptococcic infection. ...
"Gruber and Schadel insist on the frequency of periarteritis and panarteritis, and note an acute dilatation of the right heart in most cases, a finding identical with that of Hammond, Rolland and Shore (see above). Diplostreptococci were the only bacteria found by them. ...

- - - -

Eyre and Lowe October 12 1918 discuss an outbreak of 327 mild cases of measles and rubella in January 1918, followed by 124 cases in February of which 24 died. On examination it was determined these were "identical in its clinical features with the outbreak of purulent bronchitis investigated by the same observers in the Aldershot Command during the early part of 1917 as per Abrams Sept 1917] ... In the recent and severe cases cyanosis was pronounced ...
"Speaking generally, the bacteriological findings were very similar. B. influenzae was present on one or more occasions in 12 of the 14 sputa examined, usually associated with Streptococous longus and various types of Micrococcus catarrhalis.
"In the fatal cases the heart blood and spleen showed the presence of Streptococcus pyogenes longus with marked haemolytic properties. Thus the **analogy with the cases of purulent bronchitis observed the preceding year [as per Abrams Sept 1917] was complete**; there was evidence of a primary infection of the respiratory tract by Bacillus influenzae, which so lowered the resistance of the individual that secondary infection by the Streptococcus pyogenes longus (and not the pneumococcus, as in the Aldershot epidemic) ensued, and in many instances resulted in an **acute and rapidly fatal streptococcic septicaemia."**

Accordingly, March 15 to August 18, control group for Eyre and Lowe 1918; inoculations made on March 16 and March 26, resp. (first and second shots); summary results reported for influenza incidence (from June 7 to August 18) were 2 per 1000 in vaccinated compared to 28.4 (48.2 per table on p. 486) average in uninoculated New Zealanders stationed in England during the period.

This thus seems to comprise one of the first reports on the effectiveness of prophylactic vaccine in the 1918-9 pandemic, along with Cecil and Austin at approximately the same time (the latter, Feb 4 – April 15), this in reference to the first wave!

The authors provide partial fatality data for the earlier outbreak of a severe outbreak of rubella and bronchitis with 21 fatalities out of 124 cases. However, fatality data is not reported for the 1000 inoculated in March.
[This study is discussed further by Eyre in April 1919 (below).]

- - - - - -

October 26, 1918: *THE LANCET*, "THE UTILISATION OF VACCINE FOR THE PREVENTION AND TREATMENT"
    "After discussing the available evidence as to the bacteriology of the present epidemic, the majority of those present were **agreed that there was considerable doubt as to the primary etiological significance of the Bacillus influenzae of Pfeiffer**,"

- - - - - - -

Leishmann, *THE LANCET*, Feb. 14, 1920:
    "THE LANCET published on Oct. 26th, 1918, the proceedings of a Conference of bacteriologists, summoned by the Director-General of the Army Medical Service to consider the advisability of employing in the army a preventive vaccine against influenza. This Conference, of which I had the honour to be chairman, agreed that such a vaccine might be expected to be of service, and made recommendations as to its constitution and use."...
    "As was naturally to be expected, in view of the divergent views held as 'to the bacteriology of the epidemic, the proposed constitution of the vaccine was subjected to a certain amount of criticism in subsequent issues of the medical press, and the points made in these communications, many of them most valuable and helpful, were duly noted. One of the principal criticisms was concerned with the dosage which had been agreed on as appropriate for the R. influenzae moiety of the vaccine., it being urged that a considerably larger dose of this might be given with safety and with the prospect of an enhanced degree of immunity. In view of this, and also of the fact that, as the bacteriological experience of the epidemic extended, the aetiological role of Pfeiffer's bacillus came more and more into prominence, I consulted my colleagues of the original Conference afresh upon this point and found them all in agreerrent with an I increased dose of Pfeiffer's bacillus, which I proposed should be

raised from 60 millions to 400 millions in 1 c.cm., it being understood that the strains employed should not have been so cultivated or so recently I, derived from cases as to be unduly toxic in their action.

> The Revised Formula.
> The formula of the vaccine as thus revised, and as now employed in the army, is therefore
> B. Influenzae 400 millions   in 1 ccm
> Streptococci   80 "   "
> Pneumococci 200 "   "

"From the first it was desired that every attempt should be made to secure clear statistical evidence of the results of the inoculations with the vaccine, and the necessary instructions to this effect were circulated by the War Office, returns in accordance with a simple 'pro forma being called for at regular intervals. In view of the opinion, widely expressed in both medical and lay journals, that we are threatened with another epidemic wave of influenza, it is felt that the results obtained in the army commands at home last winter with the vaccine in question should be made known, not only because it is proposed to advocate its employment again in the army, if we should be so unfortunate as to find ourselves in the presence of a serious recrudescence of the disease, but also because the modified vaccine now in army use has, I understand, been adopted by the Ministry of Health for employment in the civil community.

The Original Formula. -- "The vaccine formula recommended by the Conference mentioned above was as follows : Several strains and types of each organism were used, all comparatively freshly isolated from cases of the disease. Two doses were recommended, the first 0.5 c.cm., and the second, given after 10 days' interval, 1 c.cm. The statistical results recorded below apply should be taken as a complication. The returns, all of which lie within the period between November, 1918, and April, 1919, comprise all those relating to this period which conformed to the following requirements:-

1. That the vaccine used was that prepared at the Royal Army Medical College, according to the original formula.

2. That influenza should have been present in the unit during the period under review. In many stations where inoculation has been largely carried out there was a rapid cessation of the epidemic. Such returns would have swelled the total of the inoculations without throwing any light on their protective effects.

3. That only such returns are included as showed that at least one-tenth of the average strength had been inoculated, whether with one dose or two.

Information was asked for as to the interval occurring. It will be noted from the table that nearly one-half of the inoculated had received only the first dose of the vaccine, i.e., one-third of the amount which we considered essential to effective protection. It is reasonable to assume that, had all received the full dosage, the protective results would have been still more evident. No statistical evidence bearing upon this point is, however, available.

- - - - - - -

Tunnicliff, *JAMA* 71, Nov. 23, 1918, p. 1733 - Mathers died October 5.

Mathers "isolated a green-producing streptococcus from the sputum in 87 percent of 110 cases of influenza and pneumonia examined.
"The coccus appeared in the sputum smears as gram-positive diplococci, 2 microns in length, with slightly pointed ends and a capsule. In cultures they grew in pairs and long chains and showed a capsule. On human blood agar plates the colonies were large (from .25 to .5 cm. in diameter) green, flat, moist, with regular edges, and had a tendency to become confluent. The colonies often showed umbilication in 48 hours. Cultures of this organism were not soluble in bile. They grew as a flocculent growth in glucose and plain broth, the fluid generally not remaining clear. They fermented glucose, lactose and saccharose, but neither mannite nor inulin,except in one instance. Sputum injected intraperitoneally into mice was virulent, killing them within 24 hours. These cocci were not agglutinated by type pneumococcus serums."
Tunnicliff conducted experiments with antibodies (opsonins) indicating specificity for the green producing streptococcus during the course of the disease, decreasing in pneumonia following influenza and returning to normal or above upon recovery.
"It is generally recognized that opsonins are the only antibodies easily demonstrated in streptococcus infections. ... The changes in opsonic power in influenza and influenzal pneumonia are specific for the green-producing streptococcus, no fluctuations being observed with Bacillus influenzae, Micrococcus catarrhalis or Streptococcus hemolyticus. These experiments would indicate that the green-producing streptococcus is of some significance in influenza and the complicating pneumonia."

- - - - -

Unattributed Item following Tunniciff article, page 1734
"Vaccination Against Pneumonia – The experiments of Army Medical Corps with vaccinations against pneumonia due to the pneumococcus, Types I, II and III, in two of the Army camps have had so much apparent success that a memorandum has been issued to officers, enlisted men, and employees of the War Department, announcing that this prophylactic vaccination is available to all who desire it. At Camp Upton [Cecil and Austin?] during a period of ten weeks, no cases of pneumonia due to the types of peumococcus mentioned, occurred among vaccinated troops, and
The British Medical Journal, Vol. 2, No. 3018 (Nov. 2, 1918), pp. 481-486

Nov. 2, 1918]   SECONDARY PURULENT BRONCHITIS.   [THE BRITISH MEDICAL JOURNAL   481

PURULENT BRONCHITIS COMPLICATING MEASLES AND RUBELLA.

BY

TEMP. LIEUT.-COLONEL W. M. MACDONALD, B.Sc., M.D., M.R.C.P., N.Z.M.C.,
CONSULTING PHYSICIAN NEW ZEALAND EXPEDITIONARY FORCE;

MAJOR T. R. RITCHIE, M.B., N.Z.M.C.,
PATHOLOGIST — NEW ZEALAND GENERAL HOSPITAL;

LIEUTENANT J. C. FOX, M.R.C.S., R.A.M.C.;

AND

P. BRUCE WHITE, B.Sc.,
PATHOLOGIST TIDWORTH MILITARY HOSPITAL.

THIS epidemic of exanthematous disease complicated by purulent infection of the bronchi attacked several hundred men belonging to a recent draft from New Zealand; 418 cases of measles and rubella occurred between January 1st and March 8th, 1918. In the large majority there was a copious frothy or muco-purulent bronchorrhoea, in 75 of them there was a severe purulent bronchitis, and of these 26 died. If we take into consideration only the definite cases of septicaemic bronchitis the mortality amounted to one-third of the men attacked, but, as practically all the cases showed signs of a much more severe bronchial catarrh than ordinarily occurs in measles, and as the sputa in these cases contained the same organisms as in the more severe ones, it seems reasonable to regard them all as cases of multiple infection, and, by doing so, to reduce the mortality to about 7 per cent.

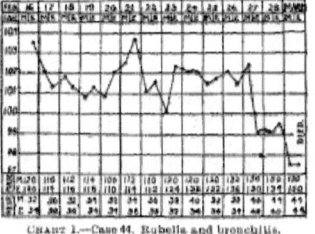

CHART 1.—Case 44. Rubella and bronchitis.

We retain the name "purulent bronchitis" as bronchitis with purulent expectoration was common to all the cases, but the severe type consisted rather of a septicaemia accompanied by various lung lesions which were not constant but ranged from bronchial catarrh to broncho-pneumonia, pleurisy, basal congestion, or lobar pneumonia. No one of these types could be said to prevail, but the serious cases which lived long enough passed through all these phases in succession, although they usually died before definite lobar pneumonia was well established.

There seems little doubt that the original infection occurred at an American port where the transports touched, as they had been free from infectious disease during the voyage, but measles and rubella broke out on board two of them just before arrival in England —that is, some fourteen days after leaving America. In the first five days after arrival at Sling Camp 77 cases developed, and thereafter the incidence was: Week ending January 19th, 60; January 26th, 125; February 2nd, 113; February 9th, 43; February 16th, 25.

During the same period 401 men suffering from febrile respiratory affections were admitted to the observation wards Sling Camp. These cases consisted largely of coryza or febricula, and 303 of them were described as "clinical influenza." It is noteworthy that none of these men developed purulent bronchitis, although most of them were respiratory cases, and had been living in the same

C .

huts as the measles and rubella cases. The complication of purulent bronchitis was limited strictly to cases of measles and rubella and to one case of scarlet fever.

Several organisms were recovered from the sputa and from the blood, and the virulence of the epidemic seems to be best explained by a symbiosis between one or more of these germs and the organisms of measles and rubella. If, as has been suggested in previous epidemics, the cause had been a symbiosis of the influenza bacillus with a pneumococcus or streptococcus, then we would certainly have expected to find some purulent bronchitis among 303 cases of clinical influenza which remained at Sling. But no single case of such a combination occurred.

Nor, again, did any purulent bronchitis arise among the 146 cases of measles and rubella occurring among British troops in the same district and at the same time, except in the case of a British motor driver who had been employed in transporting the New Zealand cases. Purulent bronchitis has only lately been clearly described and our knowledge of it is still in the mobile stage. It is undoubtedly much more widespread than is generally known. Thus, an officer (B.E.F.) died at Tidworth in February from bronchitis following some minor surgical intervention, and his lungs were found at the autopsy to show the same lesions as the cases dying from purulent bronchitis.

Further, three typical cases of purulent bronchitis complicating measles occurred in other New Zealand troops about the same time — one at Christchurch and two at Brockenhurst. These men had never associated with the draft at Sling, and they all recovered. It seems fairly certain, then, that purulent bronchitis is a condition in which there is

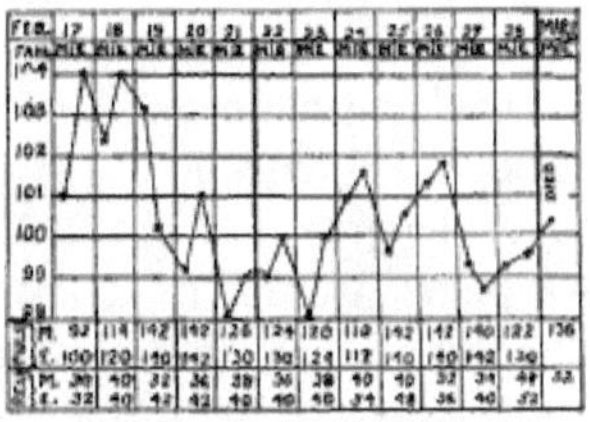

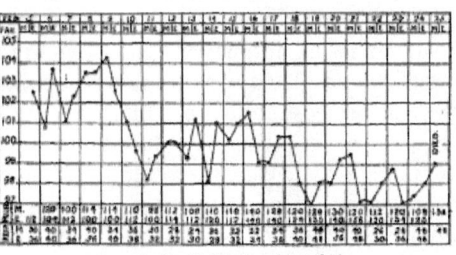

CHART 2.—Case 19. Measles and bronchitis.

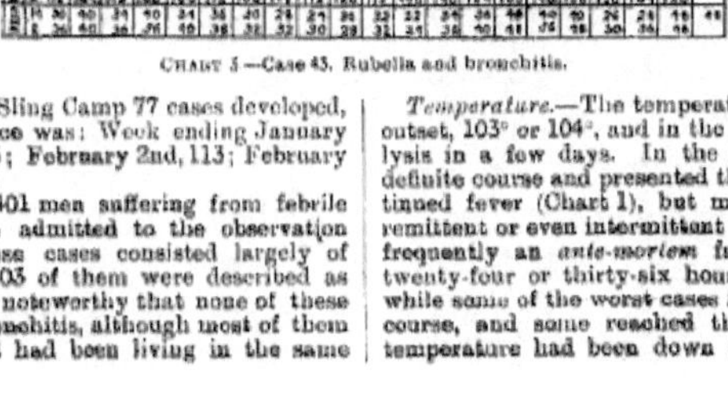

a definite symptom-complex resulting from a multiple pulmonary infection, but that the actual germs affecting this symbiosis are subject to variation. This does not necessarily lessen the stability of purulent bronchitis as a clinico-pathological entity, but seems rather to place it in the category of such conditions as haemolytic jaundice, pernicious anaemia, Banti's disease, typhoid and malignant neoplasm, in all of which a definite clinico-pathological condition is recognized as being of varied and multiple origin.

CLINICAL COURSE.

In most cases the onset was that of an ordinary cold, but in a few it was more sudden and accompanied by a slight rigor. In others there had been a bronchial or nasal catarrh for a week or longer, while in a few cases the men complained of having had a severe cough or sore throat for a month or so beforehand. Headache and pain behind the eyes were common features, and in a few cases there was profuse sweating.

Temperature.—The temperature was usually high at the outset, 103° or 104°, and in the lighter cases it dropped by lysis in a few days. In the severe cases it followed a definite course and presented the curve sometimes of a continued fever (Chart 1), but more often of an irregular remittent or even intermittent type (Chart 2). There was frequently an ante-mortem fall of temperature in the twenty-four or thirty-six hours before death (Chart 1), while some of the worst cases followed an almost apyretic course, and some reached the worst phase after the temperature had been down for several days (Chart 3).

CHART 3.—Case 45. Rubella and bronchitis.

[3018]

pneumonia due to other organisms was only one tenth as high among vaccinated as among the unvaccinated although previous to vaccination the pneumonia had occurred equally in the two groups. The vaccine employed is a lipovaccine. It is given in a single injection, containing pneumococci, Types I, II and III. Reactions from injections, etc., are, as a rule, less pronounced than after the use of antityphoid vaccination. The vaccination is not intended to cure those who are ill with pneumonia, and it is not advised for those who are suffering from acute colds or fever."

- - - - -

JAMA, Nov. 23, 1918, p. 1735 -- "Epidemic of Bronchopneumonia at Camp Brant, Ill. – Preliminary Bacteriologic Report". Edwin F. Hirsch MD (Chicago) Captain, MC US Army and Marion McKinney Chief Technician Camp Grant Rockford, Ill.

"Throat cultures were taken on Loeffler's medium from the posterior pharynx of the first 300 hospital admissions and examined after twenty-four hours' incubation. The predominating organisms growing on this medium were gram-positive, usually diplococci as such or in short chains. Following this, 159 throat cultures were taken on blood agar plates in order to differentiate the gram-positive organisms, as well as to favor the growth of the influenza bacillus whenever it would be present. Many of these plates were pure cultures of fine green colonies containing gram-positive diplococci as such or in short chains, frequently lancet shaped. In all throat cultures the occurrence of the influenza bacillus was only occasional, never in pure culture, and, when found, always with a predominating number of diplococci with tinctorial, morphologic and cultural characteristics as mentioned above. A few colonies of hemolytic streptococci were noted in twenty of the 159 blood agar plates, nonhemolytic in not more than twelve.

"The surface streaks of the blood agar plates frequently were purely fine **green** colonies containing gram positive, lancet-shaped diplococci. Organisms resembling the influenza bacillus were rarely found, and never in pure culture. Blood cultures were made on ninety patients in the hospital and forty-five of them were positive, a gram-positive diplococcus being isolated in pure strain without exception.

"Spinal fluid removed at the postmortem examinations and from patients in the hospital has yielded this organism frequently, and it has been cultivated in pure strains from the exudate in the middle ears, from the frontal, maxillary and ethmoidal sinuses. In none of the sinus infections of the head has the influenza bacillus been observed. A large number of strains of this organism have been isolated from the lungs and the heart's blood at the postmortem examinations, and from the circulating blood stream of patients in the hospital.

"Table 1 contains certain cultural, morphologic and virulence properties for a few from the heart's blood, and Table 2 the same for those isolated from the blood stream of patients in the hospital, while Table 3 lists a few from the lungs. These tables indicate that the gram-positive diplococcus recovered from these fluids and tissues has all the morphologic and cultural characteristics of a pneumococcus, at least so far as modern standards of identification permit. They further detail experiments demonstrating the exceedingly great virulence these strains possess for susceptible laboratory animals. A guinea-pig of 328 gram weight was dead ten hours after an intraperitoneal injection of half the 24-hour growth on a blood agar slant of one of the strains isolated from the heart's blood. The virulence of these strains exceeds by far that known for pneumococci usually associated with disease, and while the organisms meet all the morphologic and cultural requirements of a pneumococcus, this difference in virulence makes them distinctive.

TABLE 1.—HEART'S BLOOD CULTURES, POSTMORTEM

Culture	Inulin Fermentation	Capsule		Bile Solubility	Amount of 1-24 Hr. Blood Agar Slant Injected into W. Mouse	Dose Fatal in Hours	Type	Organism Recovered Pure from Mouse Heart's Blood
		On Blood Agar	In h. b. of Mouse					
1024	+	—	+	+	0.0231	38	II	+
1029	+	—	+	+	0.0231	26	II	+
1030	+	—	+	+	0.0231	31	II	+
1031	+	+	+	+	0.0231	25	II	+
1032	+	—	+	+	0.0231	25	IV	+
1033	—	—	+	+	0.0231	25	IV	+
1034	+	+	+	+	0.0231	25	IV	+
1035	+	+	+	+	0.0231	31	II	+
1037	—	—	+	+	0.0231	27	II	+
1038	+	+	+	• +	0.0231	25	II	+
1039	+	—	+	+	0.0231	25	II	+
1040	+	—	+	+	0.0231	24	IV	+
1041	—	+	+	+	0.0231	30	IV	+
1050	+	—	+	+	0.0231	28	II	+
1053	+	—	+	+	0.0231	43	II	+
1056	+	—	+	+	0.0231	21	IV	+

TABLE 2.—BLOOD CULTURES

Culture	Inulin Fermentation	Capsule		Bile Solubility	Amount of 1-24 Hr. Blood Agar Slant Injected into W. Mouse	Dose Fatal in Hours	Type	Organism Recovered Pure from Mouse Heart's Blood
		On Blood Agar	In h. b. of Mouse					
604	+	—	—	+	0.0231	18	II	+
605	+	—	+·	+	0.0231	22	II	+
606	+	—	+	+	0.0231	22	II	+
608	+	—	+	+	0.0231	24	IV	+
610	+	—	—	+	0.0231	18	IV	+
611	+	—	+	+	0.0231	30	IV	+
614	+	—	+	+	0.0231	12	II	+
615	+	—	+	+	0.0231	16	II	+
630	+	—	+	+	0.0231	32	II	+
636	—	+	+	+	0.0231	22	II	+
638	+	—	+	+	0.0231	16	II	+
640	+	—	+	+	0.0231	22	IV	+
646	+	—	+	+	0.0231	18	II	+
651	+	—	+	+	0.0231	68	I	+
654	+	—	+	+	0.0231	22	II	+
655	+	—	+	+	0.0231	14	II	+
660	+	—	+	+	0.0231	30	IV	+
663	+	—	+	+	0.0231	16	II	+
664	+	—	+	+	0.0231	22	IV	+
665	—	—	+	+	0.0231	16	II	+
666	—	—	+	+	0.0231	36	II	+

"To control these investigations, throat cultures were taken from fifty of the German prisoners confined at Camp Grant. This group of men has escaped entirely the infection, although they have been in the camp since last spring. Colonies of pneumococci were found in 20 of these cultures and isolated in pure culture. White mice were inoculated with half the growth of these organisms on blood agar slants after 24 hours' incubation without the slightest effect on these animals.

"CONCLUSIONS

1. The epidemic of bronchopneumonia at Camp Grant is due to infection by a virulent strain of pneumococcus.

2. The virulence of this organism exceeds greatly that of strains usually identified in pneumonia.

3. This virulence is such as to explain the epidemic of bronchopneumonia.

4. Bacillus influenzae played no role in the epidemic at Camp Grant.

TABLE 3.—LUNG CULTURES, POSTMORTEM

| Cul- ture | Inulin Fer- menta- tion | Capsule | | Bile Solu- bility | Amount of 1-24 Hr. Blood Agar Slant Injected Into W. Mouse | Dose Fatal in Hours | Type | Organ- ism Re- covered Pure from Mouse Heart's Blood |
		On Blood Agar	In h. b. of Mouse					
265	+	—	+	+	0.00555	30	IV	+
276	+	—	+	+	0.00555	24	IV	+
287	+	—	+	+	0.00555	18	IV	+
288	+	—	+	+	0.00555	24	II	+
291	+	—	+	+	0.00555	24	II	+
293	+	—	+	+	0.00555	18	II	+
294	+	—	+	+	0.00555	29	II	+
295	+	—	+	+	0.00555	32	II	+
343	+	—	+	+	0.00185	36	II	+
358	+	—	+	+	0.00185	30	IV	+
309	+	—	+	+	0.00185	36	II	+
384	+	—	+	+	0.00555	14	IV	+
398	+	—	+	+	0.00555	23	II	+

- - - -

JAMA 71, December 7, 1918, p. 1899

Barnes describes the experience with Leary's influenza baccilus (Pfeiffer's bacillus) vaccine at the state sanitorium, during the last two weeks of September 1918. In his Table, he gives comparative numbers of persons and cases, vaccinated and unvaccinated, as reflected in Chien's Table 3. Regarding mortality, he states that of 25 vaccinated patients with influenza, 4 died, compared to 9 of 57 unvaccinated patients with influenza, and that "the influenza incidence was 20 percent among both vaccinated and unvaccinated"; however, this data is not consistent with, and thus cannot be compared with, the totals he gives for numbers of persons versus numbers of cases, e.g., his table only lists a total of 23 unvaccinated cases of influenza, versus the figure of 57 given as per above. Barnes makes no mention of pneumonia at all.

Overall, he concludes that "mortality among those who developed influenza was practically the same whether vaccinated or unvaccinated.|"

- - - - -

McCoy Dec. 14, 1918, *JAMA* Volume 71, No. 24, p. 1997

In this one-column, detail-deprived report, McCoy claims to refute the effectiveness of Rosenow's vaccine. Aside from a number of other problems that would invalidate McCoy's claim as discussed further below, the basic problem is that McCoy's premise is based on the effectiveness of the vaccine against influenza, whereas Rosenow was very clear from the outset that his vaccine was not directed at influenza; rather, it was directed against pneumonia and pneumonia death, and McCoy makes absolutely no reference to pneumonia or death. Beyond this fundamental issue, there are a number of other problems with the McCoy position. He states the vaccine used was from F. O. Tonney of the Chicago Health Department. [A report by Tonney below gives high marks for this vaccine when used in Chicago.]

No information is given on the location of the investigation, and it is noted: "we are not intimately acquainted with the process of the preparation of the vaccine ...",

It seems clear the particular vaccine used was not produced locally (as was emphasized as necessary by Rosenow and others) specifically for the test, but rather was in the form as received from Chicago.

We learn from an entirely separate report (Kelley) that the McCoy "test" was conducted in Napa Valley, Ca, (July 1919, *California State Journal of Medicine*, Vol. XVII, No. 7 -- W. H. Kellogg, MD) not anywhere in Illinois where it was produced, in contraindication to the instructions of Rosenow et al. It is further notable that Kelley refers to Milton Rosenau, with whom McCoy otherwise had work relative to influenza, primarily trying (and failing) to transmit influenza to human subjects (guinea pigs). Also, Kelley refers to McCoy's use of a "Rosenau-type" vaccine, possibly a misspelling on the assumption that McCoy states that he used a Tonney/ Chicago vaccine that may have been produced in accord with the Rosenow recipe, but in any case it was not produced by Rosenow, and again, it was produced with an Illinois strain and would not have been expected to have been effective in California.

Noting the dosages of microorganisms in the McCoy test, per cc:

B. Influenzae	500 million
Pneumococci Type I	"
Pneumococci Type II	"
Pneumococci Type III	"
Pneumococci Type IV	1,500 million
Streptococcus hemolyticus	1,500 "
Staphylococcus pyogenes-aureus	500 "

And doses used:

.5 cc first injection

1 cc second injection

1.5 cc third injection with interval between injections of 48 hours.

Injecting alternate patients, 390 vaccinated and 390 not, McCoy concludes "It appears from the evidence afforded by these observations that no protection was afforded by the vaccine.

The authorship of this article lists McCoy of Washington D.C., Murray, Asst. |Surgeon of US PHS, and Teeter, an Intern at Stanford U. Hospital in San Francisco. Apparently the "test" was conducted by an intern.

- - - - - - - - - -

JAMA 71, Dec. 21, 1918, report in "Society Proceedings", on APHA Annual Meeting held in Chicago Dec. 8-11, 1918:

Of this meeting Eyler 2010 states: *"By the beginning of 1919, Rosenow, the most vocal defender of vaccines, found himself on the defensive. During the discussion of his paper at APHA's annual meeting, he faced hostile comments from both McCoy and Victor Vaughan.* [This is absolutely not correct; see below,]

In opening comments, among others; only E.C. Rosenow and G.W. McCoy are quoted below in entirety:

p. 2097 Park opens: -- Park laments the absence of sufficient control cases to assess the efficiency of influenza bacillus vaccine, citing need to wait for results of serologic studies.

Jordan attributes cases of pandemic influenza to "an unknown or unrecognized virus which increases the susceptibility of the individual normally to infection with the various pathogenic respiratory tract organisms ..."

2098 - E. C. Rosenow - "By the use of a properly prepared vaccine it is possible to afford a definite degree of protection for individuals, including pregnant women, during an epidemic of influenza. There is no noticeable increase in the number of cases immediately following the inoculations, and protection lasts for a period of at least six weeks. The favorable results from inoculations indicate that these so-called secondary invaders, which appear to have exalted and peculiar infecting powers, bear a close etiologic relation to epidemic influenza. This relation, however, may be in merely favoring the invasion of an unknown virus. Nearly all physicians report that the attacks of influenza are milder and of shorter duration, and that convalescence is more rapid in inoculated patients as compared with uninoculated individuals. The tendency of infection of the lower respiratory tract to develop pneumonia is noticeably less in the inoculated. According to the evidence at hand, the prophylactic vaccinations have conferred a decided immunity in pregnant women. This infection has proved very fatal among the uninoculated of this class."

[and immediately following, is a section entitled "DISCUSSION", with McCoy the first entry]:

G.W. McCoy: "See the article on 'The Failure of a Bacterial Vaccine as a Prophylactic Against Influenza." *JAMA* Dec. 14, 1918, p. 1997.

That's it! That is all McCoy said in this meeting, according to this JAMA report!! Compare this to statements by PHS "spokesperson" Eyler 2009-10. This could easily be considered a horrendous conflict of interest; rather such a conclusion could hardly be avoided.

Further in the DISCUSSION section: F. O. Tonney [head of the Chicago Dept. of Health]: "The ratio of influenza patients developing pneumonia in the unvaccinated of industrial groups studied was 1 in 21, while in the vaccinated it was 1 in 184. The ratio of influenza cases terminating fatally in the unvaccinated of the industrial groups in Chicago was 1 in 48, and in the completely vaccinated there were none in the 1201 cases reported.

"The influenza in vaccinated individuals occurred almost exclusively in those who had received one vaccination. No bronchopneumonias or deaths occurred in the vaccinated group after the second or third vaccination. ...

Table constructed from the above data

	Pneumonia/Influenza	Mortality/Influenza
Unvaccinated	1/ 21 (.047619)	1 / 48 (.0208)
Vaccinated	1/184 (.0054)	0/1201 (0)
	= 8.8 times worse without vaccine	

It is notable that this data is not mentioned by **Eyler** 2009-10, but rather the McCoy comment is lauded (by Eyler). Absolutely incredible!

Also provided in this report are results by Sherman of Pittsburgh, reporting on results at the Homestead plant:

	Total	# Influenza	% Influenza	# Died	% Died
Un-inoculated	1687	588	30	42	2.5 [2.5]
One inoculation	5964	213	3.5 [3.6]	9	1.5 [.15]
Two inoculations	5222	174	3.2 [3.3]	4	0.08 [.08]
Three inoculations	4720	66	1.4 [1.4]	0	0.00 [0]
Four inoculations	4007	108	2.8 [2.7]	2	1.05 [.05]
1-4	19913	561		15	
2-4	13949	348		6	

Eyler goes on to say (totally fabricate) Vaughan also was "hostile" to Rosenow, which is simply not true. Contrary to the statement of Eyler 2010, Col. Victor Vaughan makes absolutely no mention of or reference to Rosenow or his vaccines. Vaughan, whose comments comprised about 80% of the text in the discussion section, makes a general statement asserting continued ignorance of the prevention of respiratory diseases. With reference to "vaccines for influenza", he only addresses the failure of the McCoy and Park vaccines made from the Pfeiffer bacillus, and the encouraging results of Cecil and Austin:

"We have used influenza vaccine in great quantities, all they could make in the Army laboratory, and have used all that Dr. McCoy could spare, and also have used that which Dr. Park has furnished us from the New York laboratory, and I do not hesitate to say that it has not done one bit of good. Speaking on this point with the evidence of the Pfeiffer bacillus not being the cause of influenza, I can agree with those who have spoken."

Regarding vaccines for pneumonia, although Vaughan makes no reference to Rosenow, he notes "encouraging results" of Cecil and Austin.   Summarizing Cecil and Austin's work at Camp Upton, updated to a latest report within the past day or two, Vaughan notes the same number of cases of pneumonia among the 20% of unvaccinated cases as among the 80% unvaccinated; in other words, there was a four-times greater incidence of pneumonia per person among the unvaccinated compared to the vaccinated.

It is clear from the actual report that the information provided by Eyler was fabricated.

- - - - - - - - - -

R. A. Fennel -- *JAMA* 71 December 28, 1918 -- p. 2115
"This pandemic had high incidence and mortality rates. In the great majority of cases, death was directly due to a bronchopneumonia. ... "

Fennel states it is too early to determine the cause, and possible role of Pfeiffer bacillus, virus, "or a streptococcus, S. viridans or S. hemolyticus, or a heretofore unidentified gram-positive coccus."

Fennel reviews the history if pneumonia research, from 1881to 1918, noting the preponderance of emphasis had been on therapy over prophylaxis, and positing the assertion that any microbic disease should yield to prophylaxis. Tracing the progress of classification of pneumonia from Neufeld in 1900 and 1909 through Douchez and Gillespie 1913, Lister 1913, Friedlander 1918, Olmstead 1917 and Wright 1914, noting the Type IV pneumococci implicated by Friedlander at Camp Sherman (80 % of type IV in their pneumonias) and with particular attention to Lister's extensive animal experimentation and vaccines, and classification relative to Group IV (noting this is a common mouth organism).

Fennel then proceeds to assert that: "Their true worth is practically vouched for, and the results amply confirmed by the recent work of Cecil and Austin", with a saline vaccine "much after the fashion of Lister", noting the demonstration of the antigenic effects of their vaccine through animal experiments and limited human experiments, and summarizing results of Cecil and Austin's landmark pneumonia vaccination efforts in 1918.

Fennel emphasizes the advantages of a lipovaccine over a saline vaccine, as pioneered by Le Noignic and Pinoy 1916, and elaborated by the Army Medical School by Dec. 1917, Whitmore, Fennel and Peterson 1918. [all citations are in this Fennel article], particularly: (1) the enabling of massive doses in one single inoculation, rather than the three required with a saline vaccine, and (2) eliminating the sharp reaction commonly caused by saline vaccines. "The reports following its use, and the coincidental pandemic, with the attendant pneumonias, confirmed the wisdom of adopting this vaccine as a general but voluntary measure in the Army ... It is to be emphasized that this was not a vaccine developed over night as a prophylactic against influenza; **it was a vaccine aimed at pneumococcal infections, developed systematically at a time considerably antedating the present pandemic.**"

Following a description of the method of making such a vaccine, Fennel notes "This completed vaccine is then subjected to rigorous cultural tests, and is finally injected into animals to insure sterility. It is then ampuled and distributed for use. ... **the Army Medical School has manufactured and sent out for use during October and November 1918, more than two million doses of this vaccine.**" ...

"Much had been hoped for when the tabulated results of this widespread vaccination would have been available. The abrupt cessation of the war, and the rapid demobilization that must follow, will withdraw from observation this large number of vaccinated men. ...

"Preliminary clinical reports seem to be highly satisfactory. Some of the unexpected results, such as made their appearance at Camp Upton, seem to be following the use of the lipovaccine. While a specific immunity against the three types of pneumococci in the vaccine was all that was hoped for, a certain freedom from respiratory diseases in general seems to have followed its use. **Absence of bronchial symptoms in influenza, after vaccination, was noticeable. ...**"

"That the vaccines may have had some nonspecific value, comparable with that of the vaccine used at Camp Upton, cannot be denied."

p. 2117 notes: "It will be noticed that a Type I, II and III vaccine seemed to prevent practically all cases of pneumonia due to these types, and caused an apparent protection not only against Type IV, which might have been suggestive of cross protection, but also against Streptococcus hemolyticus and S. viridans."

We may also note that, from the data given, S. hemolyticus (72), S. viridans (34) and undetermined (7) accounted for a total of 113 of 172 total pneumonia cases, or 65.7 % of the total deaths, nearly 2/3, in unvaccinated persons.

TABLE 2.—RESULTS IN A SERIES OF MICE INOCULATED WITH PNEUMOCOCCUS VACCINE, TESTED TO DETERMINE THEIR RESISTANCE TO HEMOLYTIC STREPTOCOCCUS TWO MONTHS AFTER VACCINATION; SEPT. 15, 1918

Series No.	Date of Vaccine Inoculation	Vaccine	Amount, C.c.	24 Hour Broth culture*	No. of Inoculations	D.	A.	D.	A.	D.	A.	Per Cent. Dead	Per Cent. Alive
1 13 mice	7/16/18 7/24/18 8/ 1/18	Saline pneumo.	⅛ ¼ ¼	1/25 1/50 1/100	5 4 4	3 1 0	2 3 4	4 3 1	1 1 8	5 3 1	0 1 3	100 75 25	0 25 75
2 12 mice	7/16/18	Lipo-pneumo., unheated	¼	1/25 1/50 1/100	4 4 4	4 2 0	0 2 4	4 3 0	0 1 4	4 3 0	0 1 4	100 75 0	0 25 100
3 7 mice	7/16/18	Lipo-pneumo., heated 53 C. (Army)	¼	1/25 1/50 1/100	2 3 2	1 1 0	1 1 2	1 2 0	1 2 2	1 2 0	1 1 2	50 66 0	50 33 100
Control 4 26 mice	.... —	.... —	—	1/50 1/100	6 20	2 1	4 19	3 3	3 17	3 4	3 16	50 20	50 80

* Twenty-four hour culture, low virulence Streptococcus hemolyticus.

- - - - - - -

Ely, Lloyd et al, *JAMA* Jan 4, 1919, p. 24

"One of us (Lloyd) observed in 1915, 1916, and 1917 the hemolytic streptococci, fatal to rabbits in pure culture (intravenously), could usually be found in certain types of influenza." They discuss here one patient with severe **cholecystitis,** after operation and recovery, subsequently became ill with fever, collapse, **pulmonary edema and intense jaundice,** dying 21 days after operation and 48 hours after the last illness began, noting also that some fatal cases of influenza also involved jaundice.

In the then-current influenza epidemic, the polymorphic nature of the organism was noted, "Never did blood cultures show anything but diplococcal or streptococcal forms ... . Lt. Henry reports that in a few case studied by him at the Seattle training camp he obtained only diplococcal forms, which he regards as pneumococci."

In discussion of clinical data, "The cough is usually loose, and an abundant frothy, greenish fluid, pink with blood is brought up. ... In severe and fatal cases delirium is present, the facial expression is anxious, and there is often marked cyanosis."

In discussion of bacteriological findings, "Sputum examinations were made in 49 early cases, and 25 late cases with these results: Smears were made from selected portions. Gram positive cocci were found in pairs and chains, streptococci predominating throughout all examinations. ... A total of 52 attempts at blood culture on living patients gave 24 positive results, all streptococci except one, which gave only a diplococcus, which would not chain … ."

[POLYMORPHIC DISCUSSION] Cultural and staining characteristics: "On tubed solid mediums the organism we are describing grows in small, discrete colonies. On blood agar plates the colonies are usually larger, and when recently from the human body are surrounded by a well marked hemolytic zone. Hemolytic properties are quickly lost in subcultures, but may be restored by passage through rabbits or white mice. The microscopic appearance in smears from human and animal tissues is that of a coccus occurring in short or long chains; once a diplococcus only was obtained from a blood culture. In the mouse the organism may show as mixed diplococci and streptococci. On agar the growth may also show mixed diplococci and streptococci, or there may be chains of diplococci, and after a few generations bouillon cultures may show diplococci predominating and even groups suggesting staphylococci, though when grown in bouillon direct from human and animal tissues, chain formation is the rule …The size of the organisms varied from 0.3 to 1 micron; they were usually true spheres, but occasional were somewhat elongated. The development of the organism in broth produces diffuse cloudiness accompanied by varying amounts of sediment "

p. 27 The authors describe the technic of preparation of vaccine, using mixed virulent strains of hemolytic streptococci.

Regarding incidence of influenza, it is noted that influenza was introduced by a group from Philadelphia, many of whom arrived ill or became ill shortly after arrival.

"It is fair to say that no unit was divided into two parts for the purpose of running experimental subjects and controls side by side. Circumstances were such that this could not well be done." It is also noted that in this group and in the seaman's barracks many cases occurred before vaccination, how many was not known. However, for the rest, vaccination was initiated prior to outbreak.

	Vaccinated					Not Vaccinated					
	Total	Cases	%	Deaths	%	Total	Cases	%	Deaths	% cases || % total
Philadelphia Unit	131	37*	28.2	0	0	855	168	19.6	21	12.5	
Seaman's barracks	2800	57*	2.03	0	0	3472	428	12.3	42	9.8	
Subtotals	[2931]	[94]	[3.2]	[0]	[0]	[4327]	[596]		[63]		
Seattle Training Camp 1	---	---	---	---	---	4159	813	19.5	33	4.1%	0.79%
Seattle Training Camp 2	662	11	1.60	0	0						
Marines, Yard & Depot	425	5	1.2	0	0						
Filipino Unit	111	2	1.8	0	0						
Aviation Unit	83	32*	38.5	0	0						
Subtotals	[1281]	[50]		[0]		[4159]	[813]		[33]		
Totals	4212	144*		0		8486	1409		96	6.8%	1.13%

*26 of 37 before vaccination completed; 55 of 57 and 31 of 32 after only one injection; or, out of 144 vaccinated who became ill, 86 received only one injection before, and an additional 26 did not complete vaccination; thus only 32 fully vaccinated persons became ill, and none died.

p. 27 "Of 4212 men who were vaccinated, not one man died."

Of 8486 men not vaccinated, 96 died,

p. 28 "Our findings failed to show that the influenza bacillus was in any way connected with the production of the disease at the Puget Sound Navy Yard.

"We believe that the use of killed cultures as described prevented the development of the disease in many of our personnel and modified its course favorably in others. We at first used a single strain, but later mixed two or more strains. We do not know that the latter is advantageous.

"Attention is invited to the fact that a vaccine made from streptococci apparently protected 662 blue jackets [marines] in a camp where Henry found what he considered pneumococci only."

- - - - - - `

In this same issue of JAMA: Rosenow Preliminary Report, Influenza and Pneumonia #1, wherein he states: " ... we put aside the debated question as to the cause of the initial symptoms and considered primarily the possibility of immunizing persons against the ... causes of death in this disease ... particularly pneumonia."

- - - - - - -

JAMA editorial jan 1919 - [This editorial was decisively influenced if not written by McCoy. Notably, **Eyler** refers to this as an "unsigned" editorial; as such it would presumably have been written by the editor, Simmons, a close associate of McCoy]

This editorial adopts at the outset the critical perspective of a recent report of the Committee of the APHS, asserting even before commenting on the work at hand that data on prophylactic inoculation "are simply too inadequate to permit a competent judgment." Specifically regarding the immediately preceding report of Rosenow, the editorial asks for details regarding communities, population, incidence, mortality, and numbers, location and results of vaccines (all items which Rosenow responded to in detail in subsequent articles). Seemingly indicative that the editorial was more polemic than legitimate, two paragraphs down, under the guise of calling for "other points of detail", the author again calls for "dates, places, ages and population inoculated and uninoculated ..." etc.

Particularly exemplary of the intrinsically negative perspective are comments relative to the effect of Rosenow's vaccines on initial attacks of influenza. As Rosenow had stated at the outset, his intention was to reduce the severe effects of pneumonia and death, rather than the initial influenza; however as Rosenow reported, somewhat to his surprise, the vaccines did in fact seem to reduce the incidence of influenza as well. The editorial adopts the position that this result reflected an inconsistency in Rosenow's position, i.e., that Rosenow's reporting on the fact that the vaccine had beneficial effects against the initial influenza, notwithstanding that this was not its stated intention at the outset, seemed to contradict his initial intention that had not been directed at the initial influenza. In other words, the editorial attacks Rosenow for reporting that, while not intended, the vaccine IN FACT was effective against the initial influenza. !!

- - - - - - -

Brief biographical notes, George McCoy: -- Medical Director Public Health Service; Director Hygienic Laboratory, Public Health Service (which became) National Institute of Health; and a member of the *JAMA* Council on Pharmacy and Therapeutics – 1918 to 1945 !!

- - - - - - -

Abrahams January 4, 1919, p. 11 *THE LANCET "   " ...* severe cases [of then-recognized pandemic influenzal syndome] appear definitely related to the cases of purulent bronchitis, which have been described as occurring in various parts of the country and in France. ...

"The characteristic features of the septicemic type of case are variable lung symptoms, ranging from slight bronchitis to lobar pneumonia, **very characteristic heliotrope lividity**, dyspnoelia, or rather polypnoea, and very rarely orthopnoea. These, with other so-called complications of influenza, such as pleurisy, nephritis, and others of lesser import, are evidence of the septicaemia or toxaemia referred to.

Infection takes place in the upper respiratory passages, and involves the accessory nasal sinuses, where a septic sinusitis develops. From this and possibly other foci as yet undetermined, the toxaemia or septicaemia originates.

In view of the large number of instances in which the diplostreptococcus has been isolated in pure culture from the heart's blood and internal organs immediately after death, it is concluded that this organism plays an important role in the fatal cases.

- - - - - - -

Russell   Cecil and Henry Vaughn February 15 1919 *J Exp Med,* 457-83, : "Results of Prophylactic Vaccination against Pneumonia at Camp Wheeler"

A particularly notable omission from Chien 2010 is the Cecil and Vaughn article in Feb. 1919. Not only did Cecil (and Austin) publish the key article on prophylaxis of pneumonia in 1918, and further that Cecil historically is recognized for his contributions to the field of controlled studies, but this Cecil (and Vaughn) article was written coincident with the pandemic pneumonia that was the focus of Chien 2010.

This omission may be explained by two factors Chien 2010: (1) restricted consideration to those patients already inflicted with influenza that also contracted pneumonia (this fatal flaw in Cecil 2010 is discussed thoroughly above in the Introduction and Chapters 1-3; Cecil/Vaughn focused on pneumonia and dealt with influenza separately, as discussed below; and (2) excluded studies that involved only the so-called the influenza bacillus, whereas those vaccines given for influenza within Cecil/Vaughn specifically were with the influenza bacillus. While those persons in Cecil/Vaughn that received influenza vaccines also received pneumonia vaccines at the same time, the separate effects of the pneumonia vaccines are less clear in these persons as otherwise reflected in the total results. Nonetheless:

p. 470 notes that Types I, II and III constituted 43.2% of all pneumonia cases from July 1 to October 1, 1918, but only 11.5 % from October 1 to December 20 (during the influenza pandemic), and that mortality was 15.7 % in summer and 22.4 % during the influenza pandemic. It is noted that "the influenza epidemic began to make itself felt at Camp Wheeler" between October 12 and 19; the week after, the pneumonia rate for vaccinated persons ceased to increase and then rapidly declined. This is in accord with Whitmore experiments indicating protection did not begin until the 8th day after vaccination."

p. 480 "It will be recalled that at the onset of the influenza epidemic at Camp Wheeler, the proportion of Type IV pneumonia cases greatly increased even among the unvaccinated men. This may have been due to the fact that, from that time on, pneumonia at Camp Wheeler ceased almost entirely to be a primary disease, and became a complication of influenza.   Under such circumstances infection by whatever virulent organism that happened to be in the mouth would have occurred, and as the Type IV pneumococcus is the so frequently present in the normal mouth, it would naturally play a prominent part in the etiology of secondary pneumonia. …".

While Cecil/Vaughn do not further explore the relation of this observation to implications for the etiology of the pandemic, it does correlate well with the observations of Weston Price that call attention to the suggested role of oral infections in comprising a promising link between dental infections and severity of pandemic complications (See Table 1, page 10, and associated discussion in Chapter 1 above).

As clearly indicated by its title, which made no mention of influenza, the work of Cecil/Vaughn was aimed at pneumonia. The experiment at Camp Wheeler was planned and executed independent of the influenza epidemic, specifically as an experiment on vaccination against pneumonia, a more extensive trial and based on the success of Cecil and Austin earlier in the year at Camp Upton, with the purpose of consideration of establishing Army-wide pneumonia vaccination on a permanent basis. Camp Wheeler was chosen for the experiment in that pneumonia there had infected 917 soldiers from Oct. 5, 1917 to March 29, 1918, and a second epidemic of pneumonia in August 1918 caused 216 cases and 34 deaths.

Whereas a saline vaccine had been used at Camp Upton, Cecil and Vaughn used a lipid (vegetable oil) vaccine based on the experiments of Col. Whitmore [Harvey Lecture, Jan. 11, 1919]; the oily suspension was more slowly absorbed than the suspension in saline solution, and thus the three original doses of saline vaccine could be combined into one dose (1cc) without ill effect. Col Whitmore experiments showed immunity does not begin to develop until the 8th day after injection.

Excluding inoculated persons contracting pneumonia during the first week after the first inoculation, i.e., before the vaccine became effective:
Inoculated/Pneumonia cases/deaths: 13460/155/19 versus Not: 3415/327/73, i.e.,

if vaccinated it was 8.3 times less likely for you to get pneumonia and 15.1 times less likely to die from it.

p. 483, The authors conclude "… although influenza obscured to some extent the effect of pneumococcus vaccination at Camp Wheeler, the results are sufficiently encouraging to justify its further application in civil as well as in military life."

As of the time of Cecil's death in 1965, his Textbook of Medicine had made him "the best known American physician in the world". In 2008, Neuhauser etal. [J R Soc Med 2008;**101**:381-38] praised Cecil for his "clear … methodological awareness" of the role of controlled trials throughout his career. His pioneering and contributions to the history of controlled trials began soon after joining the U.S. Army in 1917, when he was asked by the Surgeon General to study pneumonia, and "carried out two very large trials to assess the value of vaccination." Cecil was noted as "creative in conducting his vaccine trials in circumstances largely outside his control", i.e., the 1918 pandemic, given the impossibility of a "textbook" controlled trial under such circumstances.

- - - - - - -

Minaker March 22, 1919 *JAMA*

Minaker notes that they had one month to prepare for pandemic. The time frame was same for vaccinated and for controls, and serologic tests.

Mention of diplococci and hemolytic streptococci.

Refers to the foundational work of Cecil and Austin.

"The fact that the recent influenza pandemic did not reach the Pacific Coast until about October 1, or more than a month after its appearance in the East, gave time to attempt a defense against it. …"

p. 847 "… there was a general agreement as to the pneumococcus and hemolytic streptococcus being largely responsible for the fatal complications. The recent work of Cecil and Austin at Camp Upton, confirming the observations of Lister, had shown that a high degree of immunity can be produced against pneumonia by prophylactic vaccination."

p. 848 Thus, Pneumococcus I, II and III, and streptoccus hemolyticus were incorporated into the vaccine; noting "a difference of opinion" as to the possible role of the so-called influenza bacillus, a culture from a fatal case of the latter was in any case also incorporated."

Cecil and Austin are again cited as having demonstrated with pneumococcic vaccination of over 12,000 men that no ill effects were encountered with pneumococcic vaccination, and that large doses were necessary to give full protection.

Table 1 – Composition of Mixed Vaccine

	No. of bacteria
B. influenzae, Rockefeller strain	5 billion
Pneumococcus Type I, various strains	3 billion
Pneumococcus Type II, regular and	

Irregular, various strains	3 billion
Pneumococcus Type III, one strain	1 billion
Streptococcus Hemolyticus, two strains	100 million

Details are given providing method of growing organisms to be included in vaccines. Since there were no prior reports on mixed vaccines, the vaccine was tested in 100 volunteers, including examinations of temperature, urine and blood count and agglutination tests. Following satisfactory experiments, general inoculation began October 12. Vaccines were injected subcutaneously at about the insertion of the deltoid muscle in doses of 0.5, 0.8 and 1.0 cc at 3-day intervals. A careful record was kept of all inoculated persons.

p. 849 Minaker provides details of inoculations in four groups of civilians, and was clearly conservative in reporting results, at least in one category. Because the 4950 (vaccinated) men of the Naval Station "were in quarantine during the height of the epidemic", notwithstanding that "no cases of epidemic influenza occurred during this period", he **omits these (otherwise-positive results), assuming this was because they were "not exposed".**

"Inoculations of the 1080 of the civilian population were completed by October 16, twenty four days after the start of the pandemic in San Francisco, and the **incidence and mortality figures for the city represent the period of time, beginning with the inoculation and running until December 1,** when the original epidemic subsided."

The 1950 marines at Mare Island were inoculated about October 20, about a week after the epidemic began, and were immediately released in Vallejo and San Francisco where the disease was at its height, and owing to the fact that statistical reports were not submitted to the PHS, the personnel of the Mare Island Navy Yard seemed to furnish a fair comparison. Incidentally all the severe cases developed within ten days after the last inoculation." [indicating that full effects of vaccine had not yet taken place].

"The low incidence of the disease in the inoculated persons can only be appreciated when **we compare with it the morbidity and mortality of the large population with whom they associated at the same period.**"

"The 3100 men from the San Pedro Naval Camp were inoculated about November 15, at which time the epidemic was in its recrudescence in Los Angeles and vicinity, and the **figures given represent only the cases reported in Los Angeles during the period of twenty four days following the inoculation of the men.**"

p. 850 "The facts presented undoubtedly indicate that a noteworthy degree of protection against influenza and its complications was obtained by means of a mixed vaccine freshly prepared from predominating etiologic bacteria."

- - - - - - -

Eyre and Lowe, *THE LANCET* April 5 1919, 553
- Citing their October 1918 article, which cites Wright, Lister, and Cecil & Austin
- Noting "a very fatal form of septicaemic influenzal pneumonia" that had broken out

-They do not list pneumonia in table 3, but give percentages for each of several entities for influenza and a "serious cases" category
-They do not provide influenza and pneumonia data for inoculated versus not, but do provide fatality data for inoculated versus not in Tables 1 and 3.

Referring to the prior Eyre/Lowe report of 1918 (above), it is noted here that in addition to the 1000 "nominal" first-inoculated troops in the prior report, another 3000 had been inoculated at about the same time, whose subsequent course reinforced the positive results in the first 1000.

Clarifying the results from the earlier report, Eyre etal confirm that the inoculated group was comprised of the first 1000 inoculated men; the control group of 1000 was an average of all other men in addition to this 1000, totaling approximately 19,000 men. This 19000 thus included some if not all of the "other" 3000 inoculated men plus all subsequent reinforcements, which were inoculated upon arrival. **Thus the figures reported**, of 2 influenza cases per the first 1000 versus 43.2 per the remainder, **were conservative in that the latter included many inoculated which if excluded would tend to increase the incidence in uninoculated.**

It is noted that this seemingly was the first and very notable report on the effectiveness of prophylactic vaccination against influenza, notwithstanding that its intention was vaccination against pneumonia.

In this current article the authors note that the decision to prepare further supplies of "mixed catarrhal vaccine" was made in early September 1918, before the outbreak of the second wave of influenza pandemic.

p. 554 In view of the apparent effectiveness of the vaccine used in the Spring against the first wave of pandemic in the summer, the same formula was used in September, utilizing and referring to "fresh material from virulent cases ... of a very fatal form of septicaemic influenzal pneumonia".

	dosage: First dose*	Second dose*
Pneumococcus	50	100
Streptococcus	10	50
B. influenzae	10	30
Staph. aureus	200	500
M. catarrhalis	25	75
B. pneumoniae	50	100
B. septus	50	100

*millions of organisms per .5 ccm

Regarding the dosage, "based upon animal experiments as well as clinical observation, ... the antigenic value of a vaccine depends primarily upon the character of the bacterial protoplasm it contains rather than the amount. ... and we are satisfied that had we used the large doses advocated by some we should have ... reaped a large crop of 'severe reactions,' and failed entirely in the attempt to immunize."

p. 555 The authors note that the second and more severe epidemic wave began in certain units before satisfactory immunity had developed.; "in most other units, however, a longer interval elapsed ..." between inoculation and outbreak. The authors present overall notes and details in some instances. Data is presented that indicate "no definite relationship between the date of onset ... [early or late in the epidemic] and the severity or mortality percentage of cases infected ... ."

"... The types of cases which occurred were similar to those noted by all observers throughout the United Kingdom.

(A) Simple pyrexia of from 2 to 7 days' duration, accompanied by malaise, prostration, headache, body pains, coryza, and epistaxis in varying degrees.

(B) Severe infection occurring in 15.5 percent of cases, in which bronchitis, bronchiolitis, broncho-pneumonia, pleurisy, etc., in varying degree and combinations supervened upon the previous pyrexia, and, in those cases which became fatal, passed [556] rapidly into a condition of intense toxemia or septicaemia with a clinical picture similar to that described originally be Abrahams, Hallows, Eyre and French, and more recently by Abrahams, Hallows and French."

    p. 558 refers to **"typical heliotrope cyanosis"**

    It is noted that CHIEN 2010 provides:

-- in C-K-M's Table 3 only that data taken from Eyre's Table V, for Military Hospital B during October, when the epidemic commenced – incidence of influenza for vaccinated versus not; and

-- in C-K-M Figure 2, data from Eyre's Table VI, also for Military Hospital B only (for the period October 4 – December 20), pneumonia per influenza cases for vaccinated versus non-vaccinated.

-- Please note that in C-K-M Figure 3, data indentified as coming from Eyre is incorrectly identified; this data is actually from Cadham's Table 1, "Report of Military Hospital", and the actual data from Eyre that might have been placed here is totally absent from C-K-M (as discussed below).]

    In the first data set of Eyre used by C-K-M, i.e., Eyre's Table V, Eyre had provided only a total of vaccinated at Hospital B (including those receiving two inoculations plus those receiving only one). Eyre had further qualified that half of the vaccinated had received only one inoculation, asserting that the result showed some protection against contracting influenza even with one inoculation.

    However, most significantly, in the latter data set of pneumonia incidence in influenza patients, **C-K-M's "vaccinated' had included the sum of recipients of both one and two doses, whereas Eyre etal's very first point discussing this specific data, page 557-8 states: "if infected before receiving their second dose of vaccine, they are not noticeably better off than the uninoculated ..." in terms of subsequently contracting pneumonia!**

    (Rosenow and others also showed that only the full vaccine course can be expected to be effective. Rosenow & Sturdivant note "we have purposely been unfair to the vaccinated group. The protection afforded among the vaccinated patients was measured from the day of the first vaccination, whereas, judging by the agglutination experiments, it should be calculated from about one week after the third injection.)

    Thus, pneumonia incidence per influenza cases data given in Chien 2010's Figure 2, i.e., 9/92 (9.8%) vaccinated versus 17/96 (17.7%) not vaccinated; would properly be corrected to 2/47 (4.3%) fully-vaccinated versus (17.0%) 24/141 not fully vaccinated, reducing the pneumonia incidence of vaccinated to ¼ that of the vaccinated, compared to the ½ reflected in the C-K-M presentation.. This "minor" correction alone, miniscule compared to the other gross deficiencies of C-K-M etal, seemingly invalidates C-K-M's (essential) Figure 2.

Interestingly, **Eyre's second point raised relative to this data, is that even among those receiving only one dose there were no fatalities, compared to 8.3% in the uninoculated.** (This information could properly have been inserted into C-K-M's Figure 3, in place of data there now wrongly attributed to Eyre in that it is clearly from Cadham.)

- - - - - - - - -

Zingher 1919 Apr 5 *JAMA*

Zingher refers to Rosenow's *JAMA* Jan. 4, 1919 article describing "an **atypical form of Streptococcus viridans**" ("Prophylactic Inoculation ..."), which "corresponds ... closely with that of the prevalent type ... as it occurred at Camp Shelby, Miss. during the winter and spring of 1918, as discussed in the prior Lathrope article in JAMA Aug. 10, 1918, p.451, in which Zingher had described this organism.

Zingher adds that he had "recently isolated from the lungs in a case of pneumonia that came to necropsy at Savenay, France, an identical organism which had produced in the patient a fatal pneumonia complicated by an empyema.

"One of the important features of the empyemas caused by this peculiar type of Streptococcus viridans was the great tendency to the encapsulation of the pus. The pus formed pockets that were difficult to diagnose except by the roentgen ray. .."

- - - - - - -

Cadham May 24, 1919:

- Streptococci/Pandemic Pneumonia
- Diplo in several places as predominant organism
- Pleomorphic diplo or streptococcus
- ¾ of Cadham's civilian vaccines used Rosenow strains
- addresses issue of controls, noting it is not possible
- Use of opsonic index
- Had warning re pandemic; **started October 20**, including viridans.
- Flu = **mortality 4 times as high in uninoculated**

"In August [1918], previous to the outbreak of recognized cases of influenza, there had occurred at the Tuxedo Military Hospital 2 cases of pneumonia, followed by empyema. I now believe from a study of their history these cases to have been originally influenza. At the time a pure culture of streptococcus was obtained from the pus of both these cases. A small amount of vaccine was made from this culture, and four of the members of the laboratory staff were inoculated. Examination in two of those inoculated showed increased opsonic index for this streptococcus. This increased opsonic index persisted for four months in one case in which the examinations were continued."

[Cadham proceeds to describe the pleomorphism of the predominant micro-organism:] "The predominant micro-organism thus found has been a streptococcus or diplostreptococcus. This is a Gram-positive streptococcus appearing in either short or long chains. It is pleomorphic. *The same micro-organism will appear at different intervals of cultivation as either a streptococcus or a diplostreptococcus.* No capsule was demonstrated. It is haemolytic on first cultivation, but loses this power on sub-cultivation. Cultivated for some days in serum-glucose bouillon it assumes a lanceolate shape. It forms discrete colonies on haemoglobin agar and confluent colonies on agar to which the blood had been added at 80 degrees C. Grown in serum-glucose bouillon it forms a diffuse cloud. It coagulates litmus milk with acid formation in 72 hours and ferments lactose. It does not ferment inulin."

"It was in the first week of October 1918 that cases of the pandemic influenza occurred in Winnepeg – that is, the first cases recognized as typical of the disease. The epidemic progressed rapidly, it reached its peak in the second week in November, and then slowly but gradually subsided.

With the knowledge that the disease was to reach us ... It was considered adisable to use a vaccine ... as a prophylactic against respiratory infection."

The vaccine for the military was prepared from streptococci from an empyema that occurred in August and two strains of streptococci from infected soldiers arriving on Oct. 1, 1918. "From time to time strains of streptococci were added ... ." Influenza bacillus from the first cases was also incorporated. The vaccine dose was .5 ccm, containing approx. 300 million streptococci, 200 million influenza bacilli and 150 million pneumococci.

Whereas 17 pneumonia and 5 fatalities occurred of 282 inoculated (half received 2 inoculations) admissions, versus 41 and 17 of 238 uninoculated admissions (between October 1, 1918 to February 28, 1919), "No soldier died who had been admitted subsequent to the second inoculation." Thus incidence of pneumonia was less than one half and mortality less than one-third in inoculated versus uninoculated admissions to the Special Military Hospital.

Regarding the civilian population, **"The majority of these inoculations were given in the earlier stages of the epidemic,** but no attempt was made to keep accurate statistics on this point. The ages of those inoculated were not obtained. Due to the exigency of war the profession was depleted and ll branches were forced to work under a great strain; also the people were nervous, so that it was **difficult to obtain full statistics or to divide any portion of the population in two parts for the purpose of running controls."**

Three-fourths of the civilian vaccines were produced from strains provided by Rosenow. The dose quantities were the same as the military.

Reports from 108 physicians provided data for 52,999 persons receiving one or two inoculations versus 85,941 uninoculated. The uninoculated were reported as more than 3 times as likely to die as those receiving one inoculation and seven times as likely to die as those receiving two. Overall both incidence of pneumonia and mortality was four times a great in the uninoculated. 101 of the 108 physicians reported that influenza attacks appeared to have been modified by one or more injections; and 32 out of 37 responding physicians reported that vaccine apparently afforded protection to pregnant women.

- - - - - - -

McCoy on Theoretical Considerations
  [See also Chapter 7, Theoretical Considerations, for perspective on early theoretical work by Greenwood and Yule, and modern work by Orenstein, etc.]

McCoy, Public Health Report, Volume 34, May 30, 1919
"Pitfalls in Determining the Prophylactic or Curative Value of Bacterial Vaccines"

In this 2.5 page report, with not a single reference citation, McCoy issues a broad, undocumented critique of bacterial vaccines with particular reference to influenza, citing three "pitfalls" and labeling both the first and third as "commonest".
  Regarding the first: "Perhaps the commonest source of error is that due to the employment of a vaccine in an institution, or in a group not in an institution, after cases of the disease have appeared."

At the outset it may be noted that, as asserted by Rosenow and others, for a vaccine to be at its most effective it must be prepared from the strain involved in the particular outbreak. Thus McCoy has set up an impossible "catch-22" dilemma. If this is true, that you need the causative organism to make an effective vaccine, you can never develop an effective vaccine before cases of disease have appeared!
  That said, the example given by McCoy for "closer examination", without specific citation, is arguably suspicious. Per McCoy:
  "It was reported that among a large group of hospital attendants, approximately one-third had been vaccinated and all had remained free from the disease, while the remaining two-thirds of the persons had not been vaccinated, all of whom had developed influenza. This appeared to be a very striking example of the prophylactic value of the vaccine, but when the fact was brought out that the vaccinations were only begun after practically all of the two thirds mentioned had become ill, the significance attributed to these figures was nullified, while the conviction remained that only the naturally immune had been vaccinated, it being unusual for more than two thirds of the personnel in any group to develop influenza."

As to the identification of the data on which McCoy's comments are based, we find suggestively-related terminology and round numbers in a prior PHS report of Oct. 1, 1918 (above): "The South Department of the Boston City Hospital reports 46 vaccinations, none of which were followed by influenza; on the other hand, of the remaining 88 attendants and patients, 28 contracted the disease." In this report, approximately one third of the total 134 persons (suggestively "attendants", in accord with the McCoy's designation), or 46, were vaccinated and indeed did not develop influenza. Of the remaining 88, only 28, or approximately one-third, developed influenza, in contrast to the example cited by McCoy in which "all" of the remaining two-thirds had developed influenza. Nonetheless, given the lack of a citation, and the similarity in terminology and overall vaccination ratio in the PHS report, leaves one suspicious of McCoy's treatment of the data and motives.

McCoy's second example illustrating this first criticism involved "a large group of persons in a civil community", in which "half of the [unvaccinated] cases had occurred before the vaccinations were completed"; again a lack of citations makes it impossible to assess its validity, and thus must be considered inadmissible.

McCoy's "second source of error", likewise undocumented, states "the writer is acquainted with a large group, where vaccinations have been done and where a rigid quarantine has been in force, which has remained free from the disease; and he is acquainted with a number of institutions where the same result has been obtained by quarantine alone." Again, McCoy offers no references or data, so it could as well be something pulled out of the air, or out of his ... imagination.

His third, which he also designates as the "perhaps commonest pitfall is the **drawing of conclusions from too meager data.** Thus, one observer assured me that he had been exposed to influenza patients many times and had taken no precautions beyond being vaccinated and he had not developed the disease. ...

"We hear of numerous examples of the cure of cases by means of vaccine. ... When the records were scrutinized, however, it was found that these remarkable cases could be duplicated by others that had done equally well without vaccine. "In the only examples with which I am familiar in which a vaccine was used on alternate cases, no better results were secured in the vaccinated than in the control group."

Again, in this "pitfall" discussion, there are no citations. Notably, in this last paragraph, McCoy is obviously discussing his own "study", using a **Chicago vaccine in California**, on a very small sample, asserting that Rosenow's vaccine was not effective. Notably, as per above, the indicated supplier of that vaccine from Chicago, reported very favorable results with the vaccine in the location for which it was intended. And, it must be noted, **McCoy's sample size was relatively small** in any case, and further, he was **strongly criticized for his technic** of using doses that were too large and at intervals that were too close in time.

McCoy goes on to claim he "has examined numerous clinical records to support the value of vaccines in pneumonia" and asserts these were not pneumonia, again without any citations/references. He provides very specific information which could easily have been checked if only a citation were given:

"In a certain large hospital, on one service, about 60 per cent of the cases admitted were diagnosed pneumonia and all were treated with vaccine, with a mortality of about 10 percent, while in the same institution, on another service, about 15 percent of cases were diagnosed pneumonia and the mortality was 40 percent. In this instance, the actual number of deaths was approximately the same, but vaccine-treated cases showed a much lower case-mortality in the pneumonias. I am by no means sure that the higher percentage of pneumonias diagnosed may not have been more nearly accurate than the lower, but it should not be the made the basis of misleading deductions."

Again, there are no citations, only, arguably, nonsensical, misleading rhetoric. The circumstance of equal numbers of mortalities in conjunction with the unsupported suggestion that the percentage of pneumonias may be off seemingly purports to nullify the data indicating that mortality was four times as likely for unvaccinated as compared with vaccinated persons.

McCoy continues: "The only way in which we are to secure promptly acceptable evidence of the value of a bacterial vaccine is by the vaccination of only a portion of the individuals in a large group, holding the remainder as controls; age, sex, and conditions of exposure being the same in the two groups." And then as if to cover his butt, he sort of says, in a sentence that doesn't completely make sense, that there are exceptions to this rigid control scenario, and concludes that "the failure of one [vaccine] does not necessarily mean the uselessness of others.

Just how this person became the first to have the title of Director of the National Institute of Health is truly bewildering, and very depressing.

- - - - - - -

"Studies on Epidemic Influenza" … by members of the faculty of the school of Medicine, U of Pittsburgh - S. R. Haythorn, M.D.

p.102: Haythorn cites personal communication:
"McCoy outlined the requirements necessary for an ideal vaccine experiment including: "The community should be as large as possible, and should number at least 10,000 persons." and "Fifty per cent, should be vaccinated before epidemic arrives, and the other 50 per cent, should be held as controls."

In other words, by McCoy's own standards, his small-sample article in CA with the Chicago vaccine, is worthless; and all of the works of the successful anti-pneumonia investigators, from Sir Almroth Wright to the present day, are flawed from the control perspective.

But then, on page 120, Haythorn praises McCoy's bogus small-sample experiment as "an excellent example … of a completely controlled test…" Hypocrisy?

Also in the U. Pittsburgh reports we find:
W. L. Holman, B.A., M.D., Professor of Bacteriology (CHIEF), June 1919
This is the same Holman that for years prior and after had sought to subvert Rosenow's work. Indeed this writer featured Holman's deceptive 1928 work in a volume, *Medicine's Grandest Fraud PhD*" (by this writer), wherein is discussed Holman's having grossly distorted Rosenow's 1915 JAMA published focal infection results; and had also previously attacked Rosenow's important work on mutations. It may be suggested that Rosenow's highly successful curture methodology undercut Holman's sale of his namesake culture media (Holman's broth).
[see also InstituteOfScience.com/nafraud.html]

W.L. Holman pp.161-205

"B-Influenzae as the Cause of This and Other Infective Processes"

Holman wastes little time asserting that it is he, Holman, who is the greatest bacteriologist of them all:

p. 181 "In all animal experiments it is of the greatest importance that the bacteria be known which may interfere in the experiments through spontaneous infection ... Rosenow in his experiments with streptococci from cases of influenza has also apparently failed to realize the importance of the lung lesions produced by the B. bronchisepticus in guinea pigs as reported by Theobald Smith, myself and many others."

p. 190 "Hemolytic streptococci have received much attention [including] ...various ill-defined streptococci" (here Holman slams Rosenow and several British writers)... citing Rosenow *Jour. A. M. A.*, 1919; Ixxii, p. 1604.

On the contrary, these so-called (by Holman) "various ill-defined streptococci" pleomorphic organisms are described / defined at great length by numerous writers, from Mathers to Rosenow to Billings and beyond.

- - - - - - - -

July 1919, *California State Journal of Medicine*, Vol. XVII, No. 7 -- W. H. Kellogg, MD, Secretary and Executive Officer, California State Board of Health

p. 228 Kellog notes "the remarkable uniformity of the epidemic of influenza in the length of time over which it extends" independent of any of the measures of control applied, i.e., that "in every one of the eleven cities shown [in his chart], the duration of time from the first sharp rise to the subsidence to approximately the base line is nine weeks."

Kellogg reviews a number of methods used to attempt to control the epidemic, including within a 3-1/2 page 2 column article (approx 40 inches of text) a brief paragraph (approx 3 inches of text) on vaccines.

P. 230 Kellogg asserts that "Vaccines have been definitely proven to be of no value as a preventive measure ...", citing only the work of McCoy and no others: "McCoy's experiment with the Rosenau type of vaccine in the Napa State Hospital, and with the straight influenza vaccine in a Massachusetts institution definitely disposes of vaccine as a preventive measure worthy of consideration. [Noting here that Kellog confuses E.C. Rosenow with "Milton Rosenau" (ally of McCoy in human experimentation, and predecessor at the Hygienic Laboratory), whereas he is seemingly referring to McCoy's bogus California "test" in any case.

It may be noted that McCoy's core of support comes from the likes of a state board of health official, i.e., Kellog of California, and city official, i.e., Park, both of which would be be beholden to McCoy for support from the federal gov't [see also commentary in "Modern Articles" file].

- - - - - - - -

Edwin O. Jordan -- *Journal of Infectious Diseases* Vol. 25, No. 1, July1919, 28-40, "Observations on the Bacteriology of Influenza" (supports Mathers diplococcus)

p. 28 In the second paragraph in his opening statement, discussing his purpose, Jordan refers to observations of two and only two organisms, the Pfeiffer bacillus and Mathers' diplococcus:

"One object especially in view was the determination of the relative frequency and abundance of the Pfeiffer bacillus in the upper respiratory tract of persons suffering from influenza and from common non-specific respiratory tract infections. Another was a series of similar observations on the diplo-streptococcus described by Mathers [(1. citing Tunnicliff, *JAMA* 1918, 71, p. 1733]

p. 29, in a description of the method of study:

"In the present series particular attention has been paid to the occurrence of the Pfeiffer bacillus and of the green-producing streptococcus isolated by Mathers."

p. 30 "**The Mathers Coccus**. – This organism was isolated by the late Captain Mathers during the influenza epidemic in September, 1918 at Camp Meade. A culture kindly furnished me by Dr. Tunnicliff possessed the characters described in her paper. (3) It **resembles the ordinary mouth streptococcus in some of its characters**, but the colonies on blood agar are much like those of the pneumococcus, although as a rule, larger, moister and more confluent. It is gram-positive, usually with pointed ends and in pairs. It is not soluble in bile, and most strains ferment neither inulin nor mannite. Morphologically and in colony growth it is closer to the pneumococcus than to the streptococcus, but the **fermentation characters are those of the ordinary mouth streptococci**.

"A coccus with these characters was found in a large percentage of the cases examined, not infrequently in practically pure culture especially in cultures from nasopharyngal swabs. One hundred and eight strains obtained at different times from 44 different cases were subjected to careful examination. All were gram-positive, had the morphology described above and gave a heavy, moist, green, confluent growth on blood agar. Table 1 shows their close relationship to strains of Streptococcus buccalis (Blake's classification) isolated in this same series of cases, although in morphology and in appearance of the growth on blood agar the difference is sharp."

TABLE 1

Showing the Close Relationship Between the Different Strains

No. of Strains	Bile Solu-bility		Fermentation						
			Lactose		Inulin		Mannit		
	+	–	+	–	+	–	+	–	
108	0	108	105	3	4	104	5	103	Mathers' coccus
85	0	64	84	1	2	62	1	63	Streptococcus buccalis
27	27	0	27	0	22	5	22	5	Pneumococcus IV

p. 32 "Attempts to differentiate the Mathers coccus and S. buccalis by testing their fermentation powers on a large number of carbohydrates have given negative results. ..." 47 cases were studied in detail. "... there is no doubt that Pfeiffer bacilli occurred more frequently and more abundantly in the uncomplicated influenza cases than in those in which pneumonia developed.

"In the October group in Table 1 (Groups A-1 and A-2), the distribution of bacteria found in uncomplicated and pneumonia-related influenza cases are as follows:

Type	No. of cases	No. with Pfeiffer bacteria	No. with Mathers cocci
Uncomplicated Influenza	11	8	4
Influenza-Pheumonia	8	3	8

"... Whereas in the earlier cases Pfeiffer bacillus colonies were relatively infrequent compared with the numbers of other bacteria, in the later cases there were many plates in which the Pfeiffer bacillus and the Mathers coccus were practically the only organisms present."

p. 37 **TONSILS** "**The association of large numbers of hemolytic streptococci (var. beta) with cases of tonsillitis and generally with cases of severe throat inflammation was markedly evident in this series. This corresponds with the relative scarcity of this organism in the cases of true influenza** in which, as a rule, sore throat was not observed. ... The term simple influenza is here used to designate those cases not showing signs of clinical pneumonia.", referring here leukocyte counts in "simple influenza" and similar counts (drops) in influenza-pneumonia cases, but which in the latter was "followed in each of the cases here observed by a moderate leukocytosis (14,000-15,000). ..."

p. 38   In the Summary: "... The two organisms most commonly and abundantly present in this series were the Pfeiffer bacillus and the diplococcus or streptococcus found by Mathers at Camp Meade.(This is apparently very similar to, if not identical with, the organism described by Zingher, JAMA, 1919, 72, p. 1020)."

p. 39   "... the Pfeiffer bacillus and the Mathers coccus often had the field almost to themselves. In a few cases the Pfeiffer bacillus was present in ... overwhelming numbers in cultures from nose, nasopharyns and throat that participation in a pathologic process was strongly suggested. These cases, however did not differ clinically in any appreciable way from other cases in which the Pfeiffer bacillus was found scantily.

"**The Mathers coccus was found about as frequently** and abundantly as the Pfeiffer bacillus, although its occurrence was quite independent of that of the latter. **Its association with the pneumonia cases seemed to be closer than that of the Pfeiffer bacillus**, but it was also found in all the later cases of simple influenza. ... Practically pure cultures of the Mathers coccus were obtained from the nasopharynx of some patients."

- - - - - - - -

July 28,1919 Duval and Harris, *J. Immunol.* Vol. 4, No. 4, 317-330

There is no mention of fatalities in this article, and it employed only B. influenzae (Pfeiffer's bacillus). There is no discussion of pneumonia perse, with only a single brief mention of the absence of "pneumonic complications" among vaccinated persons who contracted influenza.

The authors used only B. influenzae (Pfeiffer's bacillus); they acknowledged the role of other organisms in the disease, but considered them secondary invaders. Accordingly they chose to not use a mixed vaccine as they did not wish to cause simultaneous interference with the mechanism of stimulating maximum antibody production against B. influenzae. They exclusively used "a strain of B. influenzae (Wollstein) obtained from the Rockefeller Institute which had been in our possession for a number of years", based on favorable agglutination tests with this strain relative to other B. influenzae strains obtained from recent cases.

Contrary to virtually all reports that attempted use of B. influenzae, and all others included in the Chien 2010 article, Duval and Harris authors reported success in reducing influenza with the use of their vaccine, with 102 cases out of 3702 vaccinated persons versus 375 of 865 unvaccinated persons. Additional detail is provided for 2 groups, in which 27 of 981 vaccinated versus 130 of 338 unvaccinated, with no pneumonia in the vaccinated versus 41 pneumonia among the unvaccinated. There is no mention of fatalities anywhere in the article.

- - - - - - -

Public Health Journal July 1919, Volume 10, No. 7, p. 309, as reported in *JAMA* 73, August 2, 1919, p. 368, A.B.Wadsworth, "Results of preventive Vaccination Against Influenza" (one of items in Chien 2010)

Wadsworth reports on the use of influenza vaccine in New York state comprising scattered reports from different physicians and health officers, general reports from all the state institutions, and report of special selected institutions. The vaccine was prepared by suspending in physiologic sodium chloride solution the growth of fifteen different strains of the influenza bacillus on the surface of a coagulated blood glycerin veal agar. One c.c. contained one billion bacilli. Summing up the results of this study as to the practical value of [Pfeiffer's bacillus] vaccines in influenza, it is evident that the vaccines that have hitherto been used have failed to give reliable protection against influenza or influenzal pneumonia.

- - - - - - -

JAMA, August 2, 9, and 14, 1919.

In June 1919, the American Medical Association conducted a Symposium on Influenza, with eight papers read before the joint meeting of the Sections on Pharmacology and Therapeutics, Pathology and Physiology, and Preventive Medicine and Public Health at its Seventieth Annual Session in Atlantic City, N.J. The papers were published in three issues of *JAMA*, August 2, 9, and 14.

August 2 1919:

Milton Rosenau;
W. H. Frost;
William H. Park;
Lewis A. Conner
August 9 1919:
E.C. Rosenow;
C.W. McCoy
August 16 1919:
Henry F. Stoll;
James R. Herrick

- - - - - - -

August 2, 1919 – *JAMA* 73, Number 5, p. 311

Milton Rosenau, "Experiments to Determine Mode of Spread of Influenza."

Milton Rosenau conducted experiments with human volunteers, attempting to infect them with influenza using various methods: (a) 13 different strains of the Pfeiffer bacillus, sprayed into nose, eyes and throat; (b) transfer of material and mucous secretions of mouth and nose and throat and bronchi from patients, sprayed into nostrils and throat; (c) injections of blood; (d) direct coughing into the face of the volunteer. None of these efforts were successful. Rosenau also mentions a similar series of experiments on Goat Island, San Francisco, by Dr. McCoy and a Dr. Richey, also with negative results.

- - - - - - -

W.H. Frost, p. 313, "The Epidemiology of Influenza"

Frost reviews historical records, noting that "even in nonepidemic periods, there may be some intimate and constant relation between the prevalence of influenza and the mortality from pneumonia." He discussed the epidemic of 1889-92, which developed in 3 distinct phases – January 1890, April-May 1891, and January 1892, with mortality increasing in each year. Absent an epidemic in 1893, the pneumonia mortality was higher still. He then discusses the 1918-9 pandemic, noting outbreaks of pneumonia in March-May 1918 that "were definitely associated with coincident epidemics of a mild type of influenza. The rise in mortality from this group ... is so sudden, so marked and so general throughout the United States as to point very clearly to... a single definite and specific cause... [which was the] largely unnoticed ... beginning in this country of the great pandemic which developed in the autumn."

p. 318 "In general, this epidemic has been quite similar to that of 1889-1890 in its early development, first in mild, scattered outbreaks, later in a severe world-wide epidemic ... [with] much higher frequency of pneumonia and consequently much higher mortality, especially among young adults."

In his concluding paragraph he notes "It seems hardly logical to expect that any measure short of effective specific immunizations will afford lasting protection to the general population ... "

- - - - - - -

William H. Park, p. 318, "Bacteriology of Recent Pandemic of Influenza and Complicating Infections"

Park refers to the bacillus implicated by Pfeiffer in 1889, noting that "Investigations since then have thrown considerable doubt on this assumption, and many have now come to consider the bacillus as only one of several varieties of bacteria which have a special selective tendency to attack the mucous membranes of the upper respiratory tract." He notes that only in some circumstances, whereas "In their place, pneumococci, streptococci and gram-negative micrococci were found. Frequently, several varieties occurred together."

p. 319 "Even well trained bacteriologists frequently fail to realize that an epidemic strain is alike everywhere in cases belonging to the epidemic."

"The most delicate test that we have for identity of strains is that animals injected with them produce identical antibodies.

"The resemblance between the agglutinins produced is usually selected as the best evidence of identity or dissimilarity. With the filterable viruses we have to depend on finding some susceptible animal, or revert to human volunteers and if successful in producing infection, test for specific immunity."

Park asserts "that isolations from different cases from different localities are practically identical. He reviews "some representative investigations" as to the cause, involving Pfeiffer's bacillus, and various streptococci and pneumococci "which are under suspicion" and concludes "that the microorganism causing this epidemic has not yet been identified."

- - - - - - -

Lewis A. Conner, p. 321, "The Symptomatology and Complications of Influenza"

Conner notes that "there can be no possible doubt that, among the soldiers at least, the disease in its march across the country ... preserved a remarkable uniformity in its clinical picture." He discusses conditions of onset; and symptoms of prostration, respiratory, circulatory, nervous, gastro-intestinal, cutaneous, urinary and cutaneous manifestations in detail. Complications given particular attention were pneumonia and its onset and **outstanding clinical features** including cough, sputum variations and an exceptional cyanosis, elsewhere referred to as **heliotrope cyanosis**. He notes that leucopenia was present throughout pneumonia in the majority of cases, and cites other complications that may be associated, some rare, including respiratory, pulmonary abscess, pleurisy and empyema, subcutaneous emphysema, thrombophlebitis, meningitis, arthritis, inner ear, and accessory sinuses. Having been a hospital intern during the epidemic of 1889-90, he notes "striking similarity" in modes of onset, symptoms and in particular pneumonia of an unusual type, but that "The virulence of the recent epidemic was unquestionably greater."

- - - - - - -

August 9 1919: JAMA Volume 73, No. 6

E.C. Rosenow and B. F. Sturdivant, p. 396, "Studies in Influenza and Pneumonia --
IV. Further Results of Prophylactic Inoculations"
    This is the fourth in a series of eleven articles by Rosenow, incorporating detailed
discussions of the composition, testing and results of prophylactic vaccine in the
current pandemic.   Extensive data is provided, including formula, agglutinating
power, and results of large series of prophylactic vaccinations.   These included
approximately questionnaires returned to the Mayo Clinic by 530 physicians, totaling
approximately ½ million persons, of which about 30% were vaccinated; plus an
additional 62,500 persons in 19 counties, of which 42.2% were vaccinated, with
comparative data for influenza and deaths for the total population of 472,584 in these
counties; plus an additional 60,000 total of persons in another county plus 53 small
institutions, of which 35% were vaccinated.   Additionally results of prophylactic
inoculation in pregnancy were provided, for 997 persons vaccinated 3 times
compared with 3656 unvaccinated persons; plus additional results from hospitals in
Rochester, Minnesota.   In all cases, incidence of   pneumonia and deaths were
greatly reduced in vaccinated persons.   In summary, te mortality rate in persons
inoculated three times is about one-fifth of that in the uninoculated, and a definite
degree of protection was seen in vaccinated pregnant persons.

- - - - - - -

G. W. McCoy, p. 401, "Status of Prophylactic Vaccination Against Influenza"
    At the outset, McCoy notes that regarding Pfeiffer's "influenza bacillus", "there
has never been convincing evidence of its relation to influenza" and that data from
here or abroad during the pandemic "has not contributed any confirmation to the
view" that this is the cause.   He offers that a number of varying organisms may be
grouped under the name Pfeiffer's bacillus, noting "great differences that exist in
other groups, in which organisms having "common cultural and morphological
characteristics vary greatly in disease producing properties ..." In other words,
McCoy is seemingly acknowledging pleomorphism.
    "French and English workers have claimed to have produced influenza by means
of a filterable virus; this would, indeed, definitely eliminate Pfeiffer's bacillus ... "
but goes on to assert that efforts to produce the disease in man with secretions have
in most instances failed, as has been the case with the influenza bacillus.

    **McCoy proceeds to consider, first, vaccines made from the influenza bacillus
alone, intended to address the primary disease (influenza), and then, vaccines
intended to prevent pneumonia and its sequel.**

    p. 402 He erroneously proceeds to state regarding "views on the etiology and
pathology of influenzal pneumonia, we find a rather general opinion that the
pneumonia is due to Pfeiffer's bacillus or to the secondary invasion by organisms of
acknowledged pathogenicity, particularly the various types of pneumococci [and]

streptococci ..." – albeit a bit weasel-worded, insofar as the possible role of Pfeiffer's was clearly not established by then (or ever).

McCoy acknowledges that a few observers opine that "the original cause of the influenza ... is also an essential factor in ... the pneumonia. This view would appear to be entitled to much respect" considering the general pathological opinion that influenzal pneumonia is distinctly different from ordinary pneumonia. On this point he cites Rosenow as having demonstrated the unique character of the bronchopneumonia following influenza.

McCoy proposes to discuss first influenza bacillus vaccines, and secondly those directed at pneumonia.

McCoy's main critique of these influenza bacillus vaccines was that they involved inoculations during the epidemic as compared with general incidence from the beginning of the epidemic. He then proceeds with a theoretical discussion of how this works.

In his article, McCoy clearly raised this issue of vaccinations starting after the epidemic only in relation to attempts to use Pfeiffer's bacillus; absolutely no reference was made in this connection to the others:

"A vaccine made from the influenza bacillus alone seems not to have appealed sufficiently to European workers to induce them to try it when the epidemic prevailed abroad. In this country, its use has been **confined largely to New England**. The early reports on this vaccine were very encouraging; figures were presented which, if taken at their face value, would convince any one of the efficiency of the agent; but, when these figures were submitted to careful analysis, much doubt remained as to whether the vaccine was of any service whatsoever. The chief source of error lay in the fact that the inoculations had been done during the progress of the epidemic, and that the case incidence among the vaccinated was compared with the case incidence in the general population or in the control groups from the beginning of the epidemic."

McCoy lays out a theoretical discussion of how this skews the results in favor of the vaccinated persons. Simply stated, he asserts that a percentage of disease will have occurred prior to vaccination, particularly including the most susceptible, and totals including these will be compared with results in vaccinated. It must be emphasized that he is talking specifically and only about the influenza bacillus.

Resuming his discussion of the influenza bacillus, McCoy properly points out "that a vaccine can scarcely be expected to exert any appreciable prophylactic effect before from 7 to 10 days after the vaccine is given, since a week or more is required for immunity to develop. ...

"When the influenza bacillus was submitted to such critical tests as the inoculation of approximately half of the individuals in institutions, or in other large groups, its failure became apparent. A few examples of this are worth citing. Hinton and Kane (2) were able to vaccinate about half of the patients at an epileptic colony long enough before the disease became prevalent in the institution to justify the drawing of conclusions from their data. The vaccine used contained 800,000,000 organism per mil. And a total of 2,000,000,000 were administered to each person." **Results were 461 vaccinated, 123 influenza, and 68 deaths, versus 518 unvaccinated, 178 influenza, 24 deaths. ... "On the basis of this experiment the authors reach the obvious conclusion that the vaccine was without value."** *[As noted above, the Hinton article involved only the "Pfeffer's Bacillus", generally discredited by most investigators as of 1919 as not implicated in Pandemic pathology; and moreover not figuring in Chien 2010 calculations.]*

McCoy also mentions Pelham Bay Training Center (9% influenza of 554 vaccinated, versus 5% of 800 not vaccinated), and "similar failure" at Paris Island, South Carolina. And "A number of controlled vaccinations, in which influenza bacillus was used, carried out in institutions by the Public Health Service, gave the paradoxical result of showing an increased percentage of attacks among the vaccinated, but more deaths among non-vaccinated. **Results are shown in a table, of 484 vaccinated and 842 unvaccinated controls, with the notation "These figures illustrated the fallacy of giving much weight to the results of a small set of observations in work of this sort."** *[Again, while does not provide the citations enabling identification of the source of this data, the acknowledgment that this article involves the discredited "Pfeiffer's Bacillus" establishes it as being outside of the scope of Chien 2010, in any case.]*

Ironically, **McCoy's own** seemingly "landmark" work, cited by Chien 2010 as the "best" in their study, **reportedly involved 390 vaccinated and 390 unvaccinated**; thus McCoy himself would have pointed out "the fallacy" of Chien 2010 giving so much weight to McCoy's "small set of observations in work of this sort"!

Following this discussion of influenza bacillus vaccines, McCoy turned to: Vaccines from Streptococcus and other organisms

McCoy discusses the work of Ely et al [JAMA Jan. 4, 1919], directed at a hemolytic streptococcus in the blood and lungs, it is noted: "From the fact that the organisms with which these observers worked soon lost their chain-forming properties and, in some instances, the power to hemolyze promptly, they express some doubt as to whether they should be classed as streptococci ... .. McCoy notes that "The results of the use of a vaccine prepared from the organisms isolated from the cases were apparently most encouraging, though none of the experiments was controlled in a manner that would definitely establish the value of the preparation."

Regarding the work of Eyre and Lowe with a mixed vaccine, McCoy refers to their noting a negative phase following vaccination, and their stress "on the necessity of preparing a vaccine from cultures but recently isolated." Beyond this, they assert that the facts and figures given by the authors "are difficult of interpretation and permit of almost any conclusion ... ."

Thus did McCoy manage to ignore the reported results of Eyre and Lowe, involving some 16,000 vaccinated and 5700 unvaccinated persons, with the incidence of death 7 times greater in the unvaccinated as compared with vaccinated one or two times, and 32 times greater in unvaccinated as compared with vaccinated two times. Admittedly, the incidence of death in unvaccinated was only 1.5 times greater than that in those vaccinated only once. Perhaps this is what McCoy meant as "difficult of interpretation".

Coupling this with his total omission of reference to the unadulterated data indicating a far greater incidence of death in inoculated, even including those with only one inoculation, and **the true legacy of McCoy seems indisputably tarnished**.

Moving on … to "the polyvalent vaccine of Rosenow",:
At the top, McCoy properly acknowledges "Dr. Rosenow felt that this vaccine should be prepared for use in any community from the strains of organisms there prevailing, and that a vaccine adjusted to meet the needs of one locality might not meet those of another. The figures given for protection are encouraging, but do not lend themselves to critical analysis." McCoy asserts that despite "alleged good results" [in the Middle West] … it was not used until the epidemic was at, or beyond, the crest, and the records are not convincing [and that] … the practical difficulties of preparing it from locally prevailing strains and adjusting it to meet the changing flora of the respiratory tract in a disease that spreads as rapidly as influenza are obvious."

Comment: As to timing, it is noted that Leishmann was discussing the threat of a second wave in England in late October 1919, which was followed by the second wave in the U.S.; Rosenow's vaccinations began in October, thus for the most part we may attribute McCoy's negativity to standard rejection of anything that occurs after the start of an epidemic. And further, we have the "catch 22" of attempting to start a vaccination regimen prior to the proper identification of the causative organism, a total waste of time and effort. Add to this Rosenow's admonition that notwithstanding the acknowledged shortfalls of a single vaccination rather than a full course, that he felt a worthwhile vaccination of any sort must properly yield benefits even after one inoculation.

As to the "practical difficulties of preparing it", here we have a clear admission by McCoy that he was not competent to do so. Rosenow (and others) was able to do so, and did. McCoy clearly acknowledges "Dr. Rosenow felt that this vaccine should be prepared for use in any community from the strains of organisms there prevailing, and that a vaccine adjusted to meet the needs of one locality might not meet those of another." And then McCoy issues his typical back-handed unsupported/unsupportable critique: "The figures given for protection are encouraging, but do not lend themselves to critical analysis." Indeed, McCoy's incompetence is evident relative to not merely preparation but also analysis.

Incredibly, McCoy proceeds to describe his own bogus attempt to use a vaccine received from Chicago in California, contraindicated by location and time, and further in a small sample, both circumstances which McCoy himself had acknowledged as limiting:

"A specimen of the vaccine which was being used in Illinois was tried in California, under rigidly controlled conditions, without success. … Tests made in other institutions gave similar results, though we need not take the time to consider the details here."

No citations are given; however, it may be noted that this writer, following a thorough review of the literature, finally encountered a substantiating citation: W. H. Kellogg, MD, Secretary and Executive Officer, California State Board of Health, in July 1919, *California State Journal of Medicine*, Vol. XVII, No. 7, asserted that "Vaccines have been definitely proven to be of no value as a preventive measure" citing "McCoy's experiment with the [Rosenow] type of vaccine in the Napa State [Mental] Hospital"

McCoy then further illustrates his limitations here, following up with "There are several other reports of the use of vaccines prepared somewhat along the lines of Dr. Rosenow's, but the data are not presented in a manner to permit of analysis." Again, there are no details or citations provided to support this allegation. (see p. 218 and elsewhere in this volume, McCoy et al JAMA 71. 24, 1/4/1919).

On page 404, McCoy attempts to merge a discussion of Rosenow's Polyvalent vaccine into three-fourths of a column on stock vaccines, beginning with "stock commercial vaccines made from about the same organisms that went into the vaccines prepared by Dr. Rosenow", proceeding to trash the stock vaccines and by implication Rosenow. *(Of course, this directly contradicts Rosenow's omnipresent assertion that vaccines be made locally etc., i.e., Rosenow had by definition excluded the possibility of a "stock" vaccine "from about the same organisms" insofar as they had to be local and specific.)* This is followed by brief reference to Lister and lobar vaccines as different (rather than part and parcel of the body of pneumonia vaccines being addressed by Rosenow et al,), then derogatorily at Fennel on pneumococcal vaccine, to conclusion.

McCoy's conclusion, quoted here in entirety, is anything but objective:

"The general impression gained from uncontrolled use of vaccines is that they are of value in the prevention of influenza; but, in every case in which vaccines have been tried under **perfectly controlled conditions** *[e.g. impossible conditions]*, they have failed to influence in a definite manner either the morbidity or the mortality." In the first clause, "the general impression ... of value" is torpedoed with the qualifier of "uncontrolled"; and regarding the second clause, there are no citations, *and on review of the literature one may easily conclude that there was only one case that would fit McCoy's definition of "perfectly controlled conditions", i.e. his own bogus report of December 1918*, above.`

- - - - - - -

August 16 1919: Henry F. Stoll; James R. Herrick

Henry F. Stoll, "Value of Convalescent Blood and Serum in Treatment of Influenzal Pneumonia" p. 478

Stoll's summary, p. 482:

"56 patients with influenzal pneumonia, in 70 percent of whom the prognosis was poor, were treated with the blood or serum of convalescent with a mortality of approximately 45 %."

-- Of those treated within 48 hours, 10 of 12 "showed prompt improvement and recovered."

-- Of 32 treated within an average of 3.9 days of getting pneumonia, "72% showed distinct improvement; of 24 ill 5.4 days, 17% showed distinct improvement."

-- Overall, "when used early, within the first three days, a distinct improvement in all symptoms is to be noted in the majority of cases."

- - - - - - - -

James R. Herrick, "Treatment of Influenza by Means Other than Vaccines and Serums"   p. 482

Herrick herein reviews his own experiences in the 1889-90 epidemic, the years following, and the current epidemic, with such measures as drugs ("no drug is known to prevent the occurrence of influenza"), gauze masks, importance of bed rest (universally agreed as beneficial), and the likes of sunlight, fresh air, light diet, liberal amount of liquids, and opening of bowels, digitalis ("of greatest value"), as well as opium and morphine. "I think I saved one life by bleeding."

Of particular interest is the "Abstract of Discussion" following Herrick:

Dr. Anna W. Williams: "The important thing is to decide whether or not we have one type among the strains isolated. Until this point is settled in the affirmative we need not pay any attention to the so-called postulates of Koch. ... Of course, we have to determine what test we must choose to prove this. Up to the present, we have decided that we will accept the agglutination test with the absorption of agglutinins for the test of type until somebody proves that this test is not the final test. We have shown that all the influenza strains we have isolated do not respond to this test ... ."

Dr. Alexander Lambert notes in the current epidemic, "particularly ... the serious influence of the streptococcus."

P. 486   Dr. Hyman L. Goldstein notes: "In attempting to prevent the numerous deaths which Dr. E.C. Rosenow told us resulted from the secondary complications, are we justified in using the vaccine? I think we are justified in using vaccine, even if we do not know the specific cause of influenza, as preventive and therapeutic measure against the complications.

Dr. Frederick T. Lord expressed the opinion: "Vaccines may be of use in prophylaxis, but they have never been shown to be of value in treatment.

Dr. Will Walter: "Dr. McCoy's records, so far as they relate to preventive inoculation, show a violation of the fundamental principles laid down by Wright ... [see full comments by Walter above, p. 22-23]

Dr. M. K. Wylder: "I use the prophylactic vaccine. I used it in a girls' boarding school ... There were 80 people in that institution; not a single case of influenza developed. One mother...took the girl home. In less than a week that girl was dead."

Dr. H.H Coons: Regarding the use of vaccine in therapy: "Almost uniformly within 30 to 36 hours after an injection of vaccine sufficient to get an initial rise of temperature, there was a very marked decline, better respiration, lessening of cyanosis and, in most cases, an improvement in the general condition of the patient. ... In the wards where I used vaccine the mortality rate in pneumonia was under 7 per cent.   In the wards where we did not use vaccine but used all known precautionary measures, the mortality was 18%."

Dr. E.C. Rosenow: "The vaccine which we used was made to contain as soon after isolation as possible the bacteria isolated in influenza and the accompanying pneumonia together with type pneumococci. It contained, as we found months later, a high percentage of strains of green-producing streptococci which, according to their serologic reactions, appear to bear etiologic relation to this disease and with which the picture of influenza has been closely simulated in animals. ... **The difficulties in evaluating the results, as pointed out by Dr. McCoy, have been considered and the sources of error eliminated**. ... Averaging all the results obtained, it appears that the incidence of influenza was about three times as common and the death rate five times as high among the uninoculated as among the vaccinated persons."

- - - - - - -

W. H. Watters, "Vaccines in Influenza", The Boston Medical and Surgical Journal, December 25, 1919, p. 727

Watters notes that "Early in September, 1918, the epidemic ... made its expected appearance in America. He was working with Leary at the time of the outbreak, and initially "Neither [he nor Leary] was able to isolate ... the influenza bacillus, the organism predominating being a diplococcus, doubtless of the group of of the Micrococcus catarrhalis. Very shortly, however, post-mortem examinations of fatal cases revealed the influenza bacilli in the lungs and pure cultures were obtained."

Leary decided to prepare vaccine from strains of the influenza bacilli alone; "the writer [Watters], assuming that a mixed infection was active in various phases of the disease, ... prepared a mixed vaccine of the organisms isolated from lungs postmortem:

Micrococcus catarrhalis	400 million
Pneumococcus	400 million
Streptococcus hemolyticus	400 million
Bacillus influenzae	100 million

Recommended dosage was .2 cc, .3 cc and .4 cc at 3 day intervals. 50,000 doses were distributed free of charge to physicians and boards of health, requesting they be provided free and records returned.

Waters notes that the first immunizations were given to laboratory staff, with ten of fourteen receiving inoculations, none of which contracted the disease. "Of the four others, two had influenza rather severely. This seemed rather suggestive ...".

For the nurses, records for the underclasses were lost in the stress of work, but results for the intermediate and senior classes were as follows:

		Sick	% Sick
Not vaccinated	41	33	80
Vaccinated	47	14	33

The majority of results reported from the various entities reporting are in the accompanying table. In addition, reports from 23 practicing physicians listed 1471 vaccinated persons, of which 21 contracted influenza, 2 pneumonia and none died; however, a comparative total of unvaccinated persons was not listed. Watters noted "It will be seen that there is practically a unanimity of opinion in favor of the idea that active immunization by the use of vaccines may be obtained … ."

Watters further notes that "excluding the Bridgeport Board of Health [which gave only totals of inoculations and not results] and the Lovell and Covell Company, where comparisons are indefinite, that there was a disease incidence among those inoculated of approximately 3.5%" compared to 28% among the uninoculated. Only 15 of the inoculated contracted pneumonia, with eight deaths, all at Allentown. Of these, three had received only one inoculation and three received two inoculations.

In particular, **Watters directly addresses a key objection** of McCoy:
"In preparing this paper, the writer fully realizes the fact **that epidemics afflict first those most susceptible** and that measures for immunization employed later upon those not yet infected may consist of administering them to persons already naturally immune. As such, it is **obviously unfair to compare early morbidity among a hopefully partially immunized one after the most susceptible have already become diseased.**

"In the Allentown report, however, this possibility seems to be successfully met when it is noted that of those vaccinated persons contracting the disease 36% did so within one week of the first inoculation when the immunity should be theoretically only beginning and 57% did so after the fourth week when the immunity was decreasing. It would suggest that for a period of three or four weeks, a distinct degree of resistance to infection might be produced." This albeit limited period of protection was also experienced in other instances reported, i.e., reports of a Dr. Phillips and a Dr. Leard.

- - - - - - -

General Sir William B. Leishman, Feb. 14, 1920 *The Lancet*, p. 366, Maj, "The Results of Protective Inoculation Against Influenza in the Army at Home, 1918-1919

This report follows up on a conference on October 26, 1918 which Leishman chaired, which recommended preparation of vaccine and its constitution. The formula of the vaccine used in the case of the reported results:

B. influenzae	60 million }	
Streptococci	80 million }	in 1 ccm
Pneumococci	200 million }	

"Several strains and types of each organism were used, all comparatively freshly isolated from cases of the disease. Two doses were recommended, the first of .5 ccm, and the second, given after 10 days' interval, 1 ccm.

As of the time of publication, a revised formula with a larger dose of B. influenzae, 400 millions, was being used, as a result of subsequent criticism in the medical press, with strains not so recently derived so as to be unduly toxic. However, all the results reported in this article were derived from use of the original formula.

"From the first it was desired that every attempt should be made to secure clear statistical evidence of the results of the inoculations with the vaccine ... "

Summary of Table

	Strength	Incidence of attack	Ratios per 1000 Incidence of pulmonary complications	Deaths
Inoculated	15,624	14.1	1.6	0.12
Non-inoculated	43,520	47.3	13.3	2.25

p. 368   "The returns, all of which lie within the period between November, 1918, and April 1919, comprise all those relating to this period which conformed to the following requirements:

"1. That the vaccine used was that prepared at the royal Army Medical College, according to the original formula.

"2. That influenza should have been present in the unit during the period under review. In many stations where inoculation has been largely carried out there was a rapid cessation of the epidemic. Such returns would have swelled the total of the inoculations without throwing any light on their protective effects.

"3. That only such returns are included as showed that at least one-tenth of the average strength had been inoculated, whether with one dose or two."

...

"It will be noted from the table that nearly one-half of the inoculated had received only the first dose of the vaccine – i.e., one third of the mount which we considered essential to effective protection. It is reasonable to assume that, had all received the full dosage, the protective results would have been still more evident. No statistical evidence bearing upon this point is, however, available.

"The table had best be left to speak for itself, but it will, I think, be admitted that in general the results are encouraging and that they tend to confirm, and even strengthen, our original anticipations, which were, briefly, that at least a moderate degree of protection against infection might be expected, while more decidedly beneficial effects might be hoped for in a diminution of both the frequency and the gravity of the pulmonary complications."

As seen in the summary table, incidence of influenza in the uninoculated was 3.35 times, pulmonary complications 8.31 times, and death 18.75 times that in the inoculated.

- - - - - - -

Frank A. Craig, "Progress of Medicine for the year 1919, International Clinics, Quarterly, VOLUME I. THIRTIETH SERIES, 1920 p. 205, Influenza, etc., 207-228

"In the American Expeditionary Forces, the epidemic was characterized ... by three definite outbreaks or peaks, the first occurring in April and May, 1918, was comparatively mild and was spoken of as 'three-day fever.' The second, in September and October, 1918, formed a part of the terrible pandemic. The third definite outbreak was much less severe and occurred in January and February, 1919. ... among the troops in this country about one in every five had influenza, ... of these about one in six developed pneumonia, and ... of the pneumonia patients about two out of every five died." ...

"There is still some question as to the part played by [streptococcus haemolyticus] in the acute respiratory infections, whether primary or secondary to some other infective agent, as in influenza and following measles. It has been demonstrated that they are a not uncommon finding in the tonsils of apparently healthy individuals, as well as those suffering from systemic infections or toxemias. It is important to determine whether the acute respiratory infections are the result of infection from the patient's own organisms, or by a more virulent strain from some other individual. This whole problem is very thoroughly covered by Davis (JAMA Feb. 1, 1919, 72, No. 5, p. 320) who considers it reasonable to assume that individuals are being infected from time to time with their own streptococci, especially following the contagious diseases, and that by this process the streptococci become more and more virulent and aggressive ... ."

"With a recognition of the dangers of the streptococcus haemolyticus carrier state, the methods for the eradication of this organism from the tonsils assume considerable importance. Chemical means of disinfection can never reach all of the crypts harboring these streptococci, according to Bryan (Ann. Of Ot. Rhin, and Laryng., June 1919, 28, No. 2, p. 337), who urges a complete enucleation of the tonsil of the streptococcus carriers."

"One of the most serious features of the epidemic was the effect of the infection upon pregnant women, at least in the cases which developed pulmonary involvement. The frequency with which pregnancy was interrupted was very noticeable." *[Rosenow had also highlighted this circumstance.]*

- - - - - - -

Herbert French, C.B.E., M.D., F.R.C.P., 1920, *GBR Ministry of Health Reports* #4, Chapter III. "The Clinical Features of the Influenza Epidemic of 1918-19."Page 66:

"In the June 1918 outbreak, although the cases were very numerous there was little or no mortality; there was little or no pulmonary complication; and the patients, though striken severely for the time, speedily recovered after so short an attack that it was widely spoken of as "influenza of the three-day fever type." It was in the October 1918 and in the February 1919 outbreaks that the high mortality from pulmonary and general septicæmic complications developed and gave such an entirely different clinical aspect to the disease ; and it was in this part of the epidemic that the dreaded **heliotrope cyanosis** was so pronounced a feature of the fatal cases. It is of importance, however, to emphasize the fact that the heliotrope cyanosed type of case, though it attracted chief notice during the influenza epidemic of 1918-19, was not a new phenomenon confined to this epidemic ; it had already been met with and reported upon in connection with minor epidemics during 1916 and 1917, at which time the label given to these fatal cases was **"purulent bronchitis,"** though I, personally, am strongly of the opinion that these smaller outbreaks in 1916 and 1917 with heliotrope cyanosis as a striking phenomenon of the worst cases, were of precisely the same nature as those of the enormously more widespread and serious " influenza" outbreaks of 1918 and 1919.

p. 69   Those who had experienced the minor epidemics of " purulent bronchitis with heliotrope cyanosis and fatal ending " that had occurred here and there in military camps in America, England and France during 1916 and 1917 had already become familiar with some of the worst features, especially the dreaded blueness, of what was probably the same malady under a different name; but now it was a question of seeing hundreds or even thousands of cases in districts in which the fatal " purulent bronchitis " had affected but a few. ... Broadly speaking, I should say that out of 1,000 individuals striken by the disease fully 800 had no more than an ordinary attack of uncomplicated " influenza," a little more severe perhaps than the "three-day fever " of June 1918, but not any worse than simple influenza as it may occur at any other time. It was the remaining 200 who were so much more seriously ill, with " pneumonic" symptoms added to those of simple influenza ; and of these about 80 died. The **most dreaded symptom was the heliotrope cyanosis** ; it developed in less than half of the pulmonary cases, but once it became definite the prognosis was so bad that I should say out **of every 100 " blue " cases 95 died.** ...

p. 70   "It was, however, only when any given patient had absolutely recovered that one could relegate him with certainty to the " mild " category. Even the mildest case had to be regarded as potentially grave ... A patient might have been ill a day or two with mild influenza and seem to be progressing well; in an hour or two the whole picture might change, and twenty-four hours later the patient might be dead.

"... whether the case developed into the grave type, or remained benign, *epistaxis* was a phenomenally common early symptom. It is not possible to give statistics, for in the stress and dire overstrain of those strenuous days and nights no fall records were kept; but when special inquiry was made in scores of consecutive cases, some degree of nose-bleeding had occurred in over half ...

p. 71 "The "pneumonia" was an acute infective pulmonary inflammation in which such consolidation as resulted was due not to croupous lobar pneumonia of the classical sort, but to a conglomeration of changes which included bronchitis and peribronchitis, coagulative oedema, hæmorrhage, collapse, broncho-pneumonia, abscess formation, and compression by pleuritic effusion, totally different to anything ordinarily seen in the post-mortem room.

p. 73 ...when this dreaded heliotrope cyanosis appeared [that] one knew that the prognosis had now altered so completely that the patient was almost certain to die ...

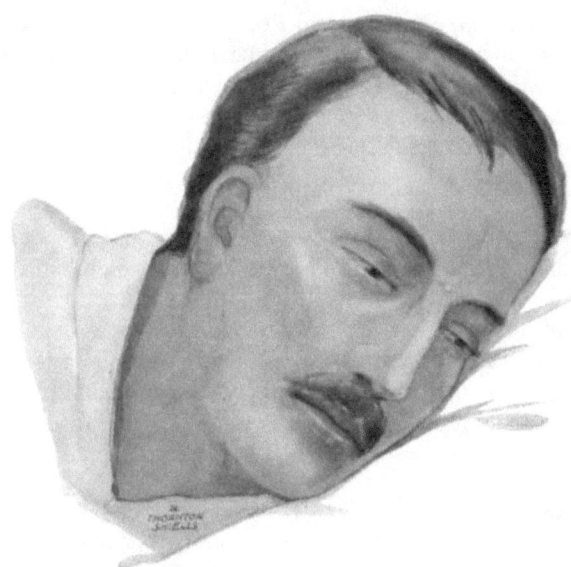

PLATE 2.—This illustrates a pronounced degree of the "heliotrope cyanosis." The patient is not in physical distress, but the prognosis is almost hopeless.

p. 75 The general conclusion was that the heliotrope cyanosis was due not to heart failure, nor to abnormal chemical changes in the blood, but to sheer anoxhæmia resulting from this widespread and extensive albuminous exudate into the alveoli and interstitial tissues of the lungs.

Bibliography: cites Mathers:
-- Mathers, G..: "Bacteriology of Acute Respiratory Infection commonly called Influenza" ; Journ. Infectious Dis., 1917, XXI., 1, 8.
-- Mathers, G.: "Etiology of Acute Respiratory Infection commonly called Influenza" ; Journ. Amer. Med. Assoc, 1917, LXVIII., 557-60.

- - - - - - -

Rosenow part v: *Journal of Infectious Diseases*, Vol. 26, No. 6 (Jun., 1920), p. 489
"The changes observed in morphology, cultural characteristics, fermentative and immunologic reactions in the **green-producing streptococci** indicate that the organism described by the English observers and designated by them as **diplostreptococcus**, the green-producing streptococcus found by Mathers as described by Tunnicliff, the diplococcus epidemicus described by Bernhardt and by Segale, the diplococcus mucosus described by Stephan, and the pleomorphic streptococcus described by Wiesner in influenza, are identical with the green-producing streptococcus isolated in this study, or modifications thereof."

- - - - - - -

Rosenow's Part VII, *Journal of Infectious Diseases*, Vol. 26, No. 6 (Jun., 1920), 542:

"These findings in general are in accord with those in human lungs described by Lord,[13] Weichselbaum,[23] Kuskow,[9] and others in previous epidemics of influenza, and by Le Count,[11,12] MacCallum,[17] Bell,[2] Chickering and Park,[5] Lucke, Wight and Kime,[15] Opie,[18] Lubarsch," Lyon,[16] and others during the recent epidemic."

- - - - - - -

Edwin O. Jordan and W. B. Sharp, *The Journal of Infectious Diseases*, Vol. 28, No. 4 (Apr. 1921), pp. 357-366

p. 357 "Approximately 6000 persons were under observation from November 1919 to June 1, 1920. About one half of these were vaccinated with the bacterial suspension to be described presently; the other half were not vaccinated ... . Three schools and two large hospitals for mental diseases were available for these observations. ... this series of observations ... was carried out in certain public and private institutions of Illinois. ...

p. 358 "All vaccinations were made with a saline suspension of a standard vaccine prepared under the direction of Dr. W.H. Park of the Influenza Commission in the Research Laboratory of the New York City Health Department. The vaccines were given subcutaneously in three doses at weekly intervals. The first dose contained: the Pfeiffer bacillus, 500 million; pneumococcus the I, 1,000 million; pneumococcus type II, 1000 million; pneumococcus type III, 500 million. The second and third doses contained double these numbers of each organism. A few of the smaller children were given only half doses. The injections were made between November 24 and Dec. 11 in 4 of the institutions and between Nov. 3 and Dec. 16 in the fifth ... ."

p. 366 The results involved small differences between vaccinated and unvaccinated persons, which "hardly warrant, although they suggest, a favorable conclusion regarding some slight prophylactic value for pneumonia."

- - - - - - -

American journal of diseases of children, Volume 23, p. 275 (January 1922)
By American Medical Association
  POLYMORPHISM- A PNEUMO-STREPTO-COCCUS
"Other Micro-Organisms in Influenza".—Tunnicliff noted that from influenza and its complications during the onset and at the height of the 1918-1919 epidemic, various investigators had isolated peculiar green-producing cocci with the characteristics of both a pneumococcus and a streptococcus. These green-producing cocci are oftener lanceolate than round, generally possess a capsule, and produce large moist green colonies on blood-agar plates. She herself succeeded in isolating this coccus from the edematous brain in influenzal broncho-pneumonia, usually in pure culture, but in no instance did she cultivate the Pfeiffer bacillus from the brain. From her serologic experiments she decided that these green-producing influenzal cocci form a group the members of which are closely related immunologically.

"Rosenow and his co-workers[25] also studied this green-producing streptococcus, finding it in a large series of- cases of influenza and influenzal pneumonia throughout four different epidemic waves, **more constantly and in larger numbers than any other organisms associated with the disease. Rosenow noted** [21] **that the virulency and mortality in animals increased for one or two successive intratracheal** injections of this microrganism, and on further animal passage diminished. And after a study of the four epidemic waves as, they occurred in Rochester, Minnesota, he found that a similar rise and fall in severity of symptoms, mortality and character of lung lesions occurred as the epidemic waves appeared and disappeared. Accordingly he **thought that (1) the** change in the type of the disease early and late in the epidemics, (2) the rise and fall in mortality rate in the same epidemic, and in the virulency of different epidemics, and (3) the lesser tendency to leukopenia late in epidemic waves, **may all be due, in the main, to changes in virulency and other properties of the green-producing streptococcus** isolated so constantly in influenzal infections. He further noted that whereas these **peculiar green-producing streptococci are immunologically quite homogenous at the outset of an epidemic, the strains tend to become more heterogenous after cultivation on artificial mediums,** and after repeated animal passages as well as late in influenza and influenzal pneumonia.

"Rosenow also studied the four main types of bacteria isolated in this disease as to their invasive powers following intratracheal injection of influenzal sputum. Invasion by the green-producing streptococcus group (including pneumococci), occurred in most instances even when not the predominating organism in the material injected. In some instances, invasion by hemolytic streptococci occurred, but usually only when they were present alone or in predominating numbers. Invasion by staphylococci occurred even more rarely and only when in predominating numbers; and invasion by the influenza bacillus following the injection of sputum and lung exudate did not occur in a single experiment.

"Recapitulating, Rosenow wrote,[28] 'Through a painstaking study of the infecting powers of the streptococcus in influenza and influenzal pneumonia throughout several epidemic waves, it has been **possible to reproduce in animals by various methods of injection, but particularly by intratracheal injection, the picture of influenza as seen in man.** The symptoms both of influenza and influenzal pneumonia have been grossly simulated in these animals as far as possible. Likewise the gross and microscopic changes which have come to be regarded as quite characteristic of influenzal infection have been reproduced. The same varied picture that often supervenes in the later stages of influenzal pneumonia in man such as leukocytosis as evidence of pleural involvement and pleural infection, becomes manifest and the varied pathologic picture in the lung of patients who died late has been noted in guinea-pigs injected intratracheally with these strains. The tendency to involvement of the female generative organs with a high mortality in pregnancy and a high incidence of abortion, of lesions of the heart, abscess in the rectus muscle, and interstitial emphysema, have been noted in the experimental animal quite as they occur in man."

References:

38. Williams, A. VV.; Nevin, M., and Gurley, C. R.: Studies on Acute Respiratory Infections: I. Methods of Demonstrating Microorganisms, Including "Filterable Viruses" from the Upper Respiratory Tract in "Health," in "Common Colds," and in "Influenza" with the Object of Discovering "Common Strains," J. Immunol. 6:5 (Jan.) 1921.

39. Branham. S. E., and Hall, I. C.: Influenza Studies: III. Attempts to Cultivate Filtrable Viruses from Cases of Influenza and Common Colds, J. Infect. Dis. 28:143 (Feb.) 1921.

40. Hall, I. C.: Influenza Studies: II. A Search for Obligate Anaerobes in Respiratory Infections, an Anaerobic Micrococcus, J. Infect. Dis. 28:127 (Feb.) 1921.

41. Tunnicliff, R.: Observations on Green-Producing Cocci of Influenza, J. Infect. Dis. 26:405 (May) 1920.

42. Rosenow, E. C.: Studies in Influenza and Pneumonia: X. The Immunologic Properties of the Green-Producing Streptococci from Influenza, J. Infect. Dis. 26:597 (June) 1920.

- - - - - - -

Given the prominence of Peter Olitsky in poliomyelitis research subsesquently, his exhaustive earlier work implicating a viral agent in influenza is worthy of mention. For the record, excerpts of some of these items, and a listing of his eleven part series, follow:

JAMA: April 8 1922, Volume 78, part 2, p. 1020
METHODS FOR THE ISOLATION OF FILTER-PASSING ANAEROBIC ORGANISMS FROM HUMAN NASOPHARYNGEAL SECRETIONS*
PETER K. OLITSKY, M.D. AND FREDERICK L. GATES. M.D. NEW YORK

"In November, 1918, during the pandemic of influenza, we isolated from the filtered nasopharyngeal secretions of influenza patients, and from the lung tissues of rabbits intratracheally inoculated with these secretions, a hitherto undescribed organism which we called *Bacterium pneumosintes.1* The same organism was recovered from similar sources during the recurrent wave of epidemic influenza in the spring of 1920. Within the last few weeks we have again isolated identical or similar organisms from the nasopharyngeal secretions of influenza patients. At present the identification of the recently recovered bacteria is not complete. But during our observation of the strains isolated in 1918-1919 and in 1920, we have noted certain unreported facts relating to the cultural and morphologic characters of *Bacterium pneumosintes* which have been useful in the isolation of the recently recovered strains. It is our purpose in this communication to report these facts briefly, in the hope that this information may be of use to others in the bactcriologic study of respiratory infections of obscure etiology.

"*Bacterium pneumosintes,* as originally isolated, was a minute bacilloid body of regular form, with a length about two to three times its breadth, measuring from 0.15 to 0.3 micron in the long axis. It passed V and N Berkefeld filters, multiplied slowly only under strictly anaerobic conditions in a medium composed of human ascitic fluid and a fragment of fresh rabbit kidney, and withstood glycerolation for a period of months. The organism decolorized by Gram's method, and stained with the usual basic dyes, of which Loeffler's alkaline methylene blue was the most suitable. *Bacterium pneumosintes* was identified as the cause of the characteristic clinical and pathologic effects induced in rabbits injected intratracheally with the nasopharyngeal secretions of influenza patients.

http://www.ncbi.nlm.nih.gov/pmc/articles/PMC2128379/

p. 144 "Whatever this active substance is, it seems to disappear from or to diminish in the nasopharyngeal secretions of cases of epidemic influenza so as to be no longer discoverable by inoculation tests about 36 hours after the obvious symptoms of the disease have appeared, and to be absent from healthy persons and in other pathological conditions."

Olitsky Series "EXPERIMENTAL STUDIES OF THE NASOPHARYNGEAL SECRETIONS FROM INFLUENZA PATIENTS":

I: http://www.ncbi.nlm.nih.gov/pmc/articles/PMC2128182/pdf/125.pdf
II: http://www.ncbi.nlm.nih.gov/pmc/articles/PMC2128189/pdf/361.pdf
III: http://ukpmc.ac.uk/articles/PMC2128187/pdf/373.pdf
IV: http://jem.rupress.org/content/33/6/713.full.pdf [June 1, 1921]
V: http://www.ncbi.nlm.nih.gov/pmc/articles/PMC2128067/pdf/1.pdf
VI: http://www.ncbi.nlm.nih.gov/pmc/articles/PMC2180242/pdf/1.pdf
VII: http://www.ncbi.nlm.nih.gov/pmc/articles/PMC2128118/pdf/553.pdf
VIII: http://www.ncbi.nlm.nih.gov/pmc/articles/PMC2128320/pdf/813.pdf
IX: http://www.ncbi.nlm.nih.gov/pmc/articles/PMC2128379/pdf/501.pdf
X: http://www.ncbi.nlm.nih.gov/pmc/articles/PMC2128393/pdf/685.pdf
XI: http://www.ncbi.nlm.nih.gov/pmc/articles/PMC2128364/pdf/303.pdf

Selected excerpts:

I. TRANSMISSION EXPERIMENTS WITH NASOPHARYNGEAL WASHINGS.Olitsky shows influenza "virus" disappears

IV -- p. 714 "The characteristic bodies were first observed in November, 1918, in strictly anaerobic cultures of the filtered nasopharyngeal secretions of an influenza patient in the early hours of the disease. "

-- p. 718: "Viewed with the highest powers of the microscope, the bodies were seen to be two to three times longer in one direction than in the other. They were, therefore, bacilloid rather than coccoid. Thus they were differentiated sharply from the globoid bodies of poliomyelitis, which they approached in size. Their long axis measured 0.15 to 0.3 microns.

-- 727-8 "From the filtered nasopharyngeal washings of patients in the first 36 hours of uncomplicated epidemic influenza and rarely in later stages of the disease, we have cultivated a minute bacilloid body, Bacterium pneumosintes, 0.15 to 0.3

microns in length, of constant cultural characters and capable of indefinite propagation on artificial media."

VIII, p. 813 In an earlier paper of this series [IV] Bacterium pneumosintes, derived from the nasopharyngeal washings of patients in the early hours of acute epidemic influenza, was described as a minute bacilloid body of regular form, with a length about two to three times its breadth, measuring 0.15 to 0.3.micron in the long axis.

IX "Bacterium pneumosintes appeared as a minute bacilloid body of regular morphology, measuring 0.15 to 0.3 micron in the long axis. Usually solitary, the bacteria were often found in diplo form, and occasionally in short chains of three or four members. ... [504] When grown on media containing nutrient broth, and especially in the presence of dextrose, Bacterium pneumosintes has developed larger bacillary forms up to 1 micron in length. The identity of these microorganisms with the original strains has been proved by serological reactions and by their reversion to the minute forms on transfer to the original medium.

- - - - - - -

DOCUMENTATION OF THE CONTINUING ROLES OF GEORGE MCCOY AND GEORGE SIMMONS IN THE INNER WORKINGS OF THE JAMA AND ITS OVERSIGHT OF PHARMACOLOGY IN THESE CRITICAL FORMATIVE YEARS:

McCoy is acknowledged in 1922 JAMA as comprising, with George Simmons, the "standing committee of the Board of Trustees, both with terms through 1925. McCoy served on the COUNCIL ON PHARMACY AND CHEMISTRY : Vice-Chairman 1918 through at least 1922 and serving on council through (e.g. 1939 JAMA Vol.113) 1945

Simmons was Editor and General Manager 1922 of JAMA, Chair of Board of Trustees as of 1925 -- JAMA "EDITED FOR THE ASSOCIATION UNDER THE DIRECTION OF THE BOARD OF TRUSTEES BY
GEORGE H. SIMMONS, M.D., LL.D.
VOLUME 71 : : i : : : JULY—DECEMBER, 1918

Chapter 6 – A Brief Survey of Additional Modern Pandemic Articles

Some internet sites discussing the 1918-1919 Pandemic:

http://en.wikipedia.org/wiki/1918_flu_pandemic
This internet source cites nothing on Rosenow or the Mayo Foundation

- - - - - - -

http://1918.pandemicflu.gov/the_pandemic/index.htm
"As a viral infection, influenza can be prevented by a vaccine and during the early weeks of the pandemic, many people believed that a vaccine against influenza was forthcoming. Although vaccines have been developed before scientists have ascertained the exact cause of a disease, medical researchers' failure to ascertain and isolate the influenza virus did not bode well for the development of an influenza vaccine at this time.

"During the fall of 1918, researchers from the Public Health Service, including the renowned Joseph Goldberger, began looking for a vaccine. They were joined by researchers in many other countries. These researchers developed a range of vaccines which were then tested in communities all over the world. None of these vaccines proved effective."

Here we find total dependence on the distorted historical record as maintained by the Public Health Service serves as a total dis-service to the facts of the numerous and effective bacterial vaccines in the $_{Wright}$-Leishmann-Rosenow tradition.

- - - - - - -

http://virus.stanford.edu/uda/ Molly Billings,The Influenza Pandemic of 1918, June 1997 modified RDS February 2005
NOTE: bibliography for this page (http://virus.stanford.edu/uda/flubib.html) includes listing of one Rosenow JAMA article, but not by name!!:

    Journal of the American Medical Association :
    October 5, 1918 p.1136-1137;
    October 12, 1918 p. 1220;
    December 7, 1918 p. 1928-9, 1935;
    December 14, 1918 p. 2015;
    December 21, 1918 p. 2068-73
    December 28, 1918 p. 2154, 2174-5;
    January 4, 1919, p. 31-34; {Rosenow!!}
    January 11, 1919 p. 155-59;
    January 18, 1919 p. 188;
    January 25, 1919 p. 268;
    March 1, 1919 p. 640;
    April 12, 1919 p. 1056-58

"The flu was most deadly for people ages 20 to 40. This pattern of morbidity was unusual for influenza which is usually a killer of the elderly and young children. ... "The physicians of the time were helpless against this powerful agent of influenza [NOT ALL OF THEM !!] ... A study attempted to reason why the disease had been so devastating in certain localized regions, looking at the climate, the weather and the racial composition of cities. They found humidity to be linked with more severe epidemics as it "fosters the dissemination of the bacteria," (Committee on Atmosphere and Man, 1923). Meanwhile the new sciences of the infectious agents and immunology were racing to come up with a vaccine or therapy to stop the epidemics."

- - - - - - -

http://virus.stanford.edu/uda/fluresponse.html 2005

"The American Public Health Association committee members believed that the best way to prevent infection was through the use of vaccines. Vaccines could prevent or mitigate infection with influenza and the frequently fatal complications of the illness due to the influenza bacillus [NOT] or strains of streptococci and pneumonococci. They believed that the current vaccines under development should be tested and administered if useful to prevent infection. The committee suggested the use of the experimental vaccines on susceptibles with equal subjects and controls and under proper scientific methodology. However, they acknowledged that the cause of the influenza was unknown and therefore an effective vaccine had no "scientific basis." These public health officials shared the perceptions of the scientific and medical community of the influenzal disease and its origins".

This Stanford posted article cites *JAMA*, 12/21/1918, which had in fact reported the successful results of Tonney of Chicago, Sherman in Pittsburgh, and Rosenow; **however this Stanford article excludes reference to these items, which seems to indicate that the author at Stanford did not actually read the original *JAMA* article to which it had referred**. Shame on Stanford.

Indeed, as discussed herein, there seems to have been a distinct split between opinions of the major public health officials, i.e., McCoy and Park (favoring the somewhat-already-discredited so-called "Pfeiffer bacillus), and the authoritative civilian and military scientists of the time, e.g., Rosenow, Waters, Ely, Minaker, etc. etc. (demonstrating the efficacy of bacterial vaccines).

Chalk this up as a puff piece for the PHS.

- - - - - - -

http://virus.stanford.edu/uda/fluscimed.html 2005

This Stanford posted item cites several *JAMA* items, including:

"Several experiments attempted to produce vaccines, each with a different understanding of the etiology of fatal influenza infection. A Dr. Rosenow invented a vaccine to target the multiple bacterial agents involved from the serum of patients. He aimed to raise the immunity to against the bacteria, the 'common causes of death,' and not the cause of the initial symptoms by inoculating with the proportions found in the lungs and sputum (*JAMA*, 1/4/1919). The vaccines made for the British forces took a similar approach and were "mixed vaccines" of pneumococcus and lethal streptococcus. The vaccine development therefore focused on the culture results of what could be isolated from the sickest patients [NOT CORRECT!] and lagged behind the scientific progress [NONSENSE]."

As clearly demonstrated by a proper consideration of the actual data even as presented in Chien 2010, these bacterial vaccines were effective and comprised significant "scientific progress"; shame on Stanford for this dribble.

- - - - - - -

http://www.ncbi.nlm.nih.gov/pubmed/16631551
Brundage JF., *Lancet Infect Dis.* 2006 May;6(5):303-12. Interactions between influenza and bacterial respiratory pathogens: implications for pandemic preparedness.
   "It is commonly believed that the clinical and epidemiological characteristics of the next influenza pandemic will mimic those of the 1918 pandemic. ... there is strong and consistent evidence of epidemiologically and clinically important interactions between influenza and secondary bacterial respiratory pathogens, including during the 1918 pandemic."

- - - - - - -

Jeffery K Taubenberger,[*] Johan V Hultin, David M Morens, *Antivir Ther.* 2007; 12(4 Pt B): 581–591. **"Discovery and characterization of the 1918 pandemic influenza virus in historical context"**

"... the notion that *B. influenzae* was the true cause of influenza persisted up to the time of the next pandemic in 1918 (see below), when Rockefeller scientists Peter Kosciusko Olitsky (1886–1964) and Frederick L Gates (1886–1933) provided strong evidence against a causal association, documenting **that the infective influenza agent survived passage through filters that excluded *B. influenzae* [10]**.
[10. Olitsky P, Gates F. "Experimental study of the nasopharyngeal secretions from influenza patients." *J Am Med Assoc.* 1920;74:1497–1499.]

"The majority of individuals who died during the 1918 pandemic succumbed to secondary bacterial pneumonia [43–45], caused by *Streptococcus pneumoniae, Streptococcus pyogenes, H. influenzae, Staphylococcus aureus,* and other organisms. ... In the hundreds of autopsies performed in 1918, the primary pathological findings tended to be confined to the respiratory tree: death was due to pneumonia and respiratory failure. These findings are consistent with infection by a well adapted influenza virus capable of rapid replication throughout the entire respiratory tree with little clinical or pathological evidence for systemic virus infection [45].]
[45. Winternitz M, Wason I, McNamara F. *The Pathology of Influenza.* Vol. 61. New Haven: Yale University Press; 1920.]

"By the early 1920s, ..., influenza research quieted down and further attempts to elucidate the aetiology were left to but a few investigators. ... revealing the biology of a pandemic that occurred nearly 90 years ago is not just a historical exercise. It may well help us prepare for, and even prevent, the emergence of new pandemics in the 21st century and beyond."

This article is difficult to understand, and seemingly self-contradictory. Firstly it says the cause is bacterial including H. Influenzae, but this latter one was ruled out by Olitsky and Gates as discussed earlier in the article. Then it brings back in the involvement of a virus, which could only be the case if it was related to the bacteria dicussed, e.g., Streptococci, etc. *[Which in any case is correct, as established by Rosenow in his 11-part series. See also Olitsky 1922 in Pandemic History file, above]*

- - - - - - -

http://www.ncbi.nlm.nih.gov/pmc/articles/PMC1997248/
Miles Ott, AB, Shelly F. Shaw, MPH, Richard N. Danila, PhD, MPH, and Ruth Lynfield, MD, *Public Health Rep.* 2007 Nov-Dec; 122(6): 803–810., "Lessons Learned from the 1918–1919 Influenza Pandemic in Minneapolis and St. Paul, Minnesota":
"At least two different vaccines were administered in Minneapolis-St. Paul, neither of them effective as neither actually contained influenza virus. One made by bacteriologists at the University of Minnesota was purported to prevent pneumonia.[39] The Mayo Clinic in Rochester, Minnesota, made another vaccine that was intended to prevent both pneumonia and influenza.[40] This latter vaccination was composed of *Streptococcus pneumoniae* types I, II, and III, *S. pneumoniae* group IV, hemolytic streptococci, *Staphylococcus aureus*, and "influenza bacillus."[41]
[*39.* Serum to be issued. St. Paul Pioneer Press 1918 Oct 19; 6.]
[*40.* Epidemic statistics show decline in city. Minneapolis Tribune 1918 Oct 25; 15.]
[*41.* Rosenow EC. Prophylactic inoculation against respiratory infections during the present pandemic of influenza. Preliminary report. *JAMA.* 1919;72:31–4.]

Ott etal mentions Mayo, vaccine, Rosenow, citing Rosenow's first article in this series, but ***incorrectly*** states that the vaccine was not effective. In fact Rosenow provided very favorable vaccination results in this, his preliminary report. Unfortunately these researchers did not properly review the literature cited, i.e., did not read the complete article, if at all. Incredibly, they have presented an entirely incorrect picture.
a. Rosenow's vaccine was specifically intended to combat pneumonia and pneumonia death, and he explicitly stated in the second paragraph of the first in his series of eleven articles that it was not intended to combat influenza:
"In considering prophylactic inoculations in this epidemic of influenza, we put aside the debated question as to the cause of the initial symptoms and considered primarily the possibility of immunizing persons against the bacteria, pneumonia, streptococci, influenza bacillus and staphylococci, which are conceded by all to be the common causes of death in this disease."

b. Rosenow's vaccine was highly effective against not only pneumonia and pneumonia deaths, but surprisingly (to Rosenow) also greatly reduced influenza incidence in vaccinated persons (as in item IV of his XII-article compilation, and repeated in his 1929 article included in this compilation). Of this he commented "granting that the initial symptoms in influenza may be due to an unknown virus, the lowered incidence of influenza among the inoculated may be only apparent. The attacks may have been so mild as to escape detection."

- - - - - - -

http://jama.ama-assn.org/content/298/6/644.full   2.a.   table: http://jama.ama-assn.org/content/298/6/644/T1.large.jpg

Howard Markel, MD, PhD; Harvey B. Lipman, PhD; J. Alexander Navarro, PhD; Alexandra Sloan, AB; Joseph R. Michalsen, BS; Alexandra Minna Stern, PhD; Martin S. Cetron, MD, JAMA. 2007;298(6):644-654. doi:10.1001/jama.298.6.644, "Nonpharmaceutical Interventions Implemented by US Cities During the 1918-1919 Influenza Pandemic":

Markel et al. discuss 43 cities including seemingly all the major metropolitan areas e.g. New York and Los Angeles etc. (including several Midwest cities e.g. St. Paul, Minneapolis and Chicago, where Rosenow's vaccines were used) and states that "cities that were able to … execute … classic public health interventions … appeared to have an associated mitigated epidemic" but blanketly states, *incorrectly*, that "… these urban communities had neither effective vaccines nor antivirals.

"Historical archival research, and statistical and epidemiological analyses. Nonpharmaceutical interventions were grouped into 3 major categories: school closure; cancellation of public gatherings; and isolation and quarantine." …

" … nonpharmaceutical interventions should be considered for inclusion as companion measures to developing effective vaccines and medications for prophylaxis and treatment. …"

"These findings contrast with the conventional wisdom that the 1918 pandemic rapidly spread through each community killing everyone in its path AND swept fully through the city. Although these urban communities had neither effective vaccines nor antivirals, cities that were able to organize and execute a suite of classic public health interventions before the pandemic appeared to have an associated mitigated epidemic experience."

This article does not mention Mayo or Rosenow, nor any of the other several successful vaccines. There was no mention of vaccination, except with reference to their purported absence.

- - - - - - -

http://jid.oxfordjournals.org/content/195/7/1018.full
David M. Morens and **Anthony S. Fauci**, *Journal of Infectious Diseases*, Vol. 195, No. 7 (2007), The 1918 Influenza Pandemic: Insights for the 21st Century

Morens and Fauci 2007 make no mention of Rosenow, nor Mayo, nor reference to vaccine in 1919. The article touts the need for both pneumococcal and influenzal vaccinations, adopting the common belief in viral-bacterial cogenesis of influenza-pneumonia.   [Whereas as shown by Rosenow particularly, and others, the pneumonia and influenza entities are caused by phases of the same organism.]

Some quotes from this Morens/Fauci article:

p. 1025: "Almost all 'then-versus-now' comparisons are encouraging, in theory. In 2007, public health is much more advanced, with better prevention knowledge, good influenza surveillance, more trained personnel at all levels, established prevention programs featuring annual vaccination with up-to-date influenza and pneumococcal vaccines ... We also have antibiotics to treat pneumonias caused by all of the major bacteria implicated in the 1918 pandemic ...   "

p. 1018: "... the 1918-1919 "Spanish flu" pandemic was among the deadliest public-health crises in human history, killing an estimated 675,000 people in the US and an estimated 50-100 million people worldwide. ... Sequence analysis suggests that the ultimate ancestral source of this virus is almost certainly avian."

p. 1020: "Clinical and autopsy series suggest that excess influenza deaths ... seem to have been associated with 2 overlapping clinical-pathologic syndromes. The most common appears to have been an acute aggressive bronchopneumonia featuring epithelial necrosis, microvasculitis/vascular necrosis, hemorrhage, edema, and widely variant pathology in different parts of the lung ... The second syndrome, compromising perhaps 10-15% of fatal cases was a severe [p. 1022] acute respiratory distress-like syndrome in which patients developed a peculiar "heliotrope cyanosis" characterized by blue-gray facial discoloration ..."

The authors note "a surprising excess of mortality among 20-40 year old individuals ... and lower than expected mortality among the elderly ..."

The authors devote the majority of the article to speculation regarding predicting future pandemics and preventing mortality therein.

- - - - - - -

http://jid.oxfordjournals.org/content/198/7/962.full
David M.. Morens, Jeffery K. Taubenberger and **Anthony S. Fauci**, *The Journal of Infectious Diseases* 2008;198(7):962-970. "Predominant Role of Bacterial Pneumonia as a Cause of Death in Pandemic Influenza: Implications for Pandemic Influenza Preparedness."

Morens, Taubenberger and Fauci 2008 repeat the co-genesis hypothesis and recommendations relating to vaccination with both influenza and pneumococcal vaccines, with particular emphasis on the latter (as reflected in their title).

p. 1: "*Conclusions*. The majority of deaths in the 1918–1919 influenza pandemic likely resulted directly from secondary bacterial pneumonia caused by common upper respiratory-tract bacteria. Less substantial data from the subsequent 1957 and 1968 pandemics are consistent with these findings. If severe pandemic influenza is largely a problem of viral-bacterial copathogenesis, pandemic planning needs to go beyond addressing the viral cause alone (e.g., influenza vaccines and antiviral drugs). Prevention, diagnosis, prophylaxis, and treatment of secondary bacterial pneumonia, as well as stockpiling of antibiotics and bacterial vaccines, should also be high priorities for pandemic planning."

p. 4: Mention is made of various suspect organisms: Discusses "the 96 identified military and civilian autopsy series" of which 82 reported pneumopathogens in >/= 50% of lungs examined, either alone or in mixed culture results ..." ... [In the other 14,] "pneumopathogens accounted for 37.4% of pneumonia deaths." The remainder were associated with other organisms including "viridans streptococci, 'green-producing streptococci' [here citing Ruth Tunnicliff, J. Infect. Dis 1920; 26: 405-17], probably largely corresponding to a-hemolytic streptococci, uncharacterized diplostreptococci, Mocrococcus (Moraxella) catarrhalis, Bacillus (Escherichia) coli, Klebsiella species, and complex mixed bacteria (36.1 % of cultures). ... It is noteworthy that ... many of the cultured ;other; bacteria were reported as 'gram-positive diplococci', 'streptococci,' or 'diplostreptococci' ...".

The authors state they attempted "to obtain all publications possibly reporting influenza pathology and/or bacteriology in 1918–1919" through a search of all major bibliographic sources, in several languages, including the Index Medicus. They "carefully examined the 1539 reports that contained human pathologic and/or bacteriologic findings" .

The authors repeat the recommendations relating to vaccination with both influenza and pneumococcal vaccines, with particular emphasis on the latter (as this in any case was the focus as per the title).

The authors adopt the common belief in viral-bacterial cogenesis of influenza-pneumonia: "Despite the availability of published data on 4 pandemics that have occurred over the past 120 years, there is little modern information on the causes of death associated with influenza pandemics. ... The majority of deaths in the 1918-1919 influenza pandemic likely resulted directly from secondary bacterial pneumonia caused by common upper respiratory-tract bacteria."

The article itself does not mention or cite Rosenow or the Mayo foundation; however, a detailed bibliography (online) cites E.C. Rosenow in multiple entries: including three citations of "Studies in Influenza and Pneumonia. Study V", one "Studies in Influenza and Pneumonia. II", and one part III, although it didn't identify it or recognize it as such.

p. 5-6 : "The pneumonia deaths during the influenza [p. 6] pandemic in 1918 proved so highly similar, pathologically, to the then-recent pneumonia deaths from the measles epidemics that noted experts considered them to be the result of one newly emerging disease: epidemic bacterial pneumonia precipitated by prevalent respiratory tract agents." [Note that Tunnicliff had asserted a role for the green streptococcus in measles; see Tunnicliff 1927.]

p. 6: "We believe that the weight of 90 years evidence ... indicates that the vast majority of pulmonary deaths from pandemic influenza viruses have resulted from poorly understood interactions between the infecting virus and secondary infections due to bacteria that colonize the upper respiratory tract."

p. 6 "The question of whether the pathogenesis of severe influenza-associated pneumonia was primarily viral (i.e., assumed to be an unknown etiologic agent in 1918) or a combination of viral and bacterial agents was carefully considered by pathologists in 1918–1919, without definitive resolution [26, 33].

> [26. Lyon MW. Gross pathology of epidemic influenza at Walter Reed General Hospital. JAMA 1919;72:924-9]
>
> [33. McIntosh J, Privy Council, Medical Research Council. Studies in the aetiology of epidemic influenza. London: Medical Research Council; 1922.]

The authors cite data from a 2008 study that "suggest that influenza vaccination may prevent bacterial disease

> [74: Lee S.E., Eick A, Bloom MS, Brundage JF . Influenza immunization and subsequent diagnoses of group A Streptococcus-illnesses among US Army trainees, 2002–2006. Vaccine 2008;26:3383-6.].

"We reviewed the late 19th- and early 20th-century literature on gross and microscopic influenza pathology and bacteriology, including evidence from 1918–1919 autopsy series with postmortem cultures of lung tissue, blood samples (usually heart blood), pleural fluid, and samples from other compartments. In an effort to obtain all publications possibly reporting influenza pathology and/or bacteriology in 1918–1919, we searched major bibliographic sources [e.g., 11–17] for papers in all languages and tables of contents of major journals in English, German, and French; in addition, we searched all of the papers we identified for additional citations."
Some of the citations listed:

> 11. Billings JS, Fletcher R, Garrison FH, editors. Index Medicus Series II (18 volumes). Washington, DC: Government Printing Office; 1903–1920.
>
> 12. Library of the Surgeon General's Office, United States Army. Index-catalogue of the Library of the Surgeon-General's Office, United States Army. Authors and Subjects. Series III (10 volumes). Washington, DC: US Government Printing Office, 1918–1932.
>
> 13. Vaughan WT. Influenza: an epidemiological study. Monograph series no.1.Baltimore, Maryland: American Journal of Hygiene; 1921.
>
> 14. Jordan EO. Epidemic influenza: a survey. Chicago, Illinois: American Medical Association; 1927.
>
> 15. Thomson D, Thomson R. Annals of the Pickett-Thomson Research Laboratory. Volume X. Influenza (Part II). With special reference to the complications and sequellæ, bacteriology of influenzal pneumonia, pathology, epidemiological data, prevention and treatment. London, Baillière: Tindall & Cox; 1934.
>
> 16. Phillips H, Killingray D, editors. The Spanish Influenza Pandemic of 1918–19New Perspectives. London: Routledge; 2003.
>
> 17. Byerly CR. Fever of War: the influenza epidemic in the U.S. Army during World War I New York: New York University Press; 2005.
> Cites "Insights into the Interaction between Influenza Virus and Pneumococcus", by Jonathan A. McCullers
> [http://cmr.asm.org/content/19/3/571.abstract?ijkey=55c57557edafde76c36 b47488c7111b61fa00b98&keytype2=tf_ipsecsha]

"From more than 2000 such publications, we carefully examined the 1539 reports that contained human pathologic and/or bacteriologic findings (the full bibliographic

list available at http://www3.niaid.nih.gov/topics/Flu/1918/bibliography.htm)
corrrected citation: http://www.niaid.nih.gov/topics/flu/documents/bibliography.pdf
The listed articles included 8 items for E.C. Rosenow, totaling 5 individual articles.

1. Rosenow EC. Studies in influenza and pneumonia. Study V. Observations on the bacteriology and certain clinical features of influenza and influenzal pneumonia. Journal of Infectious Diseases, 1920;26:469-491.

2. Rosenow EC. Influenza and pneumonia studies: bacteriology. [Abstract]. Journal of the American Medical Association 1920;75(17 July):202

3. Rosenow EC. Immunologic experiments with streptococci from influenza. Journal of the American Medical Association 1920;73(11;):861. [Volume 73 = 1919].

4. ILL-11396757-????-Rosenow EC. Studies in influenza. Med Insurance and Health Conservation 1919-1920;29:91-

1.2 85. Rosenow EC. Studies in influenza and pneumonia. Study V. Observations on the bacteriology and certain clinical features of influenza and influenzal pneumonia. Journal of Infectious Diseases 1920;26:469-491. [LH].

1.3 Rosenow EC. Studies in influenza and pneumonia. Study V. Observations on the bacteriology and certain clinical features of influenza and influenzal pneumonia. Journal of Infectious Diseases 1920;26:469-491. [LH].

5.1 Rosenow EC. Studies in influenza and pneumonia. II. The experimental production of symptoms and lesions simulating those of influenza with streptococci isolated during the present epidemic. Journal of the American Medical Association 1919;72(22; 31 May):1604-1609.

5.2 Rosenow EC. The occurrence of a pandemic strain of streptococcus during the pandemic of influenza. Journal of the American Medical Association 1919;72:1608-1609. [Same as above?].

4.2 Rosenow EC. Studies in influenza. Medical Insurance and Health Conservation 1919-1920;29:91-9

- - - - - - -

Jonathan A. McCullers· *J Infect Dis.* 2008 October 1; 198(7): 945–947., "Planning for an influenza pandemic: thinking beyond the virus"

"Theophile H. Laennec was the first to describe the pathology of pandemic influenza. The inventor of the stethoscope ... during the 1803 pandemic ... described an increase in expectoration of yellow to greenish-tinged sputum, " [Laennec RTH. Signs of peripneumonia. In: Hale-White W, editor. Translation of selected passages from De l'Auscultation Mediate. 1st. New York: Williams Wood & Co.; 1923. p. 82-95.]

"Otto Lubarsch compared preserved autopsy specimens from the 1889–1890 pandemic to fresh autopsy samples from 1918–1919 and concluded the pathologic processes were nearly identical. This homogeneity in findings reinforces the idea that the end result, death from bacterial pneumonia, is a common feature of all pandemics in the preantibiotic era." [Lubarsch O. Die anatomischen Befunde von 14 todlich verlaufenen Fallen von Grippe. Berl Klin Wchnschr 1918;55:768-9. (Fre).]

"A shift in focus is required. Pandemic planning must take into account the possibility that secondary bacterial pneumonia will be a frequent complication of pandemic influenza. Basic research into the interactions between influenza viruses and bacteria is needed."

- - - - - - -

wwwnc.cdc.gov/eid/article/14/8/07-1313.htm – Vol. 14, No.8, Aug 2008, 1193-9
John F. Brundage and G. Dennis Shanks "Deaths from Bacterial Pneumonia during 1918–19 Influenza Pandemic"

Tne authors begin with the assertion that "Deaths during the 1918-1919 pandemic have been attributed to a hypervirulent influenza strain". No citations are given. The authors "hypothesize"/adopt the "sequential-infection" alternate hypothesis whereby influenza infection with pandemic strain enabled secondary infection of bacterial pneumonias, disagreeing with view that hypervirulent virus caused fatal pneumonitis.

p. 1195 Authors note that recent arrivals at US military training camps had worse clinical outcomes than similarly aged male counterparts in the camps longer..

p. 1196 Authors note that "bacteria most often recovered from the sputum, lungs, and blood of pneumonia patients, alive or dead, were common colonizers of the upper respiratory tracts of healthy persons, i.e., Hemophilus influenzae, Streptococcus pneumoniae, S. pyogenrs and/or Staphylococcus aureus." [References 5-13 include Opie 1921, W. Vaughn 1921, EO Jordan 1921, British Ministry of Health 1920, US Sec. of Navy 1919, Hall 1928, Conner 1919, Brundage 2006, Morens and Fauci 2007]

"… correlations were stronger between mortality and pneumonia rates than between mortality and clinical [influenza] case rates." [citing Kilbourne 2006 and Frost 2008]

p. 1197 Authors note that "nonpharmeceutical interventions (e.g. isolation, quarantine, closing schools, banning public gatherings) were associated with lower influenza-related mortality rates during the autumn of 1918." [citing Markel etal 2007]

p. 1198 Implications. Authors recommend (1) prior to a pandemic decreasing barriers to receipt of S. pneumoniae vaccination (2) during pandemic, universally "vaccinate with safe and effective strain specific influenza vaccine, if available" (DUH) (3) during local epidemics "treat all serious clinical cases with an antibacterial agent that is effective against S. pneumoniae, S. pyogenes, H. influenzae, and S. aureus (including methicillin resistant S. aureus); isolate patients (DUH) (4) conduce surveillance.

Citations include the standard assortment of modern "experts", including Morens, Brundage, McCullers, Mahdi and Klugman, and Fauci.

- - - - - - -

http://articles.latimes.com/2009/aug/04/science/sci-pneumonia4
August 04, 2009|Thomas H. Maugh II

Pneumonia vaccine may help limit swine flu deaths

Most of the serious consequences linked to the virus are the result of pneumonia, and an underused vaccine called Pneumovax can prevent, or at least limit, such complications in many patients. The vaccine, made by Merck & Co., stimulates the body's ability to neutralize the bacteria responsible for many cases of pneumonia, and it has the potential to prevent an estimated one-third of pneumonia deaths linked to swine flu.

- - - - - - -

Croat Med J. 2009 August; 50(4): 412–415., **"Swine Flu"**
Charles H. Calisher

"In 1921 … Peter Olitsky and Frederick Gates of the Rockefeller Foundation published their filtration results, which demonstrated that nasal secretions from patients infected with the 1918 influenza virus (influenza A H1N1, *vide infra*), and passed it through a filter that excluded bacteria, still caused pneumonia in rabbits (4,5). Olitsky and Gates had isolated the etiologic agent of this disease but did not recognize that …

- - - - - - -

Dennis Shanks G, Mackenzie A, Waller M, Brundage JF.2011; Influenza Other Respiratory Viruses. 2011 Nov 27. doi: 10.1111/j.1750-2659.2011.00309.x. [Epub ahead of print], "Relationship between "purulent bronchitis" in military populations in Europe prior to 1918 and the 1918-1919 influenza pandemic."

Abstract
'Please cite this paper as: Shanks et al. Relationship between "purulent bronchitis" in military populations in Europe prior to 1918 and the 1918-1919 influenza pandemic. Influenza and Other Respiratory Viruses DOI: 10.1111/j.1750-2659.2011.00309.x

"Purulent bronchitis was a distinctive and apparently new lethal respiratory infection in British and American soldiers during the First World War. Mortality records suggest that purulent bronchitis caused localized outbreaks in the midst of a broad epidemic wave of lethal respiratory illness in 1916-1917. Probable purulent bronchitis deaths in the Australian Army showed an epidemic wave that moved from France to England. Purulent bronchitis may have been the clinical expression of infection with a novel influenza virus which also could have been a direct precursor of the 1918 pandemic strain."

Chapter 7. THEORETICAL CONSIDERATIONS: THEN AND NOW

A. THEN

The early thought experiments of Greenwood and Yule figured prominently into the theoretical framework used by McCoy to blanketly reject, without specific case reference, the many worthwhile studies and vaccination experiments conducted at the time. One might easily surmise, even conclude, that McCoy sought to cover his own failure to meaningfully contribute in this area by trashing everyone else who did come up with worthwhile results.

Greenwood and Yule 1915 p. 163
"Unless the number of observations is large, fluctuations of sampling are of considerable importance."
p. 111 "All the following conditions should be fulfilled by the data:
(1) The persons must be, in all material respects, alike. ... If ... no practicable care on the part of the individual can substantially reduce his risk of contracting the disease, then this particular heterogeneity [willingness to submit to inoculation] is not material and can be disregarded." ...
(2) The effective exposure to the disease must be identical in the case of inoculated and uninoculasted persons. ... Evidently, if the uninoculated have been longer at risk than the inoculated, as would be the case if inoculation is carried on throughout an epidemic, and the statistics are compiled from the totals of inoculated and uninoculated at the end of the experience, the condition is not fulfilled. ..."
(3) The criteria of the fact of inoculation and of the fact of the disease having occurred must be independent. ... when, as may quite frequently happen, doubts legitimately arise as to whether a given person had or had not been inoculated ..., it is easy to see how seriously biased statistics may be prepared without any such evil intent. ...
[(4)] ... a further condition is necessary – namely, that **the number of observations must be sufficient. ...**
Page 117 paragraph 3, through page 183, the writers review statistical theory, i.e., probabilities, deviations, calculus (?) formulas, etc. history dating from Karl Pearson 1900.
p. 114 "In Section III we develop a statistical theory of the way in which immunization results can be interpreted."
p. 133-5 "It appears that from a certain point in time, **often perhaps from the very commencement of the epidemic itself, the infectivity of the disease diminishes**. If, therefore, we were to inject persons exposed to risk with coloured water, and were so to plan our operations that the absolute number of persons inoculated in each unit of time, say each day or each week, was constant, and were finally to count up the numbers of inoculated persons and of attacks amongst them and prepare similar statistics of uninoculated persons, we should inevitably find that the attack-rate was lower in the former case. This would happen were the infectivity constant, and a declining infectivity would accentuate it.

"We can illustrate the point readily. Let us suppose that an initial population of 1,000 is exposed to risk during a period of three weeks, that during each of these weeks the chance of acquiring a disease is one in a hundred and that at the beginning of each week fifty persons receive an injection of coloured water. At the end of the first week there will be 950 uninoculated and 50 inoculated persons, and ten cases of disease will have occurred-9·5 among the uninoculated, 0'5 among the inoculated. Stopping at this point, we have identical attack-rates in the two classes-viz., 1 per cent. At the beginning of the second week, we are left with 940'5 uninoculated and 49'5 inoculated men who have not had the disease; fifty of the former are now inoculated, so that the numbers become 890'5 uninoculated, 99.5 inoculated; subjecting all to the attack-rate of 1 per cent., 8'905 uninoculated and 0'995 inoculated fall victims. Adding up from the beginning we reach 100 inoculated with 1'495 cases and 900 uninoculated with 18'405 cases-rates of 15 and 20 per mille respectively. At the end of the third week we shallhave 150 inoculated with 2'98 cases, and 850 uninoculated with 26'72 cases-rate per mille of 20 and 31; thus the relative advantage of the inoculated increases. **This error, which is inherent in the method of summation adopted,** would have been increased if the chance of infection instead of being constant had diminished as time passed -a phenomenon which we have seen reason to anticipate in practice. The conclusion is that, if we are only provided with the total number of inoculations performed during the epidemic and the allotment of attacks between inoculated and uninoculated classes, we are almost sure to find, that the inoculated have an advantage and are by no means warranted in concluding that this is any more than a necessary consequence of the manner of compilation. Of course, the explanation of the fallacy is that the **period of exposure to risk is not the same in the two classes**; the men who would perhaps have been inoculated next week have a chance of acquiring the disease this week, and if they do so will naturally be counted as unvaccinated attacked persons. **There is no way of circumventing this error on the basis of summarizing tables** and it must always, in greater or less degree, affect the statistics of inoculations performed during an epidemic. No doubt if full details as to time and place of inoculation and attack were furnished, we could isolate the true from the spurious advantage; but that, in the stress of active campaigning, such particulars are likely to be recorded is improbable."

p. 180: Approaching the end of Section III, "The reader will naturally ask if we cannot go further than this and determine in some way the true distributions and the form of the curve of chances. The answer, so far as we can see, must be in the negative."

p. 182: acknowledges, but rejects, that "the reader ... may say, that the normal distributions which we have calculated may not represent the truth ... and ... suggest that the calculation of the death-rates amongst immunized and unimmunized persons, by regarding the epidemic as eliminating all who possess less than a certain critical resistance, is a mere piece of mathematical jugglery. ..."

Acknowledging that "We think it is in all probability essentially true that the resistances of immunized and non-immunized persons vary inter se and that these distributions may largely overlap." ... and, in the final paragraph of the statistical theoretical section, "Further, we do think it is probably true that the elimination of all individuals with less than a certain resistance cannot be regarded as representing what, in fact, happens during an epidemic, ... chance must enter into the matter more or less. ... In the meantime it seems to us a distinct advantage that the element of chance may possibly be ignored, and that we may be able to determine distributions of 'pseudo-resistance' such that the elimination of individuals with pseudo resistances less than [a theoretically calculated value] ... gives the same death-rates amongst the two classes compared, as would the application of the unknown law of chances of death to the true distributions of resistance."

In other words, they seem to be saying that their theoretical construct would provide the same information as an "unknown law of chances", which by any stretch, may indeed be dismissed as "mathematical jugglery".

Section IV: The Measurement of the Relative Efficiencies of Different Immunization Processes.

"We now come to the two questions which are of interest to the practical man – vis, granted that in certain cases ... the death or incidence rates upon the uninoculated are higher than the corresponding values for the inoculated, and that these divergences cannot be dismissed as mere chance events, in which case [1] did the process of immunization produce the better result? ... [and 2] are the ... results sufficiently good to authorize taking the same step in the case of troops likely to be exposed to infection?" Here quoting Professor Pearson 1900 and his probability coefficient calculations in the case of effectiveness of diphtheria antitoxin, "that between the administration of antitoxin and recovery in laryngeal cases is substantial. But the relationship is by no means so great as in the case of vaccination, and if its magnitude justifies the use of antitoxin ... it does not justify the sweeping statements of its effectiveness which I have heard made by medical friends. It seems until wider statistics are forthcoming a case for cautiously feeling the way forward rather than for hasty generalizations." (op cit. p. 45)

P. 184 "We propose to define the advantage of an immunization process as the difference between the fatality-rates (or incidence-rates) of the unimmunized and immunized populations. The efficiency we propose to define as the ratio of the advantage to the fatality-rate (or incidence-rate) amongst the unimmunized – i.e. as the ratio of the numbers who are saved by the process to the numbers who might be saved. ..." and continuing to discuss their "imaginary illustration" assumption that fatality rates are invariable from epidemic to epidemic, which is never the case, and proceeding with additional theoretical statistical calculations (p. 185-6) and concluding on page 186, "that no coefficient of correlation or association will furnish us with answers to the questions proposed at the beginning of this section. ... In view, however, of the popularity enjoyed by certain of these coefficients and the fact that they have frequently been used in such investigations, it may be of interest to pass them in review."

Carrying on for a page with such, p. 187 continues "The correlation is, as we have stated above (p. 180), completely indeterminate."

Proceeding with additional calculations to page 189, the authors reject the coefficients under discussion: |Our condemnation of these coefficients, for the present purpose, may at least claim to be impartial, inasmuch as two of them were originally proposed by one of us. [paragraph] The results of this section are disappointing in so far as they fail to provide a simple answer to important practical questions."

In the discussion section following, p. 191, reference is made to swine fever

B. NOW

Orenstein WA, Bernier RH, Dondero TJ, et al, Field evaluation of vaccine efficacy. BullWorld Health Organ **1985**; 63:1055–1068.

[http://whqlibdoc.who.int/bulletin/1985/Vol63-No6/bulletin_1985_63%286%29_1055-1068.pdf]

page 1056   "The ideal vaccine efficacy study is a clinical trial starting with persons susceptible to disease. In a double-blind randomized placebo controlled trial, half the subjects receive vaccine and half receive placebo. To calculate the vaccine efficacy, both groups are followed prospectively to determine the attack rates for disease in vaccines and non-vaccinees. This type of study is generally not possible after a vaccine has been licensed because, **when the vaccine is of proven benefit, the use of a placebo is unethical.** In most countries today, measles vaccine has been used in a proportion of the population. These vaccines are not a randomly selected group; and their susceptibility prior to vaccination is often unknown. None the less, vaccine efficacy studies are still possible by reducing biases to a minimum and recreating as closely as possible the "ideal" conditions of the prospective clinical trial."

(2) Weinberg & Szilagyi 2010
[https://www.hidionline.com/HIDI/Documents/Vaccine_Epidemiology.pdf]

Geoffrey A. Weinberg and Peter G. Szilagyi, EDITORIAL COMMENTARY • **JID 2010:201 (1 June)** • 1607, "Vaccine Epidemiology: Efficacy, Effectiveness, and the Translational Research Roadmap"

Provides formula for calculating VE, citing Orenstein 1988 and 1985; discusses "field efficacy" and vaccine effectiveness terminology, as related. **Vaccine efficacy implies a controlled trial methodology, but it is recognized that this is not always possible, particularly in an on-going field situation.** Illustrates this in the case of **Curns et al, [citation below]** who used data from past years, prior to vaccine, to compare with results of vaccine.

See also Orenstein WA, Bernier RH, Hinman AR. Assessing vaccine efficacy in the field. Further observations. Epidemiol Rev **1988**; 10:212–241.

Aaron T. Curns, etal, *Journal of Infectious Diseases* 2010 **Volume 201, Issue 11** Pp. **1617-1624,** "Reduction in Acute Gastroenteritis Hospitalizations"
[http://jid.oxfordjournals.org/content/201/11/1617.long   ,
http://jid.oxfordjournals.org/content/201/11/1617.full.pdf+html]

Though not necessarily nationally representative of vaccine coverage in the United States, data from 6–8 population-based vaccination information system sentinel sites found that 1-dose RV5 coverage was 49% and that 3-dose coverage was 3% among age-eligible children during the 2007 rotavirus season [4 -Centers for Disease Control and Prevention . Delayed onset and diminished magnitude of rotavirus activity, United States, November 2007-May 2008. MMWR Morb Mortal Wkly Rep 2008;57:697-700; Vaccine 96% effective in preventing severe rotavirus disease   resulting   in   hospitalization   during   clinical   trials   2006 [Vesikari T, Matson DO, Dennehy P, et al, "Safety and efficacy of a pentavalent human-bovine (WC3) reassortant rotavirus vaccine". *N Engl J Med* 2006;354:23-33.]

APPENDICES A-L

* [Reprinted per provision 17 USC 107]

Efficacy of Whole-Cell Killed Bacterial Vaccines in Preventing Pneumonia and Death during the 1918 Influenza Pandemic

Yu-Wen Chien,[1] Keith P. Klugman,[1] and David M. Morens[2]

[1]Rollins School of Public Health, Emory University, Atlanta, Georgia; [2]National Institute of Allergy and Infectious Diseases, National Institutes of Health, Bethesda, Maryland

Background. Most deaths in the 1918 influenza pandemic were caused by secondary bacterial pneumonia.

Methods. We performed a systematic review and reanalysis of studies of bacterial vaccine efficacy (VE) in preventing pneumonia and mortality among patients with influenza during the 1918 pandemic.

Results. A meta-analysis of 6 civilian studies of mixed killed bacterial vaccines containing pneumococci identified significant heterogeneity among studies and estimated VE at 34% (95% confidence interval [CI], 19%–47%) in preventing pneumonia and 42% (95% CI, 18%–59%) in reducing case fatality rates among patients with influenza, using random-effects models. Using fixed-effect models, the pooled VE from 3 military studies was 59% (95% CI, 43%–70%) for pneumonia and 70% (95% CI, 50%–82%) for case fatality. Military studies showed less heterogeneity and may provide more accurate results than civilian studies, given the potential biases in the included studies. Findings of 1 military study using hemolytic streptococci also suggested that there was significant protection.

Conclusions. Despite significant methodological problems, the systematic biases in these studies do not exclude the possibilities that whole-cell inactivated pneumococcal vaccines may confer cross-protection to multiple pneumococcal serotypes and that bacterial vaccines may play a role in preventing influenza-associated pneumonia.

The 1918 influenza pandemic caused an estimated 20–100 million deaths worldwide [1]. There is growing epidemiologic, clinical, and pathologic evidence that the majority of deaths in this pandemic resulted directly from secondary bacterial pneumonia [2–5]. In the 1918 pandemic, *Streptococcus pneumoniae* was the predominant organism isolated from antemortem cultures from normally sterile sites in patients with influenza-associated pneumonia, followed by hemolytic streptococci, presumably representing *Streptococcus pyogenes* [4, 5].

Received 10 April 2010; accepted 29 June 2010; electronically published 28 October 2010.

Potential conflicts of interest: K.P.K. has received consultant fees and research support from Pfizer Vaccines and GlaxoSmithKline but received no funding from industry for this analysis. All other authors report no potential conflicts of interest.

Presented in part: 7th International Symposium on Pneumococci and Pneumococcal Disease, Tel Aviv, Israel, 14–18 March 2010 (oral presentation).

Financial support: none reported.

Reprints or correspondence: Dr Klugman, Rollins School of Public Health, 1518 Clifton Rd, Atlanta, GA 30322 (kklugma@emory.edu).

The Journal of Infectious Diseases   2010;202(11):1639–1648
0022-1899/2010/20211-0005$15.00
DOI: 10.1086/657144

The etiology of influenza was unknown at the time of the 1918 pandemic. Many contemporary investigators erroneously believed that bacteria, in particular *Bacillus influenzae* (Pfeiffer's bacillus, now known as *Haemophilus influenzae*) was the cause of influenza [6]. It was also generally believed, however, that most 1918 pandemic influenza deaths resulted from secondary bacterial pneumonia following primary influenza infections of whatever cause [2]. In attempts to prevent the primary disease of influenza, to reduce pneumonia and mortality, and to investigate the etiology of influenza, many bacterial vaccines were produced, tested, and administered during the 1918 pandemic. Here we review studies of whole-cell bacterial vaccines administered to healthy subjects during the 1918 pandemic to examine their efficacy in preventing influenza-associated pneumonia and mortality.

An important concern about such a review is that the scientific quality of 1918 vaccine studies was low by today's standards, owing to such methodological flaws as lack of subject randomization. Moreover, whereas most vaccinations were given during the declining phase of the pandemic (fall–winter 1918–1919), the incidences

Chien et al JID 2010:202 (1 December) 1639-1648

of influenza, influenza-associated pneumonia, and deaths in vaccinated individuals were usually compared with the same outcomes in unvaccinated individuals from the beginning of the epidemic [6, 7], introducing unequal observation periods more favorable to vaccinated individuals. In addition, vaccinated individuals might come from select populations with reduced exposure or susceptibility to influenza because they had not had influenza between the appearance of the pandemic and the start of vaccination. Not fully appreciating such potential design flaws, investigators studying bacterial vaccines often believed that they had demonstrated a reduction in the incidence of influenza, which is not consistent with our understanding of influenza etiology.

We reasoned that any true effect of bacterial vaccines on influenza disease might more plausibly result from reduced attack rates of secondary bacterial pneumonias and consequent reduced case fatality rates among patients with influenza. To examine this possibility while addressing methodological flaws of the original studies, we reanalyzed published data, asking whether vaccinated patients who developed influenza had lower attack rates of pneumonia or lower case fatality rates than unvaccinated patients with influenza. This approach should diminish bias caused by unequal observation periods, because these measures were less likely to be influenced by changing influenza incidence during the progress of the pandemic. In addition, the attack rate of pneumonia and case fatality rates among patients with influenza seems to be higher in the later phase of influenza epidemics [8–10]. Therefore, this approach may result in more conservative estimates of vaccine efficacy (VE), because the vaccinated individuals were more likely to be from the later phase of the 1918 pandemic.

METHODS

Search strategy and criteria. In an effort to obtain all relevant publications reporting bacterial vaccine studies in the 1918 pandemic, a literature search was performed on the Journal Storage (JSTOR) database using the search terms "influenza or flu," "vaccine or vaccination or inoculation" and "year: 1918 to 1920" in the full text, without language restriction. We also manually searched 2 bibliographic sources—*Index Medicus* and *Index-Catalogue of the Library of the Surgeon-General's Office*—for relevant articles in any language between 1918 and 1920. In addition, we examined all articles from an archive at the National Institute of Allergy and Infectious Diseases, National Institutes of Health (http://www3.niaid.nih.gov/topics/Flu/1918/bibliography.htm) [3]. The archive was originally developed to identify publications containing information on influenza pathology and bacteriology in the 1918 pandemic but was expanded to contain other topics. We examined all retrieved articles to identify additional articles.

Selection criteria and data extraction. Original reports of prophylactic administration of bacterial vaccines to humans

during the autumn 1918 or winter 1918–1919 pandemic waves were eligible for inclusion. We then searched for studies in which case fatality rates or attack rates of pneumonia among both vaccinated and unvaccinated patients with influenza could be determined. Vaccinated patients with influenza were defined as patients with clinically diagnosed influenza who had received ≥1 dose of a bacterial vaccine at any time before the onset of influenza. We excluded reports that did not provide exact denominators (numbers of vaccinated and unvaccinated patients with influenza) or in which 1 or both of the vaccine exposure denominators was <10. When multiple publications reported results from the same study population, only results from the most recent publication were included. Because these early articles did not provide much detail, we assessed the quality of study using 4 criteria: (1) whether vaccinees were randomized, (2) whether vaccination was completed before the occurrence of the first patients with influenza in the facility, (3) whether the vaccinated and unvaccinated groups were from the same population, and (4) whether the bacterial vaccine given was not reported to reduce the incidence of influenza among vaccinated subjects compared with unvaccinated subjects.

Statistical methods. For each included study, we calculated unadjusted risk ratios (RRs) comparing case fatality rates and pneumonia attack rates in vaccinated and unvaccinated patients with influenza, with 95% confidence intervals (CIs). When no pneumonia cases or deaths were recorded for a study group, a value of 0.5 was assigned. VE was calculated as $1 - RR$.

We stratified the studies according to the vaccine formula and study population (civilian or military). Meta-analysis was performed on studies of bacterial vaccines containing pneumococci. An estimate of heterogeneity across studies was assessed using Q and I^2 statistics; heterogeneity was considered significant at $P < .10$ (Q statistic) or $I^2 > 50\%$ [11]. When significant heterogeneity was found, pooled RR estimates and 95% CIs were derived using a random-effects model; otherwise, a fixed-effects model with Mantel-Haenszel weighting was used. Publication bias was assessed by using funnel plots [11]. To explore the sensitivity of the meta-analysis results, we (1) determined whether the results were strongly influenced by excluding each included study one at a time and (2) used the "trim-and-fill" method to adjust for potential publication bias [12]. Analyses were performed using free MIX software (version 1.7) [13, 14].

RESULTS

Study selection. We identified and retrieved full texts of 485 publications for assessment. Figure 1 summarizes the study selection process; 13 studies were included in the final analysis.

Characteristics and quality of included studies. Information on the vaccines in the 13 studies is shown in Table 1. Eight studies reported mixed inactivated vaccines containing

Chien et al JID 2010:202 (1 December) 1639-1648

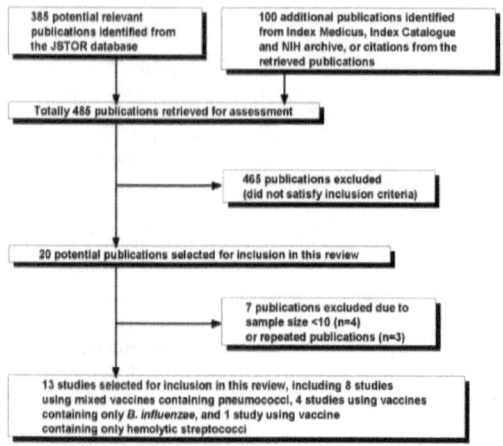

Figure 1. Selection of published studies of bacterial vaccines in the 1918 influenza pandemic. *B. influenzae, Bacillus influenzae*; JSTOR, Journal Storage; NIH, National Institutes of Health.

multiple serotypes of *S. pneumoniae* in addition to other bacteria, such as *B. influenzae*, hemolytic streptococci, or *Staphylococcus aureus* [15, 16, 18–23] . Four studies used a vaccine containing multiple strains of *B. influenzae* [24, 25, 27, 28], and the remaining study used a vaccine containing multiple strains of hemolytic streptococci [29]. The strains of bacteria used in the vaccines were usually obtained from patients during local influenza epidemics. The vaccines were whole-cell bacterial vaccines inactivated by heat, tricresol, or chloroform. The amounts of each organism and the inoculation schedules differed between studies.

The characteristics of the 13 studies are shown in Table 2. Eight studies were from civilian and 3 from military populations. Cadham reported military and civilian data separately [15]. In the study by Minaker and Irvine, vaccinated individuals were mainly from the military, and unvaccinated individuals mainly from the civilian population [21]; this study was regarded as a civilian study in our analyses.

None were double-blinded randomized trials. The studies by McCoy et al and Hinton and Kane were considered the highest quality, because vaccinated individuals were assigned randomly and vaccinations were completed before outbreaks appeared in the facilities where they were performed [20, 25]. The study reported by Minaker and Irvine was lowest in quality, because vaccinated and unvaccinated persons were from different populations [21]. For the rest of the studies, vaccinated and unvaccinated subjects were from the same military or civilian

populations, but it was not possible to fully evaluate their comparability, owing to insufficient information on potential confounders, such as age, sex, and health status, as well as on how vaccinated individuals were chosen.

Table 3 shows the incidence of influenza among vaccinated and unvaccinated subjects, as reported in the original analyses of all the studies except the Cherry study, which also used patients with influenza as the denominator in the analysis [16]. The incidence of influenza among unvaccinated subjects varied from 3.5% to 38.5%, probably reflecting differences in case identification, among other factors. According to the US house-to-house survey, ~28% of the population suffered an influenza attack during the 1918 pandemic [30]. Three studies with an influenza incidence of <10% probably used hospital admission records for case identification, whereas those with an incidence close to 28% may have included outpatients with influenza.

Except for 2 studies with random allocation [20, 25] and 1 small study [28], the included studies found a lower incidence of influenza in vaccinated subjects, presumably because vaccination usually began after the epidemic had occurred. We reanalyzed the original data including only patients with diagnosed influenza in the denominators to compare attack rates of influenza-associated pneumonia and case fatality among vaccinated and unvaccinated patients with influenza.

Effect of mixed bacterial vaccines containing pneumococci on the attack rate of pneumonia. RR estimates for the comparison of pneumonia attack rates between vaccinated and un-

Chien et al JID 2010:202 (1 December) 1639-1648

Table 1. Vaccine Contents, Dosages, and Preparation Methods in the 12 Included Studies

Study	Vaccine contents, organisms, millions/mL[a]	Dosage	Inactivation method	Sources of bacterial strains used in vaccine
Cadham [15]	Pneumococci (300 military, 600 civilian), streptococci (600 military, 300 civilian), *Bacillus influenzae* (400 for both groups)[b]	2 doses of 0.5 mL at 7-d interval	Heat	Streptococci were obtained from empyema, nasopharyngeal, blood, and portmortem lung cultures; strains of pneumococci were isolated from nasopharyngeal and sputum cultures; *B. influenzae* was isolated from nasopharyngeal cultures obtained from the first patients recognized as having typical cases of pandemic influenza in Winnipeg in October 1918. Strains of bacteria used in military studies were locally isolated; some civilian populations received vaccines containing strains obtained from E. C. Rosenow (Mayo Clinic, Rochester, MN).
Cherry [16]	Pneumococci (10, 50), streptococci (10, 50), *B. influenzae* (25, 125), *Moraxella catarrhalis* (25, 125), a gram-positive diplococcus other than the pneumococcus (10, 50)	2 doses of 1 mL at 7-d interval [17]	Tricresol	Pneumococci were not classified in Australia, but 6–15 strains were included in each batch of the vaccine; multiple strains were also used for other organisms. All included strains were isolated from patients with influenza during the epidemics in Australia and South Africa in late 1918 and early 1919; some were of postmortem origin [17].
Erye and Lowe [18]	Pneumococci (100, 200), streptococci (20, 100), *Staphylococcus aureus* (400, 1000), *B. influenzae* (20, 60), *M. catarrhalis* (50, 150), other *Bacillus* species (200, 400)	2 doses of 0.5 mL at 10-d interval	Not reported	Fresh strains of streptococci, pneumococci, and *B. influenzae* were obtained from patients with virulent infection (septicemic influenzal pneumonia) at a naval hospital and a transport ship arriving at a port in the United Kingdom.
Leishman [19]	Pneumococci (200), streptococci (80), *B. influenzae* (60)	2 doses of 0.5 and 1 mL at 10-d interval	Heat	Several strains and types of each organism, all isolated relatively freshly from case patients
McCoy et al [20]	Pneumococcal types I–IV (total, 3000), hemolytic streptococci (1000), *S. aureus* (500), *B. influenzae* (500)	3 doses of 0.5, 1, and 1.5 mL at 48-h intervals	Not reported	≥2 strains of each organism; sources were not reported.
Minaker and Irvine [21]	Pneumococcal types I–III (total, 7000), hemolytic streptococci (100), *B. influenzae* (5000)	3 doses of 0.5, 0.8, and 1 mL at 3-d intervals	Heat	*B. influenzae* was obtained not locally but from the Rockefeller Institute; sources of the other bacteria were not reported.
Rosenow and Sturdivant [22]	Pneumococcal types I–III (total, 3000), hemolytic streptococci (2000), *S. aureus* (1000), pneumococcal type IV and allied green-producing diclostreptococci (4000)[c]	3 doses of 0.25, 0.5, and 0.75 mL at 7-d intervals	Heat	Authors stressed the importance of using freshly isolated strains because of the tendency of bacteria to lose virulent properties; they also stated that the composition of vaccine should be adjusted frequently to reflect changes in the bacterial strains in circulation.
Watters [23]	Pneumococci (400), hemolytic streptococci (400), *B. influenzae* (100), *M. catarrhalis* (400)	3 doses of 0.2, 0.3, and 0.4 mL at 3-d intervals	Not reported	Organisms isolated from lungs at postmortem examinations
Barnes [24]; Hinton and Kane [25]	*B. influenzae* (800)	3 doses of 0.5, 1, and 1.5 mL at 24-h intervals	Heat	3 locally isolated strains [26]
Duval and Harris [27]	*B. influenzae*[d]	3 doses at 3-d intervals	Chloroform	Old strain obtained from Rockefeller Institute (not locally and freshly isolated)
Wadsworth [28]	*B. influenzae* (1000)	Not reported	Not reported	15 strains obtained from Research Laboratories of New York City
Ely et al [29]	Hemolytic streptococci (250)	3 doses of 0.25, 0.5, and 1 mL at 48-h intervals	Heat	Multiple virulent strains obtained from patients in the camp

[a] Except where otherwise noted, multiple numbers in parentheses represent first and second doses.

[b] In this study, the civilian population received a vaccine different from that used in military personnel; differences in composition are noted parenthetically.

[c] Vaccines used earlier in the epidemic contained *B. influenzae*.

[d] The dose for adults was 1 billion *B. influenza* organisms for the first injection, one-half this number for the second, and 1 billion for the third.

vaccinated patients with influenza ranged from 0.46 to 1.17 in 5 civilian studies (Figure 2). Three of the 5 studies showed significant vaccine protection against pneumonia, but findings of the highest-quality study, by McCoy et al, suggested no protective effect [20]. There was heterogeneity among the civilian studies ($P < .001$ for Q statistic; $I^2 = 86.23\%$). The random-effects estimate of pooled RRs was 0.66 (95% CI, 0.53–0.81),

for a VE of 34% (95% CI, 19%–47%). Combined RRs were changed most by excluding the Cherry study [16]; after exclusion of that study, no heterogeneity was indicated, and the pooled VE with a fixed-effects model was 31% (95% CI, 26%–35%). The funnel plot suggested potential publication bias, and the trim-and-fill adjusted VE was 40% (95% CI, 26%–51%) for the civilian studies.

Chien et al JID 2010:202 (1 December) 1639-1648

Table 2.   Characteristics of the 12 Included Studies

Study	Country (population type)	Study period	Remarks
Cadham [15]	Canada (civilian and military)	October 1918 to February 1919	Military and civilian data were reported separately. Military data were from soldiers in Winnipeg, and influenza case patients were among hospitalized patients; civilian data were reported by 108 physicians in Manitoba and Saskatchewan.
Cherry [16]	Australia (civilian)	December 1918 to March 1919	Unlike other studies, this study did not examine the incidence of influenza among vaccinated and unvaccinated individuals; it analyzed data from 3891 patients with influenza treated in several hospitals in Melbourne, Australia. Patients from quarantine stations or with unknown vaccination status were excluded in the current analysis.
Erye and Lowe [18]	United Kingdom (military)	October–December 1918	Data from 15 units of New Zealand troops in the United Kingdom were included. Data from hospital B and camp G were included in the current analysis because the attack rate of pneumonia or case fatality of influenza was provided.
Leishman [19]	United Kingdom (military)	November 1918 to April 1919	Data from 24 military units in the United Kingdom were combined; numbers of influenza cases, complications, and deaths were derived from hospital records.
McCoy et al [20]	United States (civilian)	15 November to 9 December 1918	Alternate patients at a mental institution were vaccinated. Vaccination was completed 11 d before the occurrence of the first influenza case in this facility. The study population was aged ≤41 years.
Minaker and Irvine [21]	United States (civilian)	October–November 1918	Vaccinated individuals were military personnel or their civilian relatives and friends. Unvaccinated subjects were from the civilian population during the same period. Data from 4 locations were combined.
Rosenow and Sturdivant [22]	United States (civilian)	15 October 1918 to end of epidemic or 1 May 1919	Data were collected by distributing questionnaires to physicians supplied with the vaccine in Minnesota; reports from 530 physicians were fairly complete and were summarized. The observation period began on the day of the first inoculation.
Watters [23]	United States (civilian)	Not reported	Data from 5 commercial firms and 1 state hospital were combined.
Barnes [24]	United States (civilian)	22 October 1918 to end of epidemic	Data were from a state sanatorium at Wallum Lake, Massachusetts.
Duval and Harris [27]	United States (civilian)	15 October 1918 to January 1919	The majority of vaccinated subjects were employees in the large commercial houses, banks, and factories of New Orleans. Control subjects were those who refused to be vaccinated in these firms. Persons who had been sick before vaccination were excluded. Only individual groups A and B reported pneumonia data and were included in our analysis.
Hinton and Kane [25]	United States (civilian)	6 October to 30 November 1918	In an experiment at a state hospital for epileptics, patients in every other bed of a ward or room were vaccinated; vaccination was completed 6 d before the first influenza case occurred in this facility.
Wadsworth [26]	United States (civilian)	Not reported	Data included were from 146 laboratory staff of the New York State Department of Health.
Ely et al [29]	United States (military)	17 September to 21 October 1918	Data were combined from 7 military units at Puget Sound Navy Yard.

RR estimates from 3 military studies ranged from 0.35 to 0.55, statistically significant in 2 studies (Figure 2). There was no heterogeneity for the military studies ($P = .627$ for Q statistic; $I^2 = 0\%$). The pooled VE using a fixed-effect model was 59% (95% CI, 43%–70%). After exclusion of the Cadham study, the pooled VE was 57% (95% CI, 37%–70%), and the trim-and-fill adjusted VE was 60% (95% CI, 46%–70%).

Effect of mixed bacterial vaccines containing pneumococci on case fatality rates.   Four of 6 civilian studies showed a significant protective effect of the bacterial vaccines for reducing influenza case fatality rates, but the best-quality study, by McCoy et al, did not suggest any vaccine effect [20] (Figure 3). There was significant heterogeneity ($P < .001$ for Q statistic; $I^2 = 81.47\%$). The random-effects pooled RR among civilian studies was 0.58 (95% CI, 0.41–0.82), for a VE of 42% (95% CI, 18%–59%). After exclusion of the Cherry study [16], which had the strongest influence on meta-analysis results, no het-

erogeneity was indicated, and the fixed-effects VE estimate was 34% (95% CI, 27%–41%). The funnel plot did not suggest publication bias.

RR estimates from 3 military studies ranged from 0.19 to 0.45, all statistically significant (Figure 3). There was no heterogeneity for the military studies ($P = .360$ for Q statistic; $I^2 = 2.25\%$). The fixed-effects estimate of VE was 70% (95% CI, 50%–82%). After exclusion of the Leishman study, the combined efficacy was 65% (95% CI, 41%–79%). The trim-and-fill efficacy, adjusted for potential publication bias, was 62% (95% CI, 37%–77%).

Effect of bacterial vaccines without pneumococci.   Four civilian studies used bacterial vaccines containing pure *B. influenzae* (Table 4). The study by Hinton and Kane, with random allocation of vaccination, did not find a vaccine effect for the reduction of case fatality [25], and neither did 2 of the other studies [24, 28]. However, the remaining study, by Duval and

Chien et al JID 2010:202 (1 December) 1639-1648

Table 3. Incidence of Influenza among Vaccinated and Unvaccinated Subjects, with Estimated Risk Ratio (RR)

Study	Population type	Subjects, no. (%)		RR (95% CI)[a]	P
		Vaccinated	Unvaccinated		
Hinton and Kane [25]	Civilian	163/461 (35.4)	178/518 (34.4)	1.03 (0.87–1.22)	.788
McCoy et al [20]	Civilian	119/390 (30.5)	103/390 (26.4)	1.16 (0.92–1.44)	.233
Wadsworth [28]	Civilian	12/44 (27.3)	27/102 (26.5)	1.03 (0.58–1.84)	>.999
Barnes [24]	Civilian	25/152 (16.4)	23/113 (20.4)	0.81 (0.48–1.35)	.425
Cadham [15]	Military	282/4842 (5.8)	238/2758 (8.6)	0.67 (0.57–0.80)	<.001
Cadham [15]	Civilian	5203/52,999 (9.8)	21,285/85,941 (24.8)	0.40 (0.39–0.41)	<.001
Minaker and Irvine [21]	Civilian	111/6400 (1.7)	43,671/1,233,782 (3.5)	0.49 (0.41–0.59)	<.001
Erye and Lowe [18]	Military	25/1817 (1.4)	18/492 (3.7)	0.38 (0.21–0.68)	.002
Rosenow and Sturdivant [22]	Civilian	13,666/143,760 (9.5)	97,258/345,133 (28.2)	0.34 (0.33–0.34)	<.001
Leishman [19]	Military	221/15,624 (1.4)	2059/43,520 (4.7)	0.30 (0.26–0.34)	<.001
Ely et al [29]	Military	144/4212 (3.4)	1409/8486 (16.6)	0.21 (0.17–0.24)	<.001
Watters [23]	Civilian	89/1638 (5.4)	471/1599 (29.5)	0.18 (0.15–0.23)	<.001
Duval and Harris [27]	Civilian	27/981 (2.8)	130/338 (38.5)	0.07 (0.05–10.6)	<.001

[a] CI, confidence interval.

Harris, suggested that the VE for reducing the attack rate of pneumonia was 94% ($P < .001$) [27]. Hemolytic streptococci were the main cause of influenza-associated pneumonia in the study by Ely et al, who reported use of a vaccine containing only this pathogen [29]; none of the 144 vaccinated patients with influenza died, and the estimated RR was 0.05 ($P < .001$), corresponding to a VE of 95% (95% CI, 19%–100%).

DISCUSSION

Strengths and limitations. The quality of vaccine studies in 1918–1919 was lower than that of studies conducted today, because accepted modern approaches to study design and evaluation were unknown or not well recognized in 1918. In addition, owing to the scope of the 1918 pandemic and the exigency of war, medical personnel were forced to work under a great strain, so it was difficult to obtain complete data and perform good trials at that time [15].

Misclassification of influenza or pneumonia may have occurred in the vaccine studies we examined, because diagnosis was based largely on physical examination findings and unstandardized diagnostic criteria. Vaccinated persons suffering from constitutional adverse reactions to the vaccine might be misclassified as having influenza, although these reactions usually appeared early and were of short duration [27]. Influenza cases diagnosed late in the pandemic may have reflected respiratory illness from less virulent viral infections after influenza activity decreased, potentially introducing differential misclassification, because vaccinated persons were usually from this phase of the pandemic. Chest radiographs were available at the time, but we do not know how much they were used in these studies to diagnose pneumonia. Because death is an outcome less susceptible to misclassification, analysis of case fatality should be less

susceptible to bias. Except for 2 studies using random allocation, other studies failed to control for important confounders. Because of population homogeneity, better standardized diagnosis, and case identification, military studies should provide more valid estimates than civilian studies by controlling for factors that can influence pneumonia attack rates and case fatality rates, such as age, health status, and environmental exposure, as well as by reducing misclassification.

Subject self-selection was another potential problem in the 1918 vaccine studies, because vaccination was usually given voluntarily. However, the direction of potential "volunteer bias" is difficult to determine and might differ among studies. One vaccine study conducted shortly after the pandemic found that high-risk individuals were more likely to be vaccinated [31], which would have resulted in bias toward the null. On the other hand, "healthy vaccinee bias" is well described in observational influenza vaccine studies today and could have played a role in the 1918 studies [32]. It is unlikely that vaccination self-selection based on health status occurred in military populations, because the military population is fairly homogeneous and selected for excellent health.

Finally, although we sought to identify all existing articles, there may be studies that we did not find. However, we believe that missing reports would not have biased our results in a specific direction, because most contemporaneous vaccine studies did not use patients with influenza as the denominators in their analyses, as we did. Although we searched only reports published until the end of 1920, we believe that the time window we selected would have covered vaccine trials pertinent to the pandemic years, because clinical studies were published much more quickly than happens now. The latest study included in our analysis was published in February 1920 [19].

Chien et al JID 2010:202 (1 December) 1639-1648

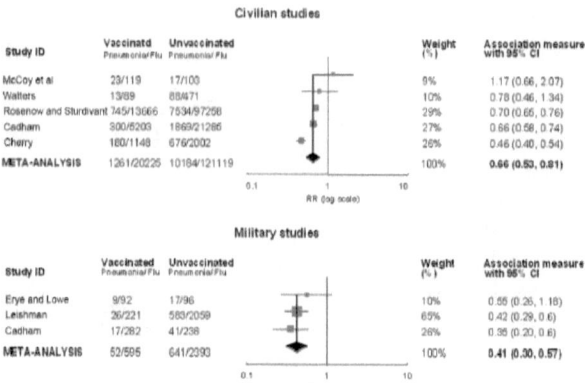

Figure 2. Random-effects meta-analysis of 8 risk ratio (RR) estimates comparing attack rates of pneumonia among vaccinated and unvaccinated patients with influenza in studies of bacterial vaccines containing pneumococci, stratified by study population (civilian or military). RRs of <1 indicated that the vaccine was protective. Point estimates and 95% confidence intervals (CIs) are shown for each study and for pooled results. Data are plotted on a log base 10 scale.

Despite these limitations, we believe that our method of analysis could remove biases caused by unequal observation periods and that the subgroup analysis of military studies may be less susceptible to other sources of bias. The estimated VE of bacterial vaccines containing pneumococci for preventing case fatalities in the military studies (70%) may be the most accurate figure in our analyses, because of less confounding, misclassification, and self-selection.

We hesitate to interpret findings in civilian studies, because residual biases could still be large in some civilian studies even with our method of analysis. Studies of *B. influenzae* provide a chance to examine this possibility, because that organism was not an important cause of secondary pneumonia in 1918 [4, 5]. Our analyses seemed to completely remove biases in the Barnes study [24]; using our method, we found no protective effect of *B. influenzae* vaccines, whereas the original analysis showed a significant protective effect. However, in our analysis of the study by Duval and Harris [27], the VE of this vaccine in preventing pneumonia was still estimated to be high. This study found a very high attack rate of pneumonia among unvaccinated patients with influenza (32%), suggesting that these patients were a very special population in this study and probably not a fair comparison group. This also reminds us of the limitations of observational vaccine studies; we need to be cautious in interpreting these results, because biases may not be completely removed, even with good statistical analyses.

Biologic plausibility. It has been suggested that most of the US Army training camps in ~1918 experienced "colonization epidemics" with specific pathogenic bacteria, either pneumococci or hemolytic streptococci, resulting in a huge number of pneumonia cases caused by these 2 bacteria during epidemics of measles (winter 1917–1918) and influenza (fall 1918 and winter 1918–1919) [3, 33]. The effect of locally produced bacterial vaccines thus depended on the bacteria circulating locally. It is very likely that ≥70% of military deaths were caused by secondary pneumonia, because soldiers were healthy adults unlikely to die because of deterioration of underlying medical conditions caused by influenza. In addition, 1 military study published in 1989 found a pneumococcal carriage rate of 1% among healthy men entering military service, compared with 13% among healthy recruits already in service [34], suggesting higher colonization prevalence and higher transmission of the pneumococcus in barracks.

Such a high VE might be less plausible if these whole-cell vaccines provided only type-specific protection, owing to the diversity of serotype distribution of pneumococci in 1918 [4]. Some of these vaccines included multiple pneumococcal strains known to be causing local epidemics and commonly isolated from pneumonia or fatal cases, but no systematic attempt could be made to identify and include strains beyond serotypes I–III, because the serologic tools to identify these strains were in their infancy. Findings of recent animal studies also support the possibility that whole-cell pneumococcal vaccines induce cross-protective (ie, broader than serotype-specific) immunity [35, 36]. Despite the likely diversity of hemolytic streptococcal strains in the 1918 pandemic, 1 small military study used a

Chien et al JID 2010:202 (1 December) 1639-1648

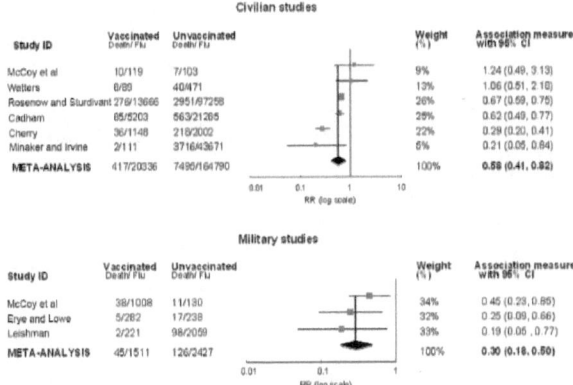

Figure 3. Random-effects meta-analysis of 9 risk ratio (RR) estimates comparing case fatality rates among vaccinated and unvaccinated patients with influenza in studies of bacterial vaccines containing pneumococci, stratified by study population (civilian or military). RRs of <1 indicated that the vaccine was protective. Point estimates and 95% confidence intervals (CIs) are shown for each study and for pooled results. Data are plotted on a log base 10 scale.

hemolytic streptococcal vaccine alone; if that vaccine used the dominant strain of group A streptococcus causing disease in the camp at that time, a high level of efficacy may be biologically plausible. Epidemics caused by a single M-type group A streptococcus have been shown in later military studies [37, 38]. Although it is important to consider the possibility of unappreciated biases, and the best-quality study (by McCoy et al [20]) with a small sample size suggested no vaccine effect, the data are generally consistent with a protective effect for the 2 types of bacterial vaccines designed to prevent infection with what are now accepted as the major causes of pneumonia and death in the 1918–1919 pandemic: pneumococci and hemolytic streptococci [4, 5].

Implications. This review supports the idea that although secondarily infecting bacteria played a major role in influenza-

associated pneumonia and mortality in the 1918 pandemic, bacterial vaccines containing pneumococci could potentially reduce influenza-associated pneumonias and deaths in modern pandemics. Few contemporary studies have evaluated bacterial vaccinations in seasonal or pandemic influenza. In a double-blind randomized trial, a 9-valent pneumococcal conjugate vaccine given to young infants had a 45% efficacy in reducing seasonal influenza-associated pneumonia [39].

Even with the current availability of antibiotics, findings of autopsy studies using modern molecular techniques from the 2009–2010 H1N1 pandemic suggest that bacterial infections, particularly pneumococcal infections, were implicated in 29%–55% of deaths [40–42]. The current H1N1 pandemic has led to a shift in the age distributions for hospitalization, severe pneumonia, and death, from the expected elderly age groups to older children

Table 4. Attack Rates of Pneumonia and Case Fatality Rates among Vaccinated and Unvaccinated Patients with Influenza and Corresponding Risk Ratios (RRs) in Studies Using Vaccines Not Containing Pneumococci

Study	Population	Formula	Outcome	Patients, no.		RR (95% CI)[a]	P
				Vaccinated	Unvaccinated		
Duval and Harris [27]	Civilian	*Bacillus influenzae*	Pneumonia	0/27	41/130	0.06	<.001
Hinton and Kane [25]	Civilian	*B. influenzae*	Death	28/163	24/178	1.27 (0.77–2.11)	.368
Barnes [24]	Civilian	*B. influenzae*	Death	4/25	9/57	1.01 (0.34–3.98)	>.999
Wadsworth [28]	Civilian	*B. influenzae*	Death	1/12	0/27	4.6 (0.16–165)	>.999
Ely et al [29]	Military	Hemolytic streptococci	Death	0/144	96/1409	0.05 (0.003–0.81)	<.001

[a] CI, confidence interval.

Chien et al JID 2010:202 (1 December) 1639-1648

and young adults, who have been at low risk of influenza-associated complications in most other influenza pandemics and in seasonal influenza, [43, 44]. A recent study of this age group showed that the presence of pneumococcus was strongly correlated with severe disease and death (odds ratio, 126) [45], consistent with the possibility that unexplained deaths in otherwise healthy young people in 1918 could also have been due to dual infections with influenza and pneumococci.

It is a challenge to review these old vaccine studies, but we believe our method of analysis and the examination of bias have made these early data more interpretable. Although these analyses cannot provide conclusive evidence of the efficacy of whole-cell pneumococcal and group A streptococcal vaccines in preventing bacterial superinfections in patients with influenza, we believe they do support further investigation of killed bacterial vaccines in the prevention of pneumococcal pneumonia, influenza-associated pneumonia, and mortality. The 1918 VE data presented here suggest to us the possibility that cheap whole-cell pneumococcal vaccines eliciting cross-protection against multiple pneumococcal serotypes may be worthy of reconsideration.

References

1. Johnson NP, Mueller J. Updating the accounts: global mortality of the 1918–1920 "Spanish" influenza pandemic. Bull Hist Med 2002; 76:105–115.
2. Brundage JF, Shanks GD. Deaths from bacterial pneumonia during 1918–19 influenza pandemic. Emerg Infect Dis 2008; 14:1193–1199.
3. Morens DM, Taubenberger JK, Fauci AS. Predominant role of bacterial pneumonia as a cause of death in pandemic influenza: implications for pandemic influenza preparedness. J Infect Dis 2008; 198:962–970.
4. Klugman KP, Chien YW, Madhi SA. Pneumococcal pneumonia and influenza: a deadly combination. Vaccine 2009; 27(suppl 3):C9–C14.
5. Chien YW, Klugman KP, Morens DM. Bacterial pathogens and death during the 1918 influenza pandemic. N Engl J Med 2009; 361:2582–2583.
6. Eyler JM. The fog of research: influenza vaccine trials during the 1918–19 pandemic. J Hist Med Allied Sci 2009; 64:401–428.
7. McCoy GW. Status of prophylactic vaccination against influenza. JAMA 1919; 73:401–404.
8. Brundage JF. Interactions between influenza and bacterial respiratory pathogens: implications for pandemic preparedness. Lancet Infect Dis 2006; 6:303–312.
9. Elyer JM. The state of science, microbiology, and vaccines circa 1918. Public Health Rep 2010; 125(suppl 3):27–35.
10. Centers for Disease Control and Prevention. 2009–2010 influenza season: week 14 ending April 10, 2010. FluView: a weekly influenza surveillance report prepared by the Influenza Division. Atlanta, GA: Centers for Disease Control and Prevention, 2010.
11. Higgins JPT, Green S, eds. Cochrane handbook for systematic reviews of interventions. Version 5.0.2. http://www.cochrane-handbook.org. Updated September 2009. Accessed 20 March 2010.
12. Duval S. The trim and fill method. In: Rothstein HR, Sutton AJ, Borenstein M, eds. Publication bias in meta-analysis: prevention, assessment and adjustments, West Sussex, United Kingdom: John Wiley & Sons, 2005:128–144.
13. Bax L, Yu LM, Ikeda N, Tsuruta H, Moons KG. Development and validation of MIX: comprehensive free software for meta-analysis of causal research data. BMC Med Res Methodol 2006; 6:50.
14. Bax L, Yu LM, Ikeda N, Tsuruta H, Moons KGM. MIX: comprehensive free software for meta-analysis of causal research data. Version 1.7. http://mix-for-meta-analysis.info. Accessed 20 March 2010.
15. Cadham FT. The use of a vaccine in the recent epidemic of influenza. Lancet 1919; 193:885–886.
16. Cherry TM. The value of inoculation: a statistical inquiry. In: Cumpston JHL, ed. Influenza and maritime quarantine in Australia. Vol 18. Melbourne, Australia: Australian Quarantine Service, 1919:89–113.
17. Penfold WJ. Influenza vaccine and inoculation. In: Cumpston JHL, ed. Influenza and maritime quarantine in Australia. Vol 18. Melbourne, Australia: Australian Quarantine Service, 1919:73–88.
18. Erye J, Lowe C. Autumn influenza epidemic (1918) as it affected the N.Z.E.F. in the United Kingdom. Lancet 1919; 193:553–560.
19. Leishman WB. The results of protective inoculation against influenza in the army at home, 1918–19. Lancet 1920; 195:366–368.
20. McCoy GW, Murray VB, Teeter AL. The failure of a bacterial vaccine as a prophylactic against influenza. JAMA 1918; 71:1997.
21. Minaker AJ, Irvine RS. Prophylactic use of mixed vaccine against pandemic influenza and its complications. JAMA 1919; 72:847–850.
22. Rosenow EC, Sturdivant BF. Studies in influenza and pneumonia. IV. Further results of prophylactic inoculations. JAMA 1919; 73:396–401.
23. Watters WH. Vaccines in influenza. Boston Med Surg J 1919; 181:727–731.
24. Barnes HL. The prophylactic value of Leary's vaccine. JAMA 1918; 71:1899.
25. Hinton WA, Kane ES. Use of influenza vaccine as a prophylactic: an experimental study conducted by the Massachusetts State Department of Health. J Tennessee State Med Assn 1918; 11:442–446.
26. Leary T. The use of influenza vaccine in the present epidemic. Am J Public Health 1918; 8:754–755.
27. Duval CW, Harris WH. The antigenic property of the Pfeiffer bacillus as related to its value in the prophylaxis of epidemic influenza. J Immunol 1919; 4:317–330.
28. Wadsworth AB. The results of preventive vaccination with suspensions of the influenza bacillus. Public Health J 1919; 10:309–314.
29. Ely CF, Lloyd BJ, Hitchcock CD, Nickson DH. Influenza as seen at the Puget Sound Navy Yard. JAMA 1919; 72:24–28.
30. Frost WH. The epidemiology of influenza. JAMA 1919; 73:313–318.
31. Jordan EO. Influenza studies. IV. Effect of vaccination against influenza and some other respiratory infections. J Infect Dis 1921; 28:357–366.
32. Jackson LA, Nelson JC, Benson P, et al. Functional status is a confounder of the association of influenza vaccine and risk of all cause mortality in seniors. Int J Epidemiol 2006; 35:345–352.
33. MacCallum WG. Pathological studies in the recent epidemics of pneumonia. Trans South Surg Assoc 1919; 31:180–192.
34. Jousimies-Somer HR, Savolainen S, Ylikoski JS. Comparison of the nasal bacterial floras in two groups of healthy subjects and in patients with acute maxillary sinusitis. J Clin Microbiol 1989; 27:2736–2743.
35. Malley R, Lipsitch M, Stack A, et al. Intranasal immunization with killed unencapsulated whole cells prevents colonization and invasive disease by capsulated pneumococci. Infect Immun 2001; 69:4870–4873.
36. Malley R, Morse SC, Leite LC, et al. Multiserotype protection of mice against pneumococcal colonization of the nasopharynx and middle ear by killed nonencapsulated cells given intranasally with a nontoxic adjuvant. Infect Immun 2004; 72:4290–4292.
37. Centers for Disease Control and Prevention. Outbreak of group A streptococcal pneumonia among Marine Corps Recruits; California, November 1–December 20, 2002. JAMA 2003; 289:1373–1375.
38. Brundage JF, Gunzenhauser JD, Longfield JN, et al. Epidemiology and control of acute respiratory diseases with emphasis on group A beta-hemolytic streptococcus: a decade of U.S. Army experience. Pediatrics 1996; 97:964–970.
39. Madhi SA, Klugman KP. A role for *Streptococcus pneumoniae* in virus-associated pneumonia. Nat Med 2004; 10:811–813.
40. Centers for Disease Control and Prevention (CDC). Bacterial coinfec-

Chien et al JID 2010:202 (1 December) 1639-1648

tions in lung tissue specimens from fatal cases of 2009 pandemic influenza A (H1N1): United States, May-August 2009. MMWR Morb Mortal Wkly Rep 2009; 58:1071–1074.

41. Mauad T, Hajjar LA, Callegari GD, et al. Lung pathology in fatal novel human influenza A (H1N1) infection. Am J Respir Crit Care Med 2009; 181:72–79.

42. Gill JR, Sheng ZM, Ely SF, et al. Pulmonary pathologic findings of fatal 2009 pandemic influenza A/H1N1 viral infections. Arch Pathol Lab Med 2010; 134:235–243.

43. Chowell G, Bertozzi SM, Colchero MA, et al. Severe respiratory disease concurrent with the circulation of H1N1 influenza. N Engl J Med 2009; 361:674–679.

44. Louie JK, Acosta M, Winter K, et al. Factors associated with death or hospitalization due to pandemic 2009 influenza A(H1N1) infection in California. JAMA 2009; 302:1896–902.

45. Palacios G, Hornig M, Cisterna D, et al. *Streptococcus pneumoniae* coinfection is correlated with the severity of H1N1 pandemic influenza. PLoS ONE 2009; 4:e8540.

Eyler- 2009 Oct. - J Hist Med Allied Sci 64 - 401-428

The Fog of Research: Influenza Vaccine Trials during the 1918—19 Pandemic

JOHN M. EYLER*

ABSTRACT. Bacterial vaccines of various sorts were widely used for both preventive and therapeutic purposes during the great influenza pandemic of 1918—19. Some were derived exclusively from the Pfeiffer's bacillus, the presumed cause of influenza, while others contained one or more other organisms found in the lungs of victims. Although initially most reports of the use of these vaccines claimed that they prevented influenza or pneumonia, the results were inconsistent and sometimes contradictory. During the course of the debates over the efficacy of these vaccines, it became clear that the medical profession had no consensus on what constituted a proper vaccine trial. Even among those who asserted that clinical impression was not enough, there was no agreement on how a trial ought to be conducted. The American Public Health Association, through its Working Program on Influenza, sought to establish standards for the profession. The standards the APHA set in December 1918 guided American vaccine trials for a quarter century. **KEYWORDS:** influenza vaccines, vaccine trials, clinical trials, American Public Health Association, William Park, George McCoy.

IN mid-October 1918, New York City's Health Department was facing a crisis. Reported cases of influenza had risen to between four and five thousand a day. Many more cases undoubtedly went unreported. In those same weeks, the daily death toll from influenza and pneumonia hovered around six

* Professor Emeritus, University of Minnesota, 4609 Gustafson Drive, Gig Harbor, Washington 98335. Email: eyler001@umn.edu.

A version of this paper was delivered to the Beaumont History Club, Yale University, 15 February 2008. Research funding was provided by a 40th Anniversary Award in the History of Medicine or Science from the Burroughs-Wellcome Fund.

JOURNAL OF THE HISTORY OF MEDICINE AND ALLIED SCIENCES, Volume 64, Number 4
Advance Access publication on June 12, 2009   doi: 10.1093/jhmas/jrp013

Eyler- 2009 Oct. - J Hist Med Allied Sci 64 - 401-428
402   *Journal of the History of Medicine*   :   *Vol. 64, October 2009*

hundred.[1] The city's Health Commissioner, Dr. Royal S. Copeland, met regularly with reporters to issue public reassurances. As early as 2 October, he announced a new basis for hope. The Director of the Health Department's laboratories, William H. Park, was preparing a vaccine which would offer protection from this dread disease.[2] Copeland did not give details, but Park provided his colleagues in the medical profession a brief account of his work in the lead article of the 12 October issue of the *New York Medical Journal*.[3] In this article, Park explained his reasoning for developing and releasing this vaccine. The severity of the epidemic suggested one or two possibilities. Either a new and more virulent strain of the Pfeiffer's bacillus, *Haemophilis influenzae*, the presumed cause of influenza, was circulating, or an unknown agent, perhaps a filterable virus, caused the initial infection which was quickly followed by the invasion of streptococci and pneumococci.

Park argued that usually only one agent was responsible for an epidemic. Up to this point in the outbreak, he, like most of his colleagues, had been able to isolate the Pfeiffer's bacillus regularly from unambiguous cases of influenza. Acting on the assumption that this organism was the cause of the outbreak, his laboratory had cultivated the current strain of the Pfeiffer's bacillus and had shown that laboratory animals injected with this organism developed antibodies against it. He prepared a heat-killed vaccine from his cultures which he administered in three, increasingly large doses at two-day intervals. Tests on laboratory workers showed that reactions were mild. With research and testing no more extensive than this, the Health Department began to release the vaccine for use in army camps and among the workers of large companies, including the 14,000 employees of the Consolidated Gas Company and 275,000 employees of U.S. Steel Company.[4] It also made the vaccine available to private physicians who promised to report on the number of persons they vaccinated and their subsequent history of influenza. In spite of the speedy release, Park was cautious.

1. Anon., "Grip in the Y. M. C. A. Checked by Vaccine," *New York Times*, 17 October 1918, 9; Anon., "Vaccine Cuts Army Influenza Deaths," *New York Times*, 18 October 1918, 24.

2. Anon., "Tells of Vaccine to Stop Influenza," *New York Times*, 2 October 1918, 10.

3. William H. Park, "Bacteriology and Possibility of Antiinfluenza Vaccine as a Prophylactic," *N. Y. Med. J.*, 1918, *108*, 621.

4. Anon., "Big Firms Take Up Fight on Influenza," *New York Times*, 23 October 1918, 8; Anon., "Copeland Sees Grip on the Wane Here," *New York Times*, 25 October 1918, 22.

Eyler- 2009 Oct. - J Hist Med Allied Sci 64 - 401-428

"We should, therefore, in a very few weeks have on hand sufficient information to form some decision as to the protection afforded by the vaccine."[5] He evidently believed that clinical experience in the midst of a severe epidemic would provide that evidence.

Park's vaccine was an early example of the many vaccines used to prevent influenza and influenzal pneumonia during the 1918–19 pandemic in the United States. All were bacterial vaccines composed of a variety of organisms isolated from patients living or dead. Their composition reflected both the changing assessment of influenza's etiology and the phase of the pandemic in which they were developed. This article traces the use of these vaccines, the claims made for them, and the controversy surrounding those claims during and immediately after the pandemic. The use of these vaccines reflects both the changing assessments of influenza's cause and the rudimentary notion of a vaccine trial in these years. As we will see, in 1918, the American medical profession had no consensus on what constituted a valid vaccine trial. The controversy over these influenza vaccines forced it to develop one. Two public health bacteriologists, William Park and George McCoy, working through the American Public Health Association, helped forge the first professional standards.

The October 1918 issue of the *American Journal of Public Health* carried an article by the Professor of Pathology and Bacteriology at Tufts Medical School, Timothy Leary.[6] Leary described the production of his vaccine in much greater detail than Park. He used three strains of the Pfeiffer's bacillus: the Carney, Navy, and Devens, which he had recently isolated in local hospitals. His vaccine was heat-killed and chemically treated and produced under conditions intended to ensure consistency and sterility. Leary recommended his vaccine for both preventive and, in larger doses, therapeutic purposes, and he was optimistic, quite sure in fact, that his vaccine was effective. While the vaccine, he explained, could not be expected to produce protection as complete as the typhoid vaccine, "the percentage of complete protection appears to be high, and there is marked amelioration of symptoms in those who do come down, and pneumonias appear in very few cases."[7]

---

5. Park, "Bacteriology," 621.
6. Timothy Leary, "The Use of Influenza Vaccine in the Present Epidemic," *Am. J. Pub. Health*, 1918, 8, 754–55, 768.
7. Ibid., 755.

Eyler- 2009 Oct. - J Hist Med Allied Sci 64 - 401-428
404   *Journal of the History of Medicine   :   Vol. 64, October 2009*

Park and Leary produced the most widely used Pfeiffer's bacillus vaccines against the flu in 1918, but there were other vaccines and other producers, most of whom were less cautious than these two. The vaccine the Health Department of Pittsburgh released to the public was prepared by a committee from the University of Pittsburgh Medical School. The researchers isolated thirteen strains of the Pfeiffer's bacillus, prepared a vaccine by modifying the technique Park had used, tested the vaccine for toxicity in a few laboratory animals and in two humans, and turned the vaccine over to the Red Cross for distribution to the people of Pittsburgh. All this took place within one week.[8]

Private physicians also produced and distributed Pfeiffer's bacillus vaccines. Horace Greeley, a private practitioner in Brooklyn, N. Y., reported isolating the Pfeiffer's bacillus from seventeen patients, and from these seventeen "strains," he produced a heat-killed vaccine intended to be given in three increasing doses.[9] He distributed eight liters of his vaccine to his colleagues, who administered it to their patients. His vaccine was also used in the Angel Guardian Home in Brooklyn and among the workers of the Wharton Steel Company in Wharton, N. J.

Other vaccines were also in use during the great pandemic. These were most often mixed vaccines made up of organisms, known and newly discovered, that had been isolated in wards and death houses during the outbreak. Such vaccines were used more often later in the epidemic when confidence in the causal role of the Pfeiffer's bacillus waned. Such vaccines were usually defended as measures to prevent the bacterial pneumonias that so often kill influenza's victims. The vaccine produced by the Naval medical officers in San Francisco and used in the Bay Area and Los Angeles contained, besides the Pfeiffer's bacillus, types I, II, and III pneumococci and streptococci.[10] Other vaccine producers added

8. Samuel R. Haythorn, "The Prevention of Epidemic Influenza with Special Reference to Vaccine Prophylaxis," in *Studies on Epidemic Influenza Comprising Clinical and Laboratory Investigations* (Pittsburgh: University of Pittsburgh School of Medicine, 1919), 109–11.

9. Horace Greeley, "Vaccine as a Prophylactic against Influenza, and Local Reaction as a Guide to Immunity," *Med. Rec.*, 1919, *96*, 624–27.

10. A. J. Minaker and Robert S. Irvine, "Prophylactic Use of Mixed Vaccine against Pandemic Influenza and Its Complications at the Naval Training Station, San Francisco," *J. Am. Med. Assoc.*, 1919, *72*, 848.

Eyler- 2009 Oct. - J Hist Med Allied Sci 64 - 401-428

staphylococci and several other organisms to concoct witches' brews of injectable fluids.[11] In some cases, the Pfeiffer's bacillus was omitted altogether. Warren B. Stone, County Bacteriologist from Schenectady, N. Y., and President of the New York Association of Public Health Laboratories, isolated bacteria from patients' sputum and produced a vaccine containing pneumococci, streptococci, and staphylococci but no Pfeiffer's bacillus.[12] A few vaccines contained only streptococci. Maurice Katzman, a Denver physician, produced a heat-killed streptococcus vaccine which he used at City and County Hospital and distributed to his colleagues in the community.[13] Likewise, the vaccine produced by the Naval medical officers at the Puget Sound Navy Yard and used among the recruits contained only phenol-killed streptococci, because streptococci were the only organisms these investigators could isolate from influenza patients during the outbreak.[14]

The best known and most widely used mixed vaccines were those of Edward C. Rosenow of the Division of Experimental Bacteriology of the Mayo Foundation in Rochester, Minn. Rosenow's avowed target was secondary infections, since he acknowledged that the cause of influenza was in dispute. He reasoned that the composition of a vaccine designed to prevent pneumonia following influenza must match the mixture of organisms found locally in patients. Since that mixture might change during the course of an epidemic, the composition of an effective vaccine must be adjusted frequently to reflect the changing mix of bacterial strains then in circulation. His initial vaccine contained 30 percent pneumococci types I, II, and III in specified proportions; 30 percent pneumococci type IV and an organism he frequently isolated which he called a "green-producing diplostreptococcus"; 20 percent hemolytic streptococci; 10 percent staphylococcus aureus; and 10 percent of the influenza or Pfeiffer's bacillus.

---

11. W. H. Watters, "Vaccines in Influenza," *Boston Med. Surg. J.*, 1919, *181*, 727–28; Warren B. Stone, "A Prophylactic Vaccine against the So-Called Spanish Influenza," *Med. Rec.*, 1918, *94*, 979–80; John H. Kolmer, "The Value of Active Immunization with Vaccine Virus against Influenza," *Med. Rec.*, 1918, *94*, 919.

12. Stone, "Prophylactic Vaccine," 979–80.

13. Maurice Katzman, "Influenza Vaccination at the Denver City and County Hospital," *Colorado Med.*, 1919, *16*, 121–22.

14. C. F. Ely, B. J. Lloyd, C. D. Hitchcock, and D. H. Nickson, "Influenza as Seen at the Puget Sound Navy Yard," *J. Am. Med. Assoc.*, 1919, *72*, 24–25, 27.

Eyler- 2009 Oct. - J Hist Med Allied Sci 64 - 401-428
406   *Journal of the History of Medicine   :   Vol. 64, October 2009*

He eliminated the Pfeiffer's bacillus in later batches and increased the proportion of pneumococci type IV and his diplostreptococcus.

Rosenow developed his vaccine during the early phases of the outbreak in Minnesota and administered it to doctors and nurses in his own institution, and, when he was convinced that it was safe and effective, the Mayo Foundation distributed it to physicians throughout the upper mid-west.[15] Physicians were asked to return a questionnaire reporting the results of the vaccination. The number of people who received the vaccine distributed by the Mayo Foundation is unknown, but Rosenow received questionnaires reporting the results for 93,000 patients who had been vaccinated three times, 23,000 who had received two injections, and nearly 27,000 who received only one dose of the vaccine.[16] Rosenow's vaccine was used even more widely when the Chicago Health Department decided to adopt it. The director of the department's laboratories, F. O. Tonney, produced 500,000 doses of Rosenow's vaccine, some of which the department distributed to physicians in the city. The rest was turned over to the state health department for distribution throughout Illinois.[17]

The vaccines promoted during the pandemic were not always new, nor were their contents always disclosed. For several years, American drug companies had been producing proprietary flu, grippe, and cold vaccines which, when analyzed, proved to contain an assortment of common organisms. As influenza illnesses and deaths mounted and public anxiety grew, drug companies actively promoted these stock vaccines to both prevent and cure flu, and, as demand swelled, there were complaints of price gouging and kick-backs by detail men.[18] Proprietary hucksterism was not limited to the drug industry. Dr. M. J. Exner issued two glowing reports, testi-monials really, to the *New York Times* on his use of a vaccine against

15. E. C. Rosenow, "Prophylactic Inoculation against Respiratory Infections during the Present Pandemic of Influenza. Preliminary Report," *J. Am. Med. Assoc.*, 1919, 72, 31–33; E. C. Rosenow and B. F. Sturdivant, "Studies in Influenza and Pneumonia. IV. Further Results of Prophylactic Inoculations," *J. Am. Med. Assoc.*, 1919, 73, 396–98.

16. Rosenow and Sturdivant, "Further Results," 398.

17. "Report of an Epidemic of Influenza in Chicago during the Fall of 1918," *Report and Handbook of the Department of Health of the City of Chicago, 1911–1918 Inclusive* (Chicago: Department of Health of the City of Chicago, 1919), 116–23.

18. For a contemporary summary, see Haythorn, "Prevention of Epidemic Influenza," 114–16.

Eyler- 2009 Oct. - J Hist Med Allied Sci 64 - 401-428
Eyler : *Influenza Vaccine Trials*   407

pneumonia, influenza, and blood poisoning that had been developed some six years earlier by Ellis Bonime of the Polyclinic Medical School and Hospital.[19] Bonime was a late adherent of the tuberculin treatment of tuberculosis, championing its use by general practitioners, and a partisan of the oposium theory of immune response and of the therapeutic use of vaccines.[20] The contents of his vaccine were not disclosed in these public announcements. As proof of the vaccine's effectiveness, Exner trumpeted its use in immunizing 430 Y. M. C. A. workers. None of the workers who received all three injections contracted influenza. Seven of those who received only one injection got sick. The only death was among those who had refused a second and third injection. The others who had received only one injection had mild, uncomplicated cases.[21] Exner told reporters that he was sure that if this vaccine had been used last year in army camps, pneumonia would not have claimed so many victims. It was a shame that some of his colleagues were wasting time experimenting with new vaccines when a "thoroughly successful vaccine was at hand."[22] Such boosterism carried conviction in some quarters. On 25 October 1918, *The New York Times* reported that the town of Far Rockaway had announced that it would offer Bonime's vaccine to all its 7000 citizens.[23]

In 1918, there were few public or professional constraints on the use of vaccines or on claims made on their behalf, but such hucksterism did prompt responses. In the spring of 1918, the American Medical Association's Council of Pharmacy and Chemistry had refused to list in its New and Nonofficial Remedies any of the stock mixed vaccines then being marketed for a variety of conditions, including influenza, citing lack of evidence of effectiveness.[24] At the end of October, during the peak of public anxiety about the epidemic, Surgeon General Rupert Blue issued a public warning that was repeated in the nation's major newspapers.

19. Anon., "903 New Cases of Grip Reported Yesterday—Use of Vaccine Not New," *New York Times*, 3 October 1918, 24; Anon., "Grip in the Y. M. C. A.," 9.
20. Ellis Bonime, *Tuberculin and Vaccine in Tubercular Affections: A Practical Guide for the Utilization of the Immune Response in General Practice* (Troy, N. Y.: Southworth Co., 1917).
21. Anon., "Grip in the Y. M. C. A.," 9.
22. Ibid.
23. Anon., "Copeland Sees Grip on the Wane."
24. Anon., "Several 'Mixed' Vaccines Not Admitted to N. N. R.: Report of the Council on Pharmacy and Chemistry," *J. Am. Med. Assoc.*, 1918, *70*, 1967–69.

Eyler- 2009 Oct. - J Hist Med Allied Sci 64 - 401-428
408   *Journal of the History of Medicine   :   Vol. 64, October 2009*

In view of the "exaggerated and in some respects misleading statements" about influenza vaccines that had been made in the press, Blue pointed out that no evidence had been put forward proving that these vaccines were effective, and their use should be considered merely experimental.[25] The *American Journal of Public Health* editorialized that, although it might be better to err on the side of using a useless vaccine rather than to risk preventable influenza deaths, the early experience with these vaccines was contradictory; therefore, the public should be warned that they were experimental, so that should these vaccines prove ineffective, public confidence in other vaccines would not be shaken.[26]

Proof of efficacy was thus deemed essential, but by the time the Surgeon General issued his warning, it was becoming very clear that the profession had no consensus on what constituted such proof or on how the value of a vaccine should be determined. A number of reports in the medical press relied solely on clinical judgment. Typical are Dr. M. J. Exner, who concluded that the Bonime vaccine was effective because none of the 450 Y. M. C. A. workers who received all three injections developed influenza, and Horace Greeley, who concluded that his vaccine was effective because there were no reported cases among those who received it.[27] W. H. Watters, the pathologist at the Massachusetts Homeopathic Hospital, placed heavy reliance on the reports of community physicians who used his vaccine. Most reported that as far as they knew, no patient they vaccinated developed influenza.[28] A similar logic sometimes applied on a much larger scale. The Illinois Influenza Commission circulated questionnaires to community physicians and public health officers asking for the respondent's judgment on whether the influenza vaccines used in that county prevented the disease or moderated its severity, and it published the results, admittedly with some acknowledgement that such returns lacked scientific rigor.[29] For Dr. Maurice Katzman of Denver, the

25. Anon., "Vaccines against Influenza," *Pub. Health Rep.*, 1918, *33*, 1866. See also Anon., "Beware of 'Sure Cures,'" *New York Times*, 27 October 1918, 14.
26. Anon., "Weapons against Influenza," *Am. J. Pub. Health*, 1918, *8*, 788.
27. Anon., "Grip in the Y. M. C. A."; Greeley, "Vaccine as a Prophylactic," 625.
28. Watters, "Vaccines," 730–31.
29. R. A. O'Neill, C. St. Clair Drake, and J. O. Cobb, "The Work of the Illinois Influenza Commission," *Am. J. Pub Health*, 1919, *9*, 24.

Eyler- 2009 Oct. - J Hist Med Allied Sci 64 - 401-428

Eyler   :   Influenza Vaccine Trials   409

way to "scrupulously avoid prejudices and testimonials" was to rely on patient self-reporting.[30] Katzman provided each of the 980 patients he injected with his streptococcus vaccine during the peak of the epidemic with a card to report on their subsequent course. He published the numbers of cases among those who completed the full course of injections and among those who did not, but he provided no information on cases among those who received no vaccine. On this basis, he concluded that his vaccine was safe and effective.[31]

We can leave such reports, common as they are in the medical literature during and immediately following the Great Influenza, and turn our attention to those researchers who insisted that clinical impression or patient testimony were not enough and that medical science demanded that a vaccine had to prove its worth in some sort of clinical trial. Consider, for example, the trial reported by Charles W. Duval and William H. Harris of the Tulane University Department of Pathology and Bacteriology.[32] Duval and Harris were well-trained medical scientists who described the production of their killed Pfeiffer's bacillus vaccine with care and thoroughness. Their trial consisted of administrating the vaccine to 3072 employees of cooperating businesses in New Orleans. They used as controls the 866 employees of these same firms who refused the vaccine, justifying their use as controls since the unvaccinated lived and worked under the same conditions as the vaccinated. The injections took place between October 18 and 23, when the epidemic was at its peak; in fact, some of these businesses were experiencing absentee rates of 30 percent or 40 percent at the time of the vaccinations. The proof of effectiveness Duval and Harris presented was a simple comparison of incidence rates: 1.7 percent of those who received three injections contracted influenza; 8 percent of those who received two injections were reported ill with influenza, while 24 percent of those who received only one injection developed the disease. No one who was vaccinated developed pneumonia. On the other hand, a full 41.6 percent of the unvaccinated

---

30. Katzman, "Influenza Vaccination," 122.
31. Ibid., 122–23.
32. Charles W. Duval and William H. Harris, "The Antigenic Property of the Pfeiffer Bacillus as Related to Its Value in the Prophylaxis of Epidemic Influenza," *J. Immunol.*, 1919, 4, 317–30.

Eyler- 2009 Oct. - J Hist Med Allied Sci 64 - 401-428

contracted flu. These researchers were convinced that although the numbers in their trial were small, their vaccine, properly administered, was highly effective. They conceded, however, that their vaccine did produce frequent constitutional reactions. In 30 percent of the vaccinated, these were deemed severe.[33]

More often, trials took place in residential institutions. Asylums, orphanages, and similar institutions offered researchers the obvious advantages of subjects under close observations and controlled conditions. Some of these reports were very brief, little more than notices. George L. Wallace, the Superintendent of the Wrentham State School in Massachusetts, reported to the *Boston Medical and Surgical Journal* on the use of Leary's vaccine in his institution.[34] During the epidemic, there were 740 cases of influenza in the institution. Eight days into the outbreak, after 122 cases had already developed in the institution, Wallace began vaccinating. He reported very favorable results, but he gave no indication of how the vaccinated and the controls were selected. In fact, he did not even calculate incidence rates. Of the seventy-one employees who were vaccinated, only five contracted influenza, while thirty-eight of the fifty-eight employees who were not vaccinated got sick. In a building housing 156 inmates, there was only one case among the twenty-eight vaccinated, but sixty-four cases appeared among the 128 unvaccinated. On that basis, Wallace concluded that Leary's vaccine protected against influenza.

The report of Warren B. Stone, the President of the New York State Association of Public Health Laboratories whose mixed vaccine we have already discussed, was similar to Wallace's.[35] Stone began administering his vaccine on 30 September, a full two weeks after the first cases appeared in the Ellis Hospital in Schenectady. He began with the hospital's medical staff. Over the next two weeks, none of the thirty-four nurses who were immunized developed flu, while eight of the thirty-two unvaccinated succumbed. Among physicians, only one of the thirty-five vaccinated developed flu, and that was a light case, but eight of the forty-four

---

33. Duval and Harris, "Antigenic Property," 324.

34. George L. Wallace, "Report of the Influenza Epidemic and Experience in the Use of Influenza Vaccine 'B' at the Wrentham State School, Wrentham, Mass.," *Boston Med. Surg. J.,* 1919, *180,* 447–48.

35. Stone, "Prophylactic Vaccine," 979–80.

Eyler- 2009 Oct. - J Hist Med Allied Sci 64 - 401-428

Eyler   :   *Influenza Vaccine Trials*   411

unvaccinated contracted the disease. On 5 October, he released his vaccine to community physicians. They reported vaccinating 12,362 people, of whom 117 were reported as contracting influenza, half of those within twenty-four hours of being vaccinated. Stone considered his test to be "rigorous."[36]

Military installations provided another possible site for a vaccine trial, and medical officers at those installations on the West Coast had the advantage of a few weeks lead time in preparing for the epidemic. But researchers working in army and naval stations were often prevented from exercising much control over their trial by military procedures and wartime conditions. For example, in testing their streptococcus vaccine, the medical officers at the naval station on Puget Sound had seven units under observation, none of whom it could deliberately divide into experimental and control groups. It was possible to observe vaccinated and the unvaccinated men simultaneously in only two of these units.[37] Among the other five units, four were entirely vaccinated and one was entirely unvaccinated. Although the men lived in different arrangements in each of these units, the authors argued that conditions of exposure were nonetheless similar, so a direct comparison of vaccinated and unvaccinated in different units was justified. Before vaccination could begin, cases of influenza had already broken out in both of the divided units. In fact, one of those units had just arrived from Philadelphia, where the epidemic was raging, and it had many sick at the time of arrival. The authors compared rates of influenza and influenza deaths among the vaccinated and the unvaccinated, but the results were not at all consistent. In the Philadelphia unit, there were incidence rates of 28.2 percent among the vaccinated and 19.6 percent among the unvaccinated, while in the Seamen's Barracks, the other divided unit, the proportions were reversed with incidence of 2.03 percent among the vaccinated and 12.3 percent among the unvaccinated. The notes accompanying the table of results explain that most of the cases among the vaccinated occurred shortly after the first injection, suggesting to the authors that the epidemic was already on the wane before vaccination was completed. Nevertheless, they concluded that their vaccine

36. Ibid., 979.
37. Ely, Lloyd, and Hitchcock, "Influenza," 27–28.

Eyler- 2009 Oct. - J Hist Med Allied Sci 64 - 401-428
412   *Journal of the History of Medicine   :   Vol. 64, October 2009*

prevented many illnesses and mitigated the severity of the illnesses in other cases.[38]

The medical officers at the Naval Training Station in San Francisco also developed a vaccine. This one was a mixed vaccine containing the Pfeiffer's bacillus. Like their counterparts on Puget Sound, they were unable to divide naval units into vaccinated and unvaccinated groups. Instead, they used unvaccinated proxies as controls. The nurses and hospital attendants of San Francisco, all of whom were presumed unvaccinated, served as the control group for the 270 hospital corpsmen who were vaccinated and then detailed to influenza wards in San Francisco. Similarly, the civilian workers on Mare Island served as the control group for the marines on Mare Island who were vaccinated and then sent to Vallejo and San Francisco, while the entire population of Los Angeles served as a control for the 3100 men at the naval camp at San Pedro.[39] Were the use of these groups as controls not problematic enough, the researchers had to rely on published incidence rates for civilian populations, and circular letters and informal means to ascertain how many of the vaccinated sailors or marines developed flu. None of these difficulties kept the authors from concluding that their vaccine provided a "noteworthy degree of protection against influenza and its complications."[40]

Among the largest and most ambitious of these early vaccine trials was that of Edward Rosenow at the Mayo Clinic. Rosenow relied on several sources of data: clinical reports from community physicians, institutional records, and vital statistics from the State of Minnesota.[41] Since he insisted that an effective vaccine against pneumonia accompanying influenza be developed from freshly iso-lated organisms, his vaccine could not be used before the outbreak began. In fact, he saw no reason why a vaccine trial might not begin during an outbreak of the disease that vaccine was intended to prevent. "A procedure, calculated to protect against an epidemic disease, such as influenza," he insisted, "should have sufficient

---

38. Ibid., 28.
39. Minaker and Irvine, "Prophylactic Use," 849.
40. Ibid., 850.
41. Rosenow published two articles describing his vaccine and the results of the trial. See Rosenow, "Prophylactic Inoculation," 31–34; Rosenow and Sturdivant, "Further Results," 396–401.

Eyler- 2009 Oct. - J Hist Med Allied Sci 64 - 401-428
Eyler   :   Influenza Vaccine Trials   413

protective value when given after the onset of the epidemic to be measurable, for it is practically impossible to anticipate these epidemics and, moreover, persons will not present themselves for vaccination until the epidemic is at hand."[42] Once Rosenow was convinced that his vaccine raised antibody levels and produced minimal adverse reactions in the medical and nursing staff in Rochester who agreed to serve as test subjects, the Mayo Foundation distributed the vaccine gratis to physicians and hospitals who requested it and agreed to provide a record of results.

The returns, however, were disappointing. Although Rosenow knew that over 140,000 individuals had received his vaccine, he received reports from only 530 physicians which were complete enough to use in compiling his results.[43] To demonstrate the effectiveness of his vaccine, he compiled tables comparing morbidity rates for influenza, acute edema of the lungs, pneumonia, and empyema; and mortality rates for acute edema of the lungs, pneumonia, empyema and encephalitis for those receiving one, two, and three injections and for those who were unvaccinated. These tables included results for three separate geographical areas: for the whole area where his vaccine was used, which was primarily within two hundred miles of Rochester, for nineteen Minnesota counties excluding the Mayo clinic, and for Olmsted County also excluding the Mayo clinic. In all three of these tables, he used physicians' reports of the total size of their practice and the number of cases and deaths among those patients who were not vaccinated to calculate the risk of influenza without the vaccine. He also published tables for two sets of institutionalized patients who were said to be under closer observation.[44] One gave the rates for some 17,000 inmates of unidentified institutions, distinguishing those receiving three injections from the unvaccinated. The other gave incidence rates for influenza and pneumonia and deaths from pneumonia among those vaccinated one, two, or three times and among the unvaccinated in the hospitals of Rochester. In neither instance did Rosenow provide detail on how the vaccinations were conducted or the trial arranged.

42. Rosenow and Sturdivant, "Further Results," 398.
43. Ibid., 398–99.
44. Ibid., 400.

Eyler- 2009 Oct. - J Hist Med Allied Sci 64 - 401-428
414   Journal of the History of Medicine   :   Vol. 64, October 2009

Rosenow made only one attempt to determine the incidence rate for influenza in the general population. For the table of influenza in the nineteen Minnesota counties, he calculated two incidence rates for the unvaccinated. One was based, as we have seen, on physicians' reports; the other used the population of those nineteen counties and the influenza cases reported in those counties to the state board of health. The last rate was much lower than the rates calculated from the physicians' reports—65 versus 375 per thousand. It was also lower than the rate for influenza cases among those receiving one, two, or three doses of his vaccine. Rosenow discounted the rate computed on state health department records as seriously understated. Based on this evidence, Rosenow concluded that individuals who received three doses of his vaccine experienced one-third the incidence and one-quarter the mortality from influenza as the unvaccinated.[45]

Regardless of the vaccine they tested or the approach they used, most researchers who published the results of influenza vaccine trials in 1918 concluded that their vaccine was effective. But there were a few exceptions. Harry Lee Barnes, writing on the experience of a state sanatorium in Rhode Island, concluded that Leary's vaccine offered only slight protection. He reached that conclusion after excluding from his results all children in the institution and two wards of adults, who, he was convinced, were not sufficiently exposed to the infection. Were these inmates included, the vaccine offered no benefit at all.[46] August B. Wadsworth, the Director of Laboratories and Research at the New York State Department of Health, published two reports on the use of a vaccine modeled on the one Park had developed in New York City and that was widely distributed in the state. In both, he was skeptical. In his report on the outbreak in the New York State Training School for Girls at Hudson, New York, he concluded that it was unclear whether the school's light brush with the epidemic was due to the use of the vaccine or to the strict quarantine the institution had imposed.[47]

45. Rosenow, "Prophylactic Inoculation," 33; Rosenow and Sturdivant, "Further Results," 401.

46. Harry Lee Barnes, "The Prophylactic Value of Leary's Vaccine," J. Am. Med. Assoc., 1918, 71, 1899.

47. Augustus B. Wadsworth, "A Bacteriologic Investigation of an Outbreak of Influenza in an Institution," J. Am. Med. Assoc., 1919, 73, 1657–58.

Eyler- 2009 Oct. - J Hist Med Allied Sci 64 - 401-428

In his report on the work of the medical committee appointed by the Governor to investigate the influenza epidemic under Hermann Biggs's chairmanship, Wadsworth explained that the committee collected information on the use and effectiveness of the vaccine from community physicians, from twenty-eight residential state institutions which used the vaccine, from a special study the committee supervised in four such institutions, and from its use among employees of the state health department laboratories. The results were inconsistent, but it was clear that the closer subjects could be observed and the more complete and consistent the information on the vaccinated and the unvaccinated, the less benefit this vaccine appeared to offer.[48]

More definitive and provocative was the article of a single-column's length in the *Journal of the American Medical Association* by George McCoy, Director of the Hygienic Laboratory of the Public Health Service, USPHS Assistant Surgeon V. B. Murray, and an intern at Stanford University Hospital, A. L. Teeter.[49] The team tested Rosenow's vaccine, the influenza vaccine with the greatest scientific pretentions. They obtained their vaccine supply from the Chicago Health Department Laboratories, which had produced the vaccine in large quantities for use in Illinois, and they conducted the trial in a single institution, an unnamed state insane asylum. McCoy and associates concluded that Rosenow's vaccine offered no protection whatever. Their conclusion is historically less significant than the design of this trial.

From our vantage point today, we can easily recognize the fundamental methodological weaknesses in many of these influenza vaccine trials: selection bias, unequal exposure to risk, major gaps in information about health status and outcomes, and so on. We can also recognize that the closer a study was to equalizing risk and to obtaining complete information, the more likely it was to conclude that the influenza vaccines of 1918–19 were useless. The contrast between McCoy's study and many of those that concluded that a vaccine was effective serves to illustrate this point. McCoy and

---

48. Augustus B. Wadsworth, "The Results of Preventive Vaccination with Suspensions of the Influenza Bacillus," *Pub. Health J.*, 1919, *10*, 309–14.

49. G. W. McCoy, V. B. Murray, and A. L. Teeter, "The Failure of a Bacterial Vaccine as a Prophylactic against Influenza," *J. Am. Med. Assoc.*, 1918, *71*, 1997.

Eyler- 2009 Oct. - J Hist Med Allied Sci 64 - 401-428

colleagues worked in a single institution where they could keep all subjects under close observation. They completed the vaccinations eleven days before the first case appeared. And they sought to equalize risk by vaccinating on every ward alternative patients under age forty-one, the cohort they considered most likely to contract influenza.

Such retrospective methodological criticism is, of course, unfair and ahistorical. American physicians were inexperienced at conducting vaccine trials, and the circumstances in 1918–19 were certainly unfavorable to careful testing. Medical and public health facilities were stretched to the limit during the outbreak. There was often little opportunity to plan carefully and to execute a clinical trial. In fact, it may be unfair to consider many of these episodes trials. Some were clearly begun by medical superintendents who in desperation obtained a vaccine as the outbreak took hold in their institutions with the hope of saving lives. Some of the evaluations of vaccines were little more than attempts to make the most of what records could be assembled after the outbreak had passed. That such studies had flaws should be no surprise. What deserves notice, however, is how little concern the authors of these reports of 1918 showed for the design of their trials or for the circumstances in which the vaccinations took place and how certain many authors were that they had demonstrated the efficacy of the vaccine they had tested. Even more significant is the willingness of editors of some the nation's leading medical journals to publish these studies. It seems that in 1918, the profession had no standards for what constituted an adequate vaccine trial.

The controversy over the influenza vaccines forced it to formulate one. The most outspoken in this effort were George McCoy and William Park. Both had developed a Pfeiffer's bacillus vaccine early in the pandemic.[50] The disillusionment of both with their vaccines probably had its roots in their growing doubts that the Pfeiffer's bacillus really caused influenza. By late 1918, they were convinced that there was no evidence that any influenza vaccine worked, and

50. Park, "Bacteriology and Possibility," 621; McCoy apparently did not publish reports of his own vaccine, but it is referred to in discussion at the American Public Health Association in December 1918. See Anon., "American Public Health Association," J. Am. Med. Assoc., 1918, 71, 2100.

Eyler- 2009 Oct. - J Hist Med Allied Sci 64 - 401-428
        Eyler   :   Influenza Vaccine Trials   417

that no such evidence would be forthcoming unless certain basic standards were met in testing it. Both men explained the fallacy of beginning a vaccine trial during an outbreak, when disease might already have claimed the most susceptible and have selected a more resistant population for vaccination who might have escaped infection even without the vaccine. They also stressed the necessity of large vaccinated and unvaccinated control groups matched by age, sex, and exposure.[51]

Their membership on the American Public Health Association's Executive Sub-Committee on the Bacteriology of the 1918 Epidemic of Influenza gave McCoy and Park a key role in shaping the Association's "Working Program against Influenza," which appeared in January 1919.[52] The Association's Editorial Committee controversially declared, through this pamphlet, that the cause of influenza was unknown. Since that was the case, there was no "scientific basis" for a vaccine against the disease itself. There was a logical basis for a vaccine against secondary infection, but no evidence had yet come to light proving that such a vaccine was effective. The document then set down standards which the Association endorsed as adequate to test a vaccine. First, the numbers of vaccinated and unvaccinated persons should be equal; second, the vaccinated and the unvaccinated should be of equal susceptibility as determined by age, sex, and prior exposure; third, their degree of exposure during the trial should be equal in duration and intensity; and fourth, the vaccinated and the unvaccinated should be exposed concurrently to infection during the same phase of the epidemic.[53]

This is a rare document in the influenza literature in being so proscriptive about standards of evidence for vaccine trials, but it is also an important historical marker. Its publication did not signal the immediate demise of the articles that judged influenza vaccines on the basis of clinical judgment alone or those in which vaccination commenced after the outbreak had begun or in which

51. G. W. McCoy, "Pitfalls in Determining the Prophylactic or Curative Value of Bacterial Vaccines," *Pub. Health Rep.*, 1919, *34*, 1193; Anna I. von Sholly and William H. Park, "Report on the Prophylactic Vaccination of 1536 Persons against Acute Respiratory Diseases, 1919–20," *J. Immunol.*, 1921, 6, 103.
52. It was also published as Anon., "A Working Program against Influenza," *Am. J. Pub. Health*, 1919, 9, 1–13.
53. Ibid., 3. See also ibid., 11–12.

Eyler- 2009 Oct. - J Hist Med Allied Sci 64 - 401-428
418   Journal of the History of Medicine   :   Vol. 64, October 2009

proxy groups were used as controls.[54] But after its publication, authors were more likely to be cautious in drawing conclusions. Several of them specifically cited the APHA "Working Program" in explaining to readers the dangers of faulty inference from the use of vaccines during epidemics and the proper standards in designing trials.[55] Its appearance may also have caused authors to weigh their evidence differently. Consider the use of Leary's vaccine in twelve institutions in Massachusetts as reported in April 1919 by William Hinton and Edna Kane, both of the Massachusetts State Department of Health.[56] The trial was conducted in ways similar to those we have seen take place in multiple institutions during the 1918–19 epidemic. But in this case, the authors concluded retrospectively that the evidence from all but one of the institutions was unreliable either because vaccinations had begun as the outbreak had reached its peak, because there were too few cases in the institution, or because the vaccinated and the control groups were incomparable. In only one institution, an institution for epileptics, did the authors believe they had reliable data. In the Monsol State Hospital, alternate inmates in each cottage were vaccinated, and the vaccination began just as the first cases appeared. Hinton and Kane concluded that Leary's vaccine caused no harm, but it did not prevent influenza, moderate its course, or lessen its complications.

The *Journal of the American Medical Association* (*JAMA*) provided extended coverage of the annual meeting of the American Public Health Association in December 1918. In the discussion at that meeting following his paper, Rosenow found himself on the defensive.[57] The discussion began inauspiciously for Rosenow by McCoy's directing the audience's attention to his own recent paper demonstrating that Rosenow's vaccine was worthless. The tide of professional opinion was changing. *JAMA* published both Rosenow's articles, but it accompanied his first with a critical

54. See, for example, Watters, "Vaccines," 727–28; Wallace, "Report," 447–48; Katzman, "Influenza Vaccination," 121–22; Greeley, "Vaccine as a Prophylactic," 624–26.

55. Wadsworth, "Results," 310–11; Frederick P. Gay, "The Use of Vaccines in the Prevention and Treatment of Influenza and Its Sequels," *J. Am. Med. Assoc.*, 1921, 76, 244.

56. William A. Hinton and Edna Sypher Kane, "Use of Influenza Vaccine as a Prophylactic—An Experimental Study Conducted by the Massachusetts State Department of Health," *J. Tenn. State Med. Assoc.*, 1918–1919, 11, 442–46.

57. Anon., "American Public Health Association," *J. Am. Med. Assoc.*, 1918, 71, 2098–2100.

Eyler- 2009 Oct. - J Hist Med Allied Sci 64 - 401-428

Eyler   :   Influenza Vaccine Trials   419

editorial which cited as authoritative the APHA's recent conclusions about influenza vaccine trials and explicitly suggested that Rosenow was more receptive to favorable than to unfavorable evidence and that his study was vague and lacking in critical details.[58] The change in opinion can be detected in regional medical journals as well. The review article on influenza prevention in the *California State Journal of Medicine* by W. H. Kellogg, Secretary and Executive Officer of the state's board of health, devoted only one paragraph to influenza vaccines. Kellogg concluded that McCoy's study "definitely disposes of vaccine as a preventive measure worthy of consideration."[59]

Perhaps the best evidence that the profession was adopting standards for vaccine trials intended to avoid some of the fallacies present in most of the studies undertaken in the winter of 1918–19 is to be found in the trials undertaken during the following flu season. Two of these, both sponsored by the Metropolitan Life Insurance Company, serve as illustrations. William Park and his colleague at the laboratory of New York's health department, Anna Von Sholly, studied the effects of using two mixed influenza vaccines among the employees of the home office of MetLife.[60] Edwin Jordan, who was soon to become a leading authority on influenza, and his colleague at the University of Chicago, W. B. Sharp, published a study of the use of a mixed influenza vaccine in three residential schools and two large mental hospitals in Illinois and among a group of students at the University of Chicago.[61]

These studies were unprecedented in the influenza literature in the amount of detail they provided on the selection of subjects and controls and of the effect of that selection on the study's results. In the residential institutions, Jordan and Sharp assigned individuals to the experimental or control arm by an alphabetical list of inmates for each ward. People who objected to vaccination or who could not be found at the time of vaccination were moved to the control group. Those in the experimental arm who did not receive all three

58. Anon., "Prophylactic Inoculation against Influenza," *J. Am. Med. Assoc.*, 1919, *72*, 44–45.
59. W. H. Kellogg, "A Consideration of the Methods Used in the Control of Influenza," *Cal. State J. Med.*, 1919, *17*, 230.
60. Von Sholly and Park, "Report," 103–15.
61. Edwin O. Jordan and W. B. Sharp, "Effect of Vaccination against Influenza and Some Other Respiratory Infections," *J. Infect Dis.*, 1921, *28*, 357–66.

Eyler- 2009 Oct. - J Hist Med Allied Sci 64 - 401-428
420   *Journal of the History of Medicine   :   Vol. 64, October 2009*

injections were dropped from the study. In contrast, the employees of MetLife and the students at the University of Chicago volunteered to receive the vaccine. The authors of both studies recognized that this procedure might introduce selection bias. Von Sholly and Park, in fact, demonstrated that bias was at work in their study by showing not only that a higher proportion of unvaccinated in their study suffered no respiratory tract infections during the winter of 1919–20, but that those who decided to forgo vaccination were more likely to have escaped such infections in the past.[62]

Both studies also acknowledged that the differential diagnosis of influenza is difficult and therefore included morbidity and mortality data for not only influenza and pneumonia but also for other respiratory tract infections. They also considered relevant previous experience with respiratory tract infection or influenza vaccination. Jordan and Sharp even paid some attention to placebo effects. Toward the end of their article, they reported that although their statistics indicated that the vaccine offered no protection against colds and other respiratory tract infections, some University of Chicago students volunteered the information that the vaccine kept them healthier that winter.[63] In the final analysis, neither study demonstrated that the vaccine being tested offered any protection against influenza; Jordan and Sharp could not rule out the possibility that the vaccine offered some protection against pneumonia, although they cautioned that the number of cases in their study was too small to be certain.[64]

The criteria for an adequate vaccine trial that the APHA set down in its Working Program remained the profession's standards for several decades. Not only were they used to judge bacterial vaccines against influenza and pneumonia in the 1920s, they were also, as I have shown, in use in the first trials of viral influenza vaccines in the middle and late 1930s and into the early 1940s.[65] The framers of these standards were concerned primarily to equalize risk among the vaccinated and the controls and to guard against selection bias. Judged from the vantage point of the early twenty-first century, what is interesting is what the standards did not include.

62. Von Sholly and Park, "Report," 111.
63. Jordan and Sharp, "Effect," 365–66.
64. Von Sholly and Park, "Report," 112–13; Jordan and Sharp, "Effect," 361–63.
65. John M. Eyler, "De Kruif's Boast: Vaccine Trials and the Construction of a Virus," *Bull. Hist. Med.*, 2006, *80*, 417–20.

Eyler- 2009 Oct. - J Hist Med Allied Sci 64 - 401-428

There was almost no discussion in the early twentieth-century influenza vaccine controversies of observer bias, and the APHA standard makes no mention of blinding, double-blinding, or placebos. There is also no insistence on randomization. There is also no discussion of who is a proper subject for experimentation, much less of that subject's informed consent. The APHA committee assumed that most trials would take place in residential institutions and that in fact remained the norm during these decades. It was usually quite easy for researchers to gain access to such subjects wholesale in the inter-war period.[66]

The history of clinical trials is a topic which has only recently begun to receive the attention it deserves. A prominent view of the origin of the modern clinical trial points to the activities of the Therapeutic Trials Committee, established in 1931, of the Medical Research Council of Great Britain, particularly to the work of the Council's statistician Austin Bradford Hill.[67] This is a view which Hill himself helped to foster.[68] According to this interpretation, the appearance of Hill's series of articles, "Principles of Medical Statistics," in the 2 January through 24 April 1937 issues of the *Lancet* is a watershed event in trial methodology, which led, a decade later, to the first randomized clinical trial, the MRC's study of streptomycin in pulmonary tuberculosis.[69] While there is no doubt of the historic importance of the work of Hill and the Committee, my own research on influenza vaccines thus far leads me to conclude that the development of the modern vaccine trial, as Harry Marks has shown with the therapeutic trial, is a longer, more convoluted, evolutionary process.[70]

66. See, for example, the ease with which Joseph Stokes gained access to his subjects in 1935 (Eyler, "De Kruif's Boast," 412).

67. Peter Armitage, "Bradford Hill and the Randomized Controlled Trial," *Pharm. Med.*, 1992, *6*, 23–37; Richard Doll, "Clinical Trials: Retrospect and Prospect," *Stat. Med.*, 1982, *1*, 337–44.

68. Austin Bradford Hill, "Memories of the British Streptomycin Trial in Tuberculosis: The First Randomized Clinical Trial," *Control. Clin. Trials*, 1990, *11*, 77–79.

69. A. Bradford Hill, "Principles of Medical Statistics," *Lancet*, 1937, I, 41–43, 99–101, 161–63, 219–21, 281–84, 337–40, 402–05, 459–61, 527–29, 583–86, 646–48, 706–08, 771–73, 825–27, 883–85, 941–43, 1001–03; Great Britain, Medical Research Council, Streptomycin in Tuberculosis Trials Committee, "Streptomycin Treatment of Pulmonary Tuberculosis," *Br. Med. J.*, 1948, II, 769–82.

70. Harry M. Marks, "Notes from the Underground: The Social Organization of Therapeutic Research," in *Grand Rounds: One Hundred Years of Internal Medicine*, ed. Russell C. Maulitz and Diana E. Long (Philadelphia: University of Pennsylvania Press,

Eyler- 2009 Oct. - J Hist Med Allied Sci 64 - 401-428
422 *Journal of the History of Medicine : Vol. 64, October 2009*

By 1918, a number of researchers clearly recognized the need for unvaccinated controls and for equalizing exposure to risk among all experimental subjects. The studies of George McCoy and associates and Jordan and Sharp accomplished this end by vaccinating alternative inmates on a ward list.[71] This procedure was what the framers of the APHA's standards seem to have had in mind, and the practice of vaccinating alternate subjects to establish controlled conditions became more common in the 1920s, especially in trials carried out in custodial institutions. Assignment by strict randomization is one of the claims made for the special historical importance of the work of the Therapeutic Trials Committee in the 1930s and 1940s. But Bradford Hill remembers that he was not insistent at first on the assignment of subjects by random numbers, and he believed until the end of his life that, if assignments were strictly alternative, the result would be a random division.[72] He first employed randomization in the M. R. C.'s whooping cough vaccine trials which only began in 1942 and were not published in definitive form until 1951.[73] As for informed consent among the subjects before World War Two, Hill remembered in 1990, "We did not ask the patient's permission or anybody's permission. We did not tell them they were in a trial—we just did it. To tell the truth, all of the discussion today about the *patient's* informed consent still strikes me as absolute rubbish."[74] Hill's view that the subject was unfit to judge his own self-interest in this matter was undoubtedly shared by many researchers between the World Wars.

While it is comparatively easy to situate the APHA's standards for vaccine trials in the confusion and controversies over the use of bacterial vaccines during the Great Influenza Pandemic, the larger context is harder to establish. It is true that one of the authors of these standards, William Park, was at the time involved testing the

1988), 297–336; Harry M. Marks, *The Progress of Experiment: Science and Therapeutic Reform in the United States, 1900–1990* (New York and Cambridge: Cambridge University Press, 1997).

71. McCoy, Murray, and Teeter, "Failure," 1997; Jordan and Sharp, "Effect," 357–58.

72. Hill, "Memories," 77.

73. Great Britain, Medical Research Council, Whooping-cough Immunization Committee, "The Prevention of Whooping-cough by Vaccination," *Br. Med. J.*, 1951, I, 1463–71.

74. Hill, "Memories," 78. Emphasis in the original.

Eyler- 2009 Oct. - J Hist Med Allied Sci 64 - 401-428

Eyler :   Influenza Vaccine Trials   423

value of diphtheria immunization by experiments with human subjects. During the Great War, Park and his colleagues at the New York City Health Department had begun Schick-testing child patients in the scarlet fever ward of the city's Willard Parker Hospital and inmates at an orphanage. This work strengthened their confidence in the Schick test as a measure of immunity to diphtheria, and it also demonstrated the persistence of passive immunity following injections of antitoxin and of active immunity from injections of the toxin–antitoxin mixtures by using the Schick test as the measure of that immunity.[75]

However, it was only after the War and hence after the publication of the American Public Health Association's standards for vaccine trials that the diphtheria work of Park and colleagues seems to mirror the type of trials those standards assume. Beginning in 1920, the Health Department moved its diphtheria research into the city's schools by Schick-testing thousands of children whose parents gave permission for the test and for subsequent immunization with the toxin–antitoxin mixture of those found to be Schick-positive.[76] By late 1922, Park and colleagues could report on a clinical trial in which, following two years of observation, the incidence of diphtheria in a control group of 90,000 children was found to be four times the rate of 90,000 children in an experimental group.[77] On the face of it, this trial seems to conform to the standards set out a little more than two years previously. It was certainly a large trial in which the experimental and the control groups were of equal size and apparently subject to the same exposure in the same schools and neighborhoods at the same time. However, this trial did not assure the equal susceptibility of the experimental and the control arms. Included in the experimental

75. William H. Park, Abraham Zingher, and H. M. Serota, "Active Immunization in Diphtheria and Treatment by Toxin–Antitoxin," *J. Am. Med. Assoc.*, 1914, *63*, 859–61; William H. Park and Abraham Zingher, "Diphtheria Immunity—Natural, Active and Passive. Its Determination by the Schick Test," *Am. J. Pub. Health*, 1916, *6*, 431–45; William H. Park, M. C. Schroder, and Abraham Zingher, "The Control of Diphtheria," *Am. J. Pub. Health*, 1923, *13*, 26.

76. Abraham Zingher, "Diphtheria Prevention Work in the Public Schools of New York City," *J. Am. Med. Assoc.*, 1921, *77*, 835–41. See also Jeffrey P. Baker, "Immunization and the American Way: 4 Childhood Vaccines," *Am. J. Pub. Health*, 2000, *90*, 199–200.

77. William Park, "Toxin–Antitoxin Immunization against Diphtheria," *J. Am. Med. Assoc.*, 1922, *79*, 1589; Park, Schroder, and Zingher, "Control of Diphtheria," 26–28, 31.

Eyler- 2009 Oct. - J Hist Med Allied Sci 64 - 401-428

424 *Journal of the History of Medicine* : *Vol. 64, October 2009*

arm were those children initially found to be Schick-positive, and, because the control group was not Schick-tested, no one knew how many of its members had prior immunity. It seems then that one cannot look to Park's work with diphtheria immunization as the clear model for the new standard for vaccine trials. Both the timing and the nature of his large field trial of diphtheria vaccine suggest that we need to look elsewhere for the intellectual origins of these new standards.

None of the documents I have located refers to previous discussions of vaccine testing or trial design or cites earlier authoritative works on such subjects. American discussions in these years are remarkable for the absence of theory or statistical principles. It is difficult to believe, however, that the authors of the APHA Working Program, especially George McCoy and William Park, were unaware of the literature that would seem to be the most relevant to the issue they faced—the controversy over the value of Almoth Wright's typhoid vaccine ignited by its use during the Boer War. Wright's vaccine was first employed by the Army in 1899; its use was suspended in 1904; and between 1904 and 1908, its scientific legitimacy was rehabilitated by the work of a military medical commission led by William Leishman.[78] This prolonged discussion over the typhoid vaccine and the introduction of another for cholera provided ample opportunity for members of the British biometrical school to comment on published reports of the use of these vaccines.

At the outbreak of World War I, Major Greenwood and Udny Yule published in the *Proceedings of the Royal Society of Medicine* a mathematically sophisticated and lengthy article on the interpretation of statistics of the use of typhoid and cholera vaccines.[79] It could well serve as a statistical primer for those planning vaccine trials. It provides, for example, a clear illustration of how the use of a vaccine during an epidemic skews the statistical results by ensuring that the vaccinated and the unvaccinated are exposed to risk for unequal periods.[80] A section of the review article on the influenza

78. Anne Hardy, "'Straight Back to Barbarism': Antityphoid Inoculation and the Great War, 1914," *Bull. Hist. Med.*, 2000, 74, 265–90.

79. Major Greenwood and G. Udny Yule, "The Statistics of Anti-Typhoid and Anti-Cholera Inoculation, and the Interpretation of Such Statistics in General," *Proc. R. Soc. Med.*, (Sect. Epidemiol. State Med.), 1914–15, 8, 113–90.

80. Greenwood and Yule, "Statistics," 134–35.

Eyler- 2009 Oct. - J Hist Med Allied Sci 64 - 401-428
Eyler   :   *Influenza Vaccine Trials*   425

vaccine literature McCoy published in August 1919 suggests that he had read and understood Greenwood and Yule's text, because he provides a similar but not identical explanation of the statistical fallacy of vaccinating during an epidemic and of including as ill-nesses among the controls all illnesses that occurred among the unvaccinated during the course of the epidemic.[81] Both the British and American authors pose a thought experiment to the reader in which half a population of 1000 is inoculated with a useless sub-stance after the beginning of an epidemic and subjected to equal risk of illness thereafter. Greenwood and Yule hypothesize that each week, fifty persons who have not had the disease or been inoculated are inoculated and that during the week 1 percent of both the inoculated and the uninoculated become ill. At the end of three weeks, the morbidity rate among the inoculated would be twenty per thousand, and among the uninoculated it would be thirty-one per thousand. McCoy asked his reader to imagine that the inocu-lation of half the population begins one week after the outbreak begins and that each week 20 percent of all inmates are attacked. At the end of two weeks, there would be eighty sick among the inocu-lated but 280 recorded as sick among the unvaccinated "controls" (Table 1).

In their paper, Greenwood and Yule propose three principles which must be observed in designing a valid vaccine trial.[82] First, the vaccinated and the controls must be "in all material respects, alike." They mention specifically age, sex, social and racial compo-sition. Second, the "effective exposure" to the disease must be identical for the vaccinated and the unvaccinated. Third, "the cri-teria of the fact of inoculation and of the fact of the disease having occurred must be independent." The APHA's standards are thus not identical to those of Greenwood and Yule set out four years before, but there is certainly a very strong resemblance. Greenwood and Yule did not insist that the vaccinated and the controls should be equal in number, but their first principle would certainly encompass the second of the APHA, that the two groups should be of equal susceptibility. Greenwood and Yule's second principle, of equal

81. G. W. McCoy, "Status of Prophylactic Vaccination against Influenza," *J. Am. Med. Assoc.,* 1919, 73, 402.
82. Greenwood and Yule, "Statistics," 115–17.

Eyler- 2009 Oct. - J Hist Med Allied Sci 64 - 401-428
426   *Journal of the History of Medicine   :   Vol. 64, October 2009*

TABLE I

Clinical Trials of Influenza Vaccines

Examples provided by George McCoy[81]

	Vaccinated		Unvaccinated	
		Sick		Sick
Day 1	0	0	1000	0
Day 7	400	0	400	200
Day 14	400	80	400	280

Example provided by Major Greenwood and Udny Yule[79]

	Vaccinated			Unvaccinated		
	Total	Well	Sick	Total	Well	Sick
Day 1	50	50		950	950	
Day 7	100	49.5	0.5	900	940.5	9.5
		99.5	0.5		890.5	9.5
Day 14		98.5	1.495		872.095	18.405
	148.505	1.495		822.095	18.405	
Day 21	150	147.02	2.98	850	795.47	26.62
			20/1000			31/1000

Eyler- 2009 Oct. - J Hist Med Allied Sci 64 - 401-428

Eyler   :   Influenza Vaccine Trials   427

effective exposure, would seem to encompass the APHA's third principle—that exposures should be of equal duration and intensity. Greenwood and Yule do not insist that exposure take place during the same phase of the epidemic. On the other hand, their third principle, the one insisting that the fact of inoculation and the fact of disease be independent, has no counterpart in the APHA standards.

The differences in these two sets of standards can be understood as reflections of the specific problems the two sets of authors faced. Greenwood and Yule were dealing with statistics of incidence of endemic diseases primarily in military men. In these circumstances, risks of exposure were long term and the problems of correlating inoculation histories with mortality and morbidity records extreme. The American authors were preoccupied with an epidemic disease that occurred in explosive outbreaks, but in which the site of observation was frequently residential institutions, where the fact of vaccination was seldom in doubt. However, the exact phase of the epidemic when individuals faced exposure was of paramount importance. It seems entirely likely that the Americans who drafted the APHA's standards for vaccine trials were familiar with the work of Greenwood and Yule, but that they modified these British criteria to suit the circumstances they faced. The APHA criteria were a practical set of guidelines drawn up in response to a public health crisis. Under the circumstances, the authors did not burden their readers with statistical principles or citations to other authorities. They did succeed in crafting standards for vaccine trials that would be observed for a quarter century. The Army Epidemiological Board's trial of its viral influenza vaccine in 1943 became the first influenza vaccine trial to significantly tighten these standards when it insisted on randomization, double-blinding, and placebo controls.[83]

We have thus seen that during the influenza pandemic of 1918–19, American health workers developed a large number of influenza vaccines. Some of these vaccines, especially those developed by Park, Leary, and Rosenow, were very widely used. The medical literature during the pandemic contained frequent reports of the

83. Eyler, "De Kruif's Boast," 426.

Eyler- 2009 Oct. - J Hist Med Allied Sci 64 - 401-428

428   *Journal of the History of Medicine   :   Vol. 64, October 2009*

use of these vaccines claiming to prove their efficacy. Readers of the medical literature in those months faced the remarkable circumstance that all these vaccines, regardless of their composition or mode of administration, were proven to prevent influenza. By late 1918, a few skeptical voices were heard questioning the basis for these claims. A turning point was clearly the trial of Rosenow's vaccine conducted by George McCoy in a California mental institution. Using stricter standards to guard against selection bias and to ensure the equal exposure of the experimental and control arms, McCoy showed that Rosenow's vaccine offered no protection at all. McCoy and William Park also helped initiate a discussion of the design fallacies of most vaccine trials, such as beginning the trial after the epidemic it was intended to prevent had begun, and they played a leading role in formulating the standards for a valid vaccine trial that the American Public Health Association endorsed in January of 1919. Those standards would guide American vaccine trials through the inter-war period.

Eyler- 2010 - Public Health Reports - Supp 3 Vol 25, 27-36

THE SCIENCE OF INFLUENZA

The State of Science, Microbiology, and Vaccines Circa 1918

JOHN M. EYLER, PHD[a]

SYNOPSIS

The influenza pandemic of 1918–1919 dramatically altered biomedical knowledge of the disease. At its onset, the foundation of scientific knowledge was information collected during the previous major pandemic of 1889–1890.
The work of Otto Leichtenstern, first published in 1896, described the major epidemiological and pathological features of pandemic influenza and was cited extensively over the next two decades. Richard Pfeiffer announced in 1892 and 1893 that he had discovered influenza's cause. Pfeiffer's bacillus (*Bacillus influenzae*) was a major focus of attention and some controversy between 1892 and 1920. The role this organism or these organisms played in influenza dominated medical discussion during the great pandemic.
Many vaccines were developed and used during the 1918–1919 pandemic. The medical literature was full of contradictory claims of their success; there was apparently no consensus on how to judge the reported results of these vaccine trials. The result of the vaccine controversy was both a further waning of confidence in Pfeiffer's bacillus as the agent of influenza and the emergence of an early set of criteria for valid vaccine trials.

[a]Program in the History of Medicine, University of Minnesota, Minneapolis, MN

Address correspondence to: John M. Eyler, 4609 Gustafson Dr., Gig Harbor, WA 98335; tel. 253-851-7311; e-mail <eyler001@umn.edu>.

Eyler- 2010 - Public Health Reports - Supp 3 Vol 25, 27-36

When the great influenza pandemic of 1918–1919 began, the most important sources of knowledge about epidemic influenza were studies conducted during and immediately following the previous pandemic, that of 1889–1990. The 1889–1890 influenza pandemic was the first to occur in the Western world after the pandemic of 1848–1849. That meant that it was the first to have taken place since more prosperous nation states had created active, professional health departments and systems of vital statistics, and the first to be studied using the methods of modern pathology and bacteriology. The 1889–1890 pandemic generated a very large literary output and two particularly important biomedical syntheses. In 1891, Franklin Parsons, a member of the Medical Department of the Local Government Board in London, published a 300-page report on the pandemic based on surveys of all sanitary districts in England and Wales and on local studies in selected areas.[1] Five years later, drawing on continental, especially German, scientific and clinical literature, Otto Leichtenstern published the definitive scientific study of influenza in Hermann Northnagel's multi-volume handbook of special pathology.[2,3] These two major works, particularly Leichtenstern's, were the well from which American authors of medical textbooks and reference works, such as William Osler and Frederick Lord, would draw for the next two decades and the standards against which medical authorities would judge their observations and conclusions during the next great pandemic.[4–6]

It says volumes about the rudimentary state of scientific knowledge of influenza in the early 1890s that the most important and lasting conclusion of these two seminal works was that influenza was a specific, communicable disease.[1,3] (p. 51–3, 70–102) (p. 554–64, 573–5) It did spread very rapidly, more rapidly than any other known communicable disease, and it produced explosive local outbreaks. However, it never arose spontaneously, nor did it travel faster than humans travel. Close investigation easily debunked accounts of outbreaks occurring without precursor cases or in places without contact with infected individuals. Furthermore, isolated populations, such as those within prisons in heavily infected cities, sometimes escaped entirely. Although influenza occurred more often in winter and spring months, the pandemic struck in all latitudes of both hemispheres, at all altitudes inhabited by humans, and in all climates. It was clearly not caused by overt climatic or environmental factors. A serious influenza epidemic was seldom a solo event. A major epidemic was often followed within months by one or more additional outbreaks. Authorities of the early 1890s recognized that the diagnosis of influenza was difficult, and that mild cases were easily confused with other respiratory and catarrh-like disorders. They were quite certain from clinical and epidemiological records that the influenza of the great pandemic of 1889–1890 was the same disease that had caused the influenza pandemics of the past, such as that of 1848–1849. The more vexing problem was whether this pandemic influenza was the same disease as the disorder commonly known as influenza or grippe that occurred almost every year. Parsons thought they undoubtedly were distinct diseases; Leichtenstern agreed, although less adamantly.[1,3] (p. 81) (p. 530–1)

INFLUENZA TYPES

Its clinical features and its opaque identity made influenza seem an especially protean disease. Writing in 1907, Clifford Allbutt, Regius Professor of Medicine, observed "influenza is of protean diseases the most protean; more diversified even than syphilis."[7] (p. 1) Individual cases were characterized by their sudden onset and by extreme prostration, which was out of all proportion to other pathological features. The disease's regular target was the respiratory tract, and pneumonia was the most serious complication of influenza and the major cause of mortality during an outbreak. But Leichtenstern observed that cases might exhibit no respiratory symptoms at all. In addition to the typical respiratory cases, both he and Parsons passed on a division of three subtypes inherited from earlier authors: nervous, catarrhal, and gastric.[1,3] (p. 64) (p. 590–1) In succeeding years, the number of recognized clinical types swelled enormously. In 1907, when Frederick Lord wrote his chapter on influenza in Osler's multi-volume reference work, *Modern Medicine*, he described no fewer than 10 clinical types, including influenza of the circulatory system, of the genito-urinary system, of the joints, and of the skin.[6] (p. 474–83) Influenza, it seems, was having an identity crisis. This is a point to which we will return.

The generation working after the pandemic of 1889–1890 also classified influenza cases according to their occurrence and presumed cause. Leichtenstern proposed a tripartite division of influenza types: pandemic *influenza vera* (the disease that occurred in great global outbreaks), endemic-epidemic *influenza vera* (the disease having the same cause but which occurred in smaller outbreaks following a pandemic), and endemic *influenza nostras* (pseudo-influenza due to different causes).[3] (p. 531) Both Osler and Lord passed on this classification to their readers, although Lord significantly altered the third category to endemic *influenza*

Eyler- 2010 - Public Health Reports - Supp 3 Vol 25, 27-36

vera, suggesting that cases in this classification must have the same cause as those occurring in epidemics[5,6] (p. 116) (p. 473).

The experience with the 1889–1890 pandemic taught medical authorities that pandemic influenza was a disease of very high morbidity and low case fatality, although it seemed that in the outbreaks immediately following a pandemic, morbidity rates could be expected to decline and case fatality rates to rise. Given the problems of differential diagnosis and the existence of mild cases, exact statistics were difficult to obtain. Authorities concluded, however, that in 1889–1890 the infection was very widely distributed in European nations. Leichtenstern estimated that as much as 50% of the German population had been infected, while Parsons put the estimate for Greater London at 25%. Reported incidence rates for employees of British institutions ranged from 9% for troops stationed in Britain to 33% for postal employees.[1,3] (p. 3–7, 109–10) (p. 532, 564–70)

The experience of 1889–1890 suggested that pandemic influenza had distinct patterns of age-specific morbidity and mortality. Continental figures indicated that morbidity was highest between ages 20 and 40 and lowest after age 50, while case fatality rates were highest among the elderly. Deaths registered as due to influenza in England and Wales were highest in the age group 40–60 at 36%, while 24% of influenza deaths took place between the ages of 20 and 40 and 22% between the ages of 60 and 80. Parsons demonstrated that this mortality pattern was very different from that of the inter-pandemic period. Between 1876 and 1889, 33% of deaths attributed to influenza occurred in the first year of life and another 34% occurred after age 60.[1] (p. 6)

THE BACTERIOLOGY OF INFLUENZA

During the pandemic of 1889–1890, researchers used the new methods of medical microbiology in unsuccessful efforts to identify the microbial cause of influenza. An apparent breakthrough came in 1892, during a subsequent outbreak, when Richard Pfeiffer announced in a single-page preliminary publication,[8] and a year later in a more substantial article, that he had found influenza's cause.[9] Pfeiffer reported finding in every case of influenza he examined a rod-shaped organism. In uncomplicated cases he found these bacilli in overwhelming numbers and frequently in pure culture. Pfeiffer's bacillus was challenging to work with. It was very small and fastidious. It would only grow on blood argar plates. It could not be stained with Gram's stain,

but it would accept Loeffler's methylene blue stain, and it displayed characteristic polar staining, making it easy to confuse with diplococci. Pfeiffer was never able to find an animal model for influenza, although he innoculated mice, rats, guinea pigs, rabbits, pigs, cats, dogs, and monkeys. To further complicate matters, although he had focused his investigation almost exclusively on influenza cases, he reported finding in a few cases of "diphtheric bronchopneumonia" a bacillus that was indistinguishable from his own bacillus on the grounds of morphology and of culture and staining characteristics. He labeled this organism pseudo-influenza bacillus.

In retrospect, Pfeiffer's chain of evidence may seem more shaky than it did to his contemporaries. Pfeiffer, a protégé of Robert Koch, was, after all, a productive and distinguished bacteriologist. Contemporaries respected the technical skill he exhibited in isolating and characterizing his bacillus. The failure to satisfy Koch's Postulates by producing an experimental disease in animals by the inoculation of pure culture was not in itself damning. Koch, himself, had sometimes failed in this regard. The existence of the pseudo-influenza bacillus would seem to his contemporaries no more implausible than the existence of the pseudo-diphtheria bacillus. While the scientific response to Pfeiffer's discovery is difficult to characterize concisely, it does seem fair to conclude that most medical authorities believed that Pfeiffer was basically correct in his identification, even though his evidence might not be complete. (Although the organism that Pfeiffer isolated was most likely what we know today as *Hemophilus influenzae*, we refer to it in this article in the way it was referred to during the period under discussion: Pfeiffer's bacillus and *Bacillus influenzae* [*B. influenzae*]).

Parsons published before Pfeiffer's announcement, but Leichtenstern published three years after, and he endorsed Pfeiffer's discovery with only modest qualification. "Should the *Bacillus influenzae*, discovered by R. Pfeiffer in 1892, continue to maintain in future pandemics its place as the exclusive cause of the disease, as may certainly be expected, its discovery may be considered as the most important achievement of our latest influenza pandemic."[3] (p. 524)

In succeeding years there was keen interest in Pfeiffer's bacillus. In 1892, when Pfeiffer announced the discovery of *B. influenzae*, Americans had little, if anything, to add to the discussion. By 1918, on the other hand, they were active participants. By that time, laboratory courses in medical bacteriology were being taught in most American medical schools, diagnostic laboratories operated in many hospitals and in some

Eyler- 2010 - Public Health Reports - Supp 3 Vol 25, 27-36

public health departments, and in some laboratories American bacteriologists were already doing world-class research. The active participation of medical officers in the U.S. Army in 1918 and 1919 is an indication of how widely disseminated the new laboratory techniques were in the American medical profession. These laboratories may seem rudimentary by 21st century standards. Microorganisms were identified primarily by morphology and by basic culture and staining techniques. Routine clinical diagnosis, sputum examinations for tuberculosis, and throat cultures for diphtheria, for example, had begun to exploit these basic laboratory techniques. More specialized techniques, such as the Widal examination of typhoid fever and complement fixation tests such as the Wassermann test for syphilis, were early examples of the exploitation of immunological phenomena. Filterable viruses were known to exist, but very little was known about them, and there were very few techniques for working with them.

In the years immediately following Pfeiffer's discovery, many investigators confirmed his findings by isolating his bacillus from influenza cases. But there were complications. Others reported isolating organisms indistinguishable by contemporary laboratory methods from *B. influenzae* from other diseases and even from normal throats.[10] (p. 28–32) For example David J. Davis, from the Memorial Institute for Infectious Diseases in Chicago, reported in 1906 isolating Pfeiffer's bacilli from all but five of the series of 61 cases of whooping cough he studied. He also found them in 40% to 80% of a smaller number of cases of cerebro-spinal meningitis, varicella, measles, and bronchitis. Significantly, he succeeded in isolating Pfeiffer's bacilli in only three (18%) of 17 cases of influenza.[10] (p. 12–3, 25–8)

Such results suggested to some that Pfeiffer's bacillus was merely a secondary invader. But these findings might also indicate that this organism was a key player in a more complex etiology. W. D'Este Emery, clinical pathologist at King's College Hospital, London, drew attention to the fact that *B. influenzae* grew more readily in culture in the presence of other organisms and seemed to be more virulent for animals in the presence of killed streptococci. Emery wondered whether Pfeiffer's bacillus might be a "harmless saprophyte" most of the time but be capable in the presence of other pathogens of being transformed into "the pathogenic bacillus which occurred in the pandemic of the nineties."[11] (p. 110)

The confusion over the etiology of influenza on the eve of the pandemic of 1918–1919 is well illustrated in the eighth edition of Osler's textbook of 1912. In the definition of the disease he states that "a special

organism, *Bacillus influenzae*, is found," and in the section on bacteriology he also states that this organism "is recognized as the cause of the disease," but he also points out that it is commonly found in other diseases and is "probably constantly with us."[5] (p. 115–7) Despite such reservations, medical authorities recognized that Pfeiffer's bacillus was the only viable candidate for the cause of influenza. On the eve of the pandemic of 1918–1919, it was deeply implicated in the understanding and even the definition of the disease. That great expansion in clinical types of influenza identified in Frederick Lord's synthesis of scientific knowledge was made possible because *B. influenzae* had been isolated from the blood, from heart valves, from the joints, and from the urinary tract. In an age when etiological definitions of disease were of growing importance and bacteriology was beginning to provide the gold standard for differential diagnosis in infectious diseases, Pfeiffer's bacillus had become indispensable.

INFLUENZA VACCINES

The fate of Pfeiffer's bacillus as the probable cause of influenza is reflected in the use of vaccines in the United States during the pandemic of 1918–1919. By 1918, the successful use of some vaccines, especially those against rabies, typhoid fever, and diphtheria, as well as the use of diphtheria anti-toxin, had raised high expectations for a vaccine against influenza.[12] Those who already had a vaccine in hand were quick off the mark to promote their vaccines as sure preventives or cures for influenza. Drug manufacturers aggressively promoted their stock vaccines for colds, grippe, and flu. These vaccines were of undisclosed composition. As public anxiety and demand swelled, there were complaints of price gouging and kickbacks.[13] (p. 114–6) Preexisting vaccines of undisclosed composition were also endorsed by physicians such as M.J. Exner, who actively promoted in newspaper interviews and testimonials the vaccine developed some six years earlier by his colleague, Ellis Bonime.[14,15] Bonime was a late champion of the tuberculin treatment of tuberculosis and an adherent of the opsonin theory of immune response and of the therapeutic use of vaccines.[16] His vaccine was claimed to prevent pneumonia, influenza, and blood poisoning. Exner's boosterism paid some dividends. At least one municipality, Far Rockaway, New York, announced that it would provide Bonime's vaccine to all its citizens.[17]

Early in the pandemic, more highly respected and well-placed authorities developed vaccines based explicitly on Pfeiffer's bacillus. On October 2, 1918, Royal S. Copeland, Health Commissioner of New York

Eyler- 2010 - Public Health Reports - Supp 3 Vol 25, 27-36

City, sought to reassure citizens that help was on the way, because the director of the Health Department's laboratories, William H. Park, was developing a vaccine that would offer protection against this dreaded disease.[18] Park's successes in combating diphtheria with anti-toxins and vaccines developed in these same laboratories gave Copeland's announcement much weight. Park explained to his colleagues that he and his staff consistently had been able to isolate Pfeiffer's bacillus from influenza cases, and that his laboratory had isolated the current strain, shown that animals injected with it developed specific antibodies, and developed a heat-killed vaccine that was to be administered in three doses at two-day intervals.[19]

Park's was not the only Pfeiffer's bacillus influenza vaccine to make an early appearance during the pandemic. At Tufts Medical School in Boston, Timothy Leary, professor of bacteriology and pathology, developed another Pfeiffer's bacillus vaccine. His was developed from three locally isolated strains, and it was heat-killed and chemically treated. Leary promoted his vaccine as both a preventive and a treatment for influenza.[20] Other Pfeiffer's bacillus vaccines soon followed. Faculty from the Medical School of the University of Pittsburgh isolated 13 strains of the Pfeiffer's bacillus and produced a vaccine from them by modifying the techniques Park had used. In the crisis atmosphere of the pandemic, the Pittsburgh vaccine developers isolated their strains, prepared the vaccine, tested it for toxicity in some laboratory animals and in two humans, and turned it over to the Red Cross for use in humans—all in one week.[13] (p. 109–11) In New Orleans, Charles W. Duval and William H. Harris from Tulane University's Department of Pathology and Bacteriology developed their own chemically killed Pfeiffer's bacillus vaccine. Their justification for its use was the common presence of the bacillus in influenza cases and the example of the typhoid vaccine whose administration schedule they followed.[21]

It was not only heads of bacteriological laboratories who acted on the assumption that Pfeiffer's bacillus was the cause of influenza and developed vaccines on that assumption. Some private physicians did the same. Horace Greeley of Brooklyn, New York, reported isolating 17 strains of the bacillus from 17 patients, and from these "strains," he developed a heat-killed vaccine intended to be administered in three increasing doses. With it he immunized his own patients, and he distributed eight liters to colleagues who did the same.[22]

These vaccines were widely used. Park's vaccine was released to the military for use in Army camps as well as to private physicians. It was also used as corporate policy among industrial workers, including the 14,000 employees of the Consolidated Gas Company and 275,000 employees of the U.S. Steel Company.[17,19,23] Leary's vaccine was used frequently during the epidemic in state custodial institutions of the Northeast and by some private physicians.[13] (p. 105–7)[24–27] Duval and Harris reported immunizing approximately 5,000 people, most of whom were employees of large New Orleans companies.[21] (p. 320–2) Almost without exception, those reporting on the use of these Pfeiffer's bacillus vaccines reported that they were effective in preventing influenza.

THE FALTERING CASE FOR PFEIFFER'S BACILLUS

At first the apparent success of these vaccines served to increase confidence in the role played by Pfeiffer's bacillus. But other evidence was accumulating. Initially, when observers reported difficulty isolating Pfeiffer's bacillus from influenza cases, they found their technique and experience questioned.[28,29] (p. 320) But slowly the evidence against Pfeiffer's bacillus mounted, first ambiguously and then emphatically. J.J. Keegan, a naval medical officer working in the Boston area, published an early report on studies undertaken during an outbreak of 2,000 cases in the First Naval District during the two-week period between August 28 and September 11, 1918. Keegan made a special effort to study the outbreak bacteriologically. He had difficulty isolating Pfeiffer's bacillus from throat washings or from sputum in both influenza cases and from patients admitted to the hospital with other conditions. He wondered whether the organism might be harbored in the sinuses or some other place more inaccessible to him. When he resorted to lung punctures in life and lung cultures at postmortem, he succeeded in isolating Pfeiffer's bacillus in 82.6% of 23 cases.[30] (p. 1053–5)

Other ambiguous results came from Edwin Jordan, a future American influenza expert. Jordan reported on a large bacteriological study of patients diagnosed with influenza and with other diseases during and after the epidemic at the University of Chicago. He reported finding no consistent bacteriology in his cases. No microorganism was present in all influenza cases. Although he identified Pfeiffer's bacillus in 64% of influenza cases, and this was more frequent than any other organism, its relative abundance varied a great deal among cases. He also isolated *B. influenzae* in 14% of colds and other infections.[31,32]

A group from the medical staff of Cook County Hospital in Chicago undertook a careful study using 3,000 blood agar culture plates and procedures that they held should have detected *B. influenzae*, if it were present. They found that Pfeiffer's bacillus was present in only a small number of cases: in only 4% of cultures made from washed sputum samples and in only 8.7% of postmortem lung cultures. They did find the organism in near pure culture in the lungs of a soldier who had died of influenzal pneumonia. They regarded Pfeiffer's bacillus as the cause of that case of pneumonia. They found that pneumococci were the most common organisms isolated in this study, appearing in 70% of sputum cultures and in 38% of throat swab cultures. Type IV pneumococci were isolated in 50% of lung cultures made at autopsy. Types I–III were all also present but at lesser frequencies.[33]

By early 1919, evidence was running more strongly against Pfeiffer's bacillus. In February, David Davis, employing strict morphological and culture criteria, reported that he had succeeded in isolating what he identified as *B. influenzae* in only 8% of 62 cases of influenza he studied. As noted, he had earlier isolated this organism in higher percentages of cases of measles, varicella, tuberculosis, and pertussis. There was no doubt, he argued, that Pfeiffer's bacillus was pathogenic for humans. He had isolated it from the spinal fluid in all cases of meningitis accompanying bronchopneumonia where *B. influenzae* was also present in pure or nearly pure culture. He concluded that whatever the cause of influenza might be, its most serious features were due to secondary invaders including streptococci, pneumococci, and *B. influenzae.*[34] Frederick Lord and colleagues at Boston reached similar conclusions. Like Davis, Lord had already isolated *B. influenzae* from diseases other than influenza. In this pandemic, he and his colleagues isolated organisms resembling Pfeiffer's bacillus in 84% of 38 hospitalized influenza cases, but also in 41% of the throats of members of the Harvard Students' Army Training Corps, who had no record of illness for the previous three months. Lord concluded that *B. influenzae* should be regarded as a part of the normal flora of the human throat, but that there was no way to be certain whether the organisms found in normal throats and in other diseases with similar morphology and culture and staining characteristics were really identical to those found in influenza.[35]

There remained, it seemed, a possibility that would clarify recent bacteriological findings and still rescue a place for Pfeiffer's bacillus in the etiology of influenza. Perhaps, as would prove to be the case with diphtheria, there was a pseudo-influenza bacillus or different strains of *B. influenzae,* not all of which caused influenza. In that case, the finding of organisms morphologically identical to Pfeiffer's bacillus in other diseases was not evidence against the role of Pfeiffer's bacillus in influenza.

Several researchers investigated this possibility by trying to type strains of Pfeiffer's bacillus, but their findings did little to buttress faith in *B. influenzae's* role in influenza. F.H. Rapoport, a naval medical officer from Chelsea, Massachusetts, employed the complement fixation test for antibodies to *B. influenzae* in convalescent sera from cases of influenzal pneumonia and from normal control sera. He concluded that specific antibodies against Pfeiffer's bacillus were formed during convalescence from pneumonia accompanying influenza, but that these had weak complement-binding properties. He could not determine whether one or more strains of Pfeiffer's bacillus were circulating during the epidemic, although he observed that polyvalent antigens in his samples gave no better results than did monovalent ones.[36]

Park and his associates studied cultures taken from 100 cases of influenza. In some cases, cultures were taken repeatedly over time. Careful antigen typing showed that there was a large variety of types of *B. influenzae,* that the organisms taken from an individual were quite stable over time, but that there were differences among the many types isolated from different individuals. He suggested that, like pneumococcus, *B. influenzae* had over the years in the throats of healthy carriers altered into distinct types. Pfeiffer's bacillus in cases of influenza, he concluded, must be regarded as a secondary invader.[29] (p. 320–1)

ALTERNATIVE ETIOLOGIES, OTHER VACCINES

Other candidates had been proposed as the cause of influenza during the pandemic, but these were disposed of rather quickly. An Army medical officer, Captain George Mathers, who died of influenza during his investigation, isolated and characterized a streptococcus that produced a green color on blood agar plates. At Fort Mead, he isolated his green-producing streptococcus from 87% of influenza and pneumonia cases, while he was able to isolate Pfeiffer's bacillus in only 58% of these cases.[37]

The Mathers streptococcus attracted some attention during the early months of the pandemic. Jordan, for example, systematically looked for it in his study but found no evidence that made it seem a more probable cause than *B. influenzae.* Then, in both Europe and America, investigators considered the possibility that influenza might be caused by a filterable virus.[34] (p. 148–9) At issue was the disputed finding that influenza could be caused in humans by inoculation of material from the noses or throats of influenza patients that had been passed through a bacterial filter. French and Japanese investigators had reported succeeding

Eyler- 2010 - Public Health Reports - Supp 3 Vol 25, 27-36

in transferring influenza by this method.[38,39] American researchers failed to confirm these findings. The researchers from Cook County Hospital used this method to inoculate seven human volunteers without causing disease. They did the same with cultures made from the lungs of influenza pneumonia victims and inoculated two Rhesus monkeys with similar results.[33] (p. 1564–5) Other laboratory and human inoculation experiments aimed at detecting a filterable virus were also negative.[40,41] These negative findings were also confirmed by extensive human experiments with influenza sponsored by the U.S. Navy and the U.S. Public Health Service.

As confidence in the role of Pfeiffer's bacillus in influenza waned, the strategy of prevention by vaccine changed. Vaccines developed later in the pandemic—and almost all developed in the middle of the country and on the West Coast—were composed of other organisms either singly or in mixtures. Increasingly, vaccines were justified as preventing the pneumonias that accompanied influenza. Killed streptococci vaccines were developed by a physician in Denver and by the medical staff of the Puget Sound Naval Yard.[42,43] The latter was used among sailors and also among civilians in Seattle.

Mixed vaccines were more common. These typically contained pneumococci and streptococci. Sometimes staphylococci, Pfeiffer's bacillus, and even unidentified organisms recently isolated in the ward or morgue were included.[44-47] The most widely used, and historically the most interesting, was the vaccine produced by Edward C. Rosenow of the Mayo Clinic's Division of Experimental Bacteriology.[48,49] Rosenow argued that the exact composition of a vaccine intended to prevent pneumonia had to match the distribution of the lung-infecting microbes then in circulation. For that reason, he insisted that the composition of his vaccine had to be frequently readjusted. His initial vaccine consisted of killed bacteria in these proportions: 30% pneumococci types I, II, and III; 30% pneumococci type IV and a "green-producing diplostreptococcus;" 20% hemolytic streptococci; 10% staphylococcus aureus; and 10% *B. influenzae.* He later dropped Pfeiffer's bacillus entirely. The Mayo Clinic distributed Rosenow's vaccine widely to physicians in the upper Midwest. No one seems to know for sure how many people received this vaccine, but, through physicians, Rosenow received returns for 93,000 people who had received all three injections, 23,000 who had received two injections, and 27,000 who had received one.[49] (p. 398) Rosenow's vaccine received even wider distribution. It was adopted by the City of Chicago. The Laboratories of the Chicago Health Department produced more than 500,000 doses

of the vaccine. Some of it was distributed to Chicago physicians and the rest was turned over to the state health department for use throughout Illinois.[50] (p. 116–23)[51,52]

VACCINE CONTROVERSY AND STANDARDS FOR VACCINE TRIALS

As was the case with Pfeiffer's bacillus vaccines, most of the early reports on the use of these mixed vaccines indicated they were effective. Readers of American medical journals in 1918 and for much of 1919 were thus faced with the strange circumstance that all vaccines, regardless of their composition, their mode of administration, or the circumstances in which they were tested, were held to prevent influenza or influenzal pneumonia. Something was clearly wrong. The medical profession had at the time no consensus on what constituted a valid vaccine trial, and it could not determine whether these vaccines did any good at all. The lack of agreed-upon standards was exacerbated by the informal editorial procedures and the absence of peer review in scientific publication in 1918. During the pandemic of 1918–1919, the profession was forced to develop standards for vaccine trials.[53] Park and George McCoy, director of the Hygienic Laboratory of the Public Health Service, led the assault pointing out the fallacies in design or inference of current reports. Most trials began after the first cases of influenza had appeared locally, often after the epidemic peak had passed, and hence the most susceptible may already have been attacked and could not appear in the vaccinated group, and the more resistant were likely to be assigned to the vaccinated group. Little effort was usually made to minimize selection bias in assignments to experimental or control arms or to match each group by age, sex, and exposure. And too many trials operated with poor observation and imperfect data collection.[54,55] (p. 103)

McCoy arranged his own trial of the Rosenow vaccine produced by the Laboratories of the Chicago Health Department. He and his associates worked in a mental asylum in California where they could keep all subjects under close observation. They immunized alternate patients younger than age 41 on every ward, completing the last immunization 11 days before the local outbreak began. Under these more controlled conditions, Rosenow's vaccine offered no protection whatsoever. McCoy's article appeared as a one-column report in the December 14, 1918, edition of the *Journal of the American Medical Association* (*JAMA*).[56]

At the meeting of the American Public Health Association (APHA) later that month, McCoy and Park

Eyler- 2010 - Public Health Reports - Supp 3 Vol 25, 27-36

used their positions on the Executive Sub-committee on the Bacteriology of the 1918 Epidemic of Influenza to issue a manifesto that appeared in APHA's "Working Program against Influenza."[57] APHA declared that because the cause of influenza was unknown, there was no logical basis for a vaccine to prevent the disease. There was a logical basis for believing that a vaccine to prevent the secondary infections might be developed, but there was no evidence that any of the vaccines currently available were effective. The association then specified the criteria that a trial must meet, if its conclusions were to be valid. There must be a control group, the association specified, and the vaccinated and the control group must be equal in size. The relative susceptibilities of the two groups must be equivalent as determined by age, sex, and prior exposure. Their degree of exposure must be of equal duration and intensity, and should take place during the same phase of the epidemic.[57] (p. 3)

The reformers' campaign had an impact. Following its publication—although the basic design faults of many trials remained—some authors now acknowledged shortcomings in their data or qualified their conclusions, and a few cited APHA's new standards as authoritative.[55] (p. 418-9) By the beginning of 1919, Rosenow, the most vocal defender of vaccines, found himself on the defensive. During the discussion of his paper at APHA's annual meeting, he faced hostile comments from both McCoy and Victor Vaughan.[58] (p. 2098-100) The next month, *JAMA* ran an anonymous critical editorial accompanying his first article on the use of his vaccine.[59] Perhaps the best evidence that professional standards were changing is found in two studies sponsored by the Metropolitan Life Insurance Company during the 1919-1920 influenza season. Both were unprecedented in the influenza literature in the care taken in trial design and analysis. Park and his associate, Anna Von Sholly, studied the use of two mixed vaccines among the employees of the home office of Met Life.[55] Edwin Jordan and W.B. Sharp studied the effects of a single mixed vaccine in three residential schools and two large mental hospitals in Illinois.[60] While adhering to the standards APHA had set forth, both studies concluded the vaccines used were ineffective.

EPIDEMIOLOGICAL STUDIES

American epidemiologists also devoted much attention to the 1918-1919 pandemic. Some of their studies—such as the substantial study on the epidemic in Connecticut by Winslow and Rogers,[61] or the study of

trends from 1910 to 1918 that W.H. Frost prepared for the Public Health Service,[62] or Raymond Pearl's statistical analysis of the epidemic curves of major American cities[63]—were large-scale studies based on mass mortality data. Some of the more illuminating, however, were smaller-scale studies in which chains of transmission could be traced and incubation periods estimated in small, isolated populations such as inmates in a prison[64] or residents on a small island.[65] Among the most important were studies that acknowledged that accurate information on cases of influenza, rather than simply influenza and pneumonia deaths, was both lacking and critically important. The Public Health Service made a major effort to obtain records of illness through household surveys it conducted in 10 communities across the nation in which it was already doing research.[66,67] A more intensive study was undertaken by Warren T. Vaughan in a population of 10,000 in six carefully chosen districts in Boston during the 1920 flu season.[68] He also obtained information retrospectively on household illness during 1918-1919.

This epidemiological research confirmed many of the findings from 1889-1890 about pandemic influenza's rapid spread, explosive local outbreaks, and very high morbidity rates. Frost's analysis of the household returns show a range of local influenza morbidity rates ran from 150 to 530 cases per 1,000, although both he and Vaughan concluded that 200 per 1,000 was more typical for 1918-1919.[66,68] (p. 588) (p. 142) Those enormously high rates of incidence explained how a disease with case fatality rates these authors found to range from 0.8% to 3.1% could cause so many deaths.[66,68] (p. 593) (p. 165) These studies also showed that differences in case fatality rates were more important than differences in incidence rates in explaining the age group mortality patterns, including the high death rates among young adults during the pandemic.[66] (p. 588-96)

Vaughan was unusual in paying attention to the question of population immunity. Although the cause of influenza must have been widely distributed in his districts in 1918-1919, some people showed remarkable resistance to the disease. Fifty-five percent of those in his study groups who shared a bed with an influenza victim during the pandemic escaped the disease. He argued that the patterns of incidence and death during the 1918-1919 pandemic could not be explained by immunity acquired during the pandemic of 1889-1890, and he suggested, perhaps more sagaciously than he realized, that understanding of herd immunity would be the key to understanding the epidemiology of influenza. If measles produced no lasting immunity, he

Eyler- 2010 - Public Health Reports - Supp 3 Vol 25, 27-36

SCIENCE, MICROBIOLOGY, AND VACCINES IN 1918 ◊ 35

pointed out, its outbreaks in cities would be as explosive as those of the great pandemic of 1918–1919.[68] (p. 209–10, 230–2)

Perhaps the most interesting epidemiological studies conducted during the 1918–1919 pandemic were the human experiments conducted by the Public Health Service and the U.S. Navy under the supervision of Milton Rosenau on Gallops Island, the quarantine station in Boston Harbor, and on Angel Island, its counterpart in San Francisco. The experiment began with 100 volunteers from the Navy who had no history of influenza. Rosenau was the first to report on the experiments conducted at Gallops Island in November and December 1918.[69] His first volunteers received first one strain and then several strains of Pfeiffer's bacillus by spray and swab into their noses and throats and then into their eyes. When that procedure failed to produce disease, others were inoculated with mixtures of other organisms isolated from the throats and noses of influenza patients. Next, some volunteers received injections of blood from influenza patients. Finally, 13 of the volunteers were taken into an influenza ward and exposed to 10 influenza patients each. Each volunteer was to shake hands with each patient, to talk with him at close range, and to permit him to cough directly into his face. None of the volunteers in these experiments developed influenza. Rosenau was clearly puzzled, and he cautioned against drawing conclusions from negative results. He ended his article in *JAMA* with a telling acknowledgement: "We entered the outbreak with a notion that we knew the cause of the disease, and were quite sure we knew how it was transmitted from person to person. Perhaps, if we have learned anything, it is that we are not quite sure what we know about the disease."[69] (p. 313)

The research conducted at Angel Island and that continued in early 1919 in Boston broadened this research by inoculating with the Mathers streptococcus and by including a search for filter-passing agents, but it produced similar negative results.[70-72] It seemed that what was acknowledged to be one of the most contagious of communicable diseases could not be transferred under experimental conditions.

THE PANDEMIC AND BIOMEDICAL KNOWLEDGE

While the experience of the great pandemic of 1918–1919 had given American medical researchers a heightened appreciation of the dangers of pandemic influenza, and while it permitted epidemiologists to enlarge the fund of descriptive information on influenza outbreaks, it had done little to unlock the mysteries of the disease. If anything, the experience of 1918–1919 served to deconstruct existing biomedical knowledge.

This void in fundamental knowledge would not be filled soon. When Jordan published his massive, 500-page authoritative synthesis of the influenza literature in 1927, the most basic and fundamental features of influenza were still unexplained. Jordan told his readers that influenza could only be defined by its pattern of occurrence—its epidemiology. Its cause was unknown, and its pathology was indefinite. It was uncertain whether there was acquired immunity for influenza, and, if there was, how long it lasted. Why pandemics occurred when they did and why they spared some places were also unknown. It was also uncertain whether the disease called influenza that occurred every year in sporadic cases and small outbreaks was the same disease that circulated in the pandemics. He continued the practice of distinguishing "influenza" from "epidemic influenza."[73]

Jordan did suggest that changes in virulence of the still unknown agent of influenza might be important and that this agent might be filterable, but in 1927 these were still speculations for which there was no direct evidence. In short, the three decades that had passed since Leichtenstern published his major synthesis had seen remarkably little addition to the fund of basic scientific knowledge of influenza, in spite of concerted efforts by researchers employing the best available research tools.

REFERENCES

1. Parsons F. Report on the influenza epidemic of 1889–90 [C.—6387]. London: HMSO; 1891. p. 324.
2. Leichtenstern OML. Influenza and dengue. Vienna: A. Hölder; 1896. p. 222. (Northnagel H, editor. Specielle Pathologie und Therapie; Band 4)
3. Leichtenstern OML. Influenza. In: Mannaberg J, Leichtenstern OML. Malaria, influenza, and dengue. Ross R, Stephens JWW, Grünbaum AS, editors. Stengel A, translator. Philadelphia/London: W.B. Saunders; 1905. p. 523–719.
4. Osler W. Influenza. Principles and practice of medicine. 2nd ed. New York: D. Appleton; 1895: p. 92–4.
5. Osler W. Influenza. Principles and practice of medicine. 8th ed. New York: D. Appleton; 1912. p. 115–9.
6. Lord FT. Influenza. In: Modern medicine: its theory and practice. Vol. 2. Osler W, McCrae T, editors. Philadelphia/New York: Lea Brothers; 1907. p. 469–88.
7. Allbutt TC. Influenza: introduction. Practitioner 1907;78:1–10.
8. Pfeiffer R. Vorläufige Mitheilungen über die Erreger der Influenza. Deutsche med. Wchschr 1892;18:28.
9. Pfeiffer R. Die Aeteiologie der Influenza. Ztschr. f. Hyg. u. Infektionskr 1893;13:357–86.
10. Davis DJ. The bacteriology of whooping cough. J Infect Dis 1906;3:1–37.
11. Emery WD'E. The micro-organisms of influenza. Practitioner 1907;78:109–17.
12. Hansen B. New images of a new medicine: visual evidence for the widespread popularity of therapeutic discoveries in America after 1885. Bull Hist Med 1999;73:629–78.

Eyler- 2010 - Public Health Reports - Supp 3 Vol 25, 27-36

36 ◇ The Science of Influenza

13. Haythorn SR. The prevention of epidemic influenza with special reference to vaccine prophylaxis. Studies on epidemic influenza comprising clinical and laboratory investigations by members of the faculty of the School of Medicine, University of Pittsburgh. Pittsburgh: University of Pittsburgh Medical School; 1919. p. 97–153.

14. 903 new cases of grip reported yesterday—use of vaccine not new. New York Times 1918 Oct 3:24.

15. Grip in the Y.M.C.A. checked by vaccine. New York Times 1918 Oct 17:9.

16. Bonime E. Tuberculin and vaccine in tubercular affections: a practical guide for the utilization of the immune response in general practice. Troy (NY): Southworth; 1917. p. 267.

17. Copeland sees grip on the wane here. New York Times 1918 Oct 25:22.

18. Tells of vaccine to stop influenza. New York Times 1918 Oct 2:10.

19. Park WH. Bacteriology and possibility of antiInfluenza vaccine as a prophylactic. N Y Med J 1918;108:621.

20. Leary T. The use of influenza vaccine in the present epidemic. Am J Public Health 1918;8:754-5, 768.

21. Duval CW, Harris WH. The antigenic property of the Pfeiffer bacillus as related to its value in the prophylaxis of epidemic influenza. J Immunology 1919;4:317-30.

22. Greeley H. Vaccine as a prophylactic against influenza, and local reaction as a guide to immunity. Med Rec 1919;96:624-7.

23. Big firms take up fight on influenza. New York Times 1918 Oct 23:8.

24. Hinton WA, Kane ES. Use of influenza vaccine as a prophylactic—an experimental study conducted by the Massachusetts State Department of Health. J Tennessee State Med Assn 1918-19;11:442-6.

25. Barnes HL. The prophylactic value of Leary's vaccine. JAMA 1918;71:1899.

26. Hawes JB. Experience of Massachusetts State sanatoria for tuberculosis during the recent influenza epidemic. Boston Med Surg J 1919;180:35-7.

27. Wallace GL. Report of the influenza epidemic and experience in the use of the influenza vaccine "B" at the Wrentham State School, Wrentham, Mass. Boston Med Surg J 1919;180:447-48.

28. The factor of technique in the detection of the influenza bacillus. Public Health Rep 1919;34:1973.

29. Park WH. Bacteriology of recent pandemic of influenza and complicating infections. JAMA 1919;73:318-21.

30. Keegan JJ. The prevailing pandemic of influenza. JAMA 1918;71:1051-5.

31. Jordan EO. Observations on the bacteriology of influenza. Public Health Rep 1919;34:1413-25.

32. Jordan EO. Observations on the bacteriology of influenza. J Infect Dis 1919;25:28-40.

33. Nuzum JW, Pilot I, Stangl FH, Bonar BE. Pandemic influenza and pneumonia in a large civil hospital. JAMA 1918;71:1562-5.

34. Davis DJ. The bacteriology of influenza. Proc Inst Med Path 1919;2:142-50.

35. Lord FT, Scott AC Jr, Nye RN. Relation of influenza bacillus to the recent epidemic of influenza. JAMA 1919;72:188-90.

36. Rapoport FH. The complement fixation test in influenzal pneumonia: studies with serum from convalescent patients, the influenza bacillus being used as antigen. JAMA 1919;72:683-6.

37. Tunnicliff R. Phagocytic experiments in influenza. JAMA 1918;71:1783-4.

38. Nicolle C, Lebailly C. Recherches expérimentales sur la grippe. Ann De l'Inst Pasteur 1919;33:395-402.

39. Yamanouchi T, Sakakami K, Iwashima S. The infecting agent in influenza: an experimental research. Lancet 1919;1:971.

40. Branham SE, Hall IC. Attempts to cultivate filterable viruses from cases of influenza and common colds. J Infect Dis 1921;28:143-9.

41. Wahl HR, White GB, Lyall HW. Some experiments on the transmission of influenza. J Infect Dis 1919;25:419-26.

42. Katzman M. Influenza vaccination at the Denver City and County Hospital. Colorado Med 1919;16:121-3.

43. Ely CF, Lloyd BJ, Hitchcock CD, Nickson DH. Influenza as seen at the Puget Sound Naval Navy Yard. JAMA 1919;72:24-8.

44. Minaker AJ, Irvine RS. Prophylactic use of mixed vaccine against pandemic influenza and its complications at the Naval Training Station, San Francisco. JAMA 1919;72:847-50.

45. Watters WH. Vaccines in influenza. Boston Med Surg J 1919;181:727-31.

46. Stone WB. A prophylactic vaccine against the so-called Spanish influenza. Med Rec 1918;94:979-80.

47. Kolmer JH. The value of active immunization with vaccine virus against influenza. Med Rec 1918;94:919.

48. Rosenow EC. Prophylactic inoculation against respiratory infections during the present pandemic of influenza. Preliminary report. JAMA 1919;72:31-4.

49. Rosenow EC, Sturdivant BF. Studies in influenza and pneumonia. IV. Further results of prophylactic inoculations. JAMA 1919;73:396-401.

50. Report of an epidemic of influenza in Chicago during the fall of 1918. Report and handbook of the Department of Health of the City of Chicago, 1911–1918 inclusive. Chicago: Chicago Department of Health; 1919. p. 40–150.

51. Illinois Influenza Commission. Letter to the medical profession 1918 Oct 23. Ludvig Hektoen Papers, Box 5, Folder 3, Special Collections Research Center, University of Chicago Library.

52. Illinois Influenza Commission. Letter to the medical profession 1918 Oct 24. Ludvig Hektoen Papers, Box 5, Folder 3, Special Collections Research Center, University of Chicago Library.

53. Eyler JM. The fog of research: influenza vaccine trials during the 1918–19 pandemic. J Hist Med 2009;64:401-28.

54. McCoy GW. Pitfalls in determining the prophylactic or curative value of bacterial vaccines. Public Health Rep 1919;34:1193-5.

55. Von Sholly AI, Park WH. Report on the prophylactic vaccination of 1536 persons against acute respiratory diseases, 1919–20. J Immunology 1921;6:103-15.

56. McCoy GW, Murray VB, Teeter AL. The failure of a bacterial vaccine as a prophylactic against influenza. JAMA 1918;71:1997.

57. A working program against influenza. Am J Public Health 1919;9:1-13.

58. American Public Health Association. JAMA 1918;71:2097-100, 2173-7.

59. Prophylactic inoculation against influenza. JAMA 1919;72:44-5.

60. Jordan EO, Sharp WB. Effect of vaccination against influenza and some other respiratory infections. J Infect Dis 1921;28:357-66.

61. Winslow C-EA, Rogers JF. Statistics of the 1918 epidemic of influenza in Connecticut. J Infect Dis 1920;26:185-216.

62. Frost WH. The epidemiology of influenza. JAMA 1919;73:313-38.

63. Pearl R. On certain general statistical aspects of the 1918 epidemic in American cities. Public Health Rep 1919;34:1743-83.

64. Stanley LL. Influenza at San Quentin Prison, California. Public Health Rep 1919;34:996-1008.

65. Armstrong C. An epidemiological study of the 1920 epidemic of influenza in an isolated rural community. Public Health Rep 1921;36:1671-702.

66. Frost WH. Statistics of influenza morbidity with special reference to certain factors in case incidence and case fatality. Public Health Rep 1920;35:584-97.

67. Frost WH, Sydenstricker E. Influenza in Maryland: preliminary statistics of certain localities. Public Health Rep 1919;34:491-504.

68. Vaughan WT. Influenza: an epidemiological study. Baltimore: American Journal of Hygiene; 1921. p. 260.

69. Rosenau MJ. Experiments to determine mode of spread of influenza. JAMA 1919;73:311-3.

70. Rosenau MJ, Keegan WJ, Goldberger J. Experiments upon volunteers to determine the cause and mode of spread of influenza, Boston, November and December, 1918. USPHS Hygienic Lab Bull 1921;123:5-41.

71. McCoy GW, Richey DW. Experiments upon volunteers to determine the cause and mode of spread of influenza, San Francisco, November and December, 1918. USPHS Hygienic Lab Bull 1921;123:42-53.

72. Rosenau MJ, Keegan WJ, Richey DW, McCoy GW, Goldberger J, Leake JP, et al. Experiments upon volunteers to determine the cause and mode of spread of influenza, Boston, February and March, 1919. USPHS Hygienic Lab Bull 1921;123:54-99.

73. Jordan ED. Epidemic influenza. Chicago: American Medical Association; 1927.

Cadham – The Lancet – May 29 1919 885-6

THE USE OF A VACCINE IN THE RECENT EPIDEMIC OF INFLUENZA.

BY F. T. CADHAM, M.D.,
MAJOR, C.A.M.C.

IT was in the first week of October, 1918, that cases of the pandemic influenza occurred in Winnipeg—that is, the first cases recognised as typical of the disease. The epidemic progressed rapidly, it reached its peak in the second week in November, and then slowly but gradually subsided.

With the knowledge that the disease was to reach us, methods were considered of combating it. The information to be derived at the time was meagre. Quarantine and isolation methods appeared uncertain in effect and the value of prophylactic methods was not established. It seemed, however, to be an outstanding feature that infections of the respiratory tract were coincident with the disease and accounted largely for the mortality. It was considered advisable to use a vaccine prepared from micro-organisms infecting the respiratory tract of those suffering from the disease, as a prophylactic against respiratory infection.

Bacteriology.

Naso-pharyngeal.—Naso-pharyngeal swabs were taken from 123 cases at different stages of the disease. Direct smears were made and stained, and cultures were made on hæmoglobin-agar. The following were the predominant bacteria found : Streptococcus, 106 cases ; pneumococcus, 18 cases ; B. influenzæ, 23 cases ; Friedländer's bacillus, 6 cases ; staphylococcus, 24 cases.

Sputum.—Smears made from the sputum of 18 cases showed a Gram-positive diplostreptococcus in 16. Cultures from sputum taken from 6 patients suffering from pneumonia showed in 5 a diplostreptococcus, and in 1 a streptococcus and pneumococcus. Free expectoration in the cases of pneumonia that developed in the military was uncommon.

Empyema.—Examination of the pus from 5 cases of empyema showed in 4 streptococcus, and in the fifth a streptococcus and a pneumococcus.

Blood cultures.—Positive findings were obtained in 4 out of 22 blood cultures. These 4 showed a characteristic diplostreptococcus ; 2 of these positive cases were in the acute stages, 1 was a case complicated by pneumonia, and in 1 the culture was positive ten days after the acute symptoms had subsided. This patient had developed a phlebitis in the leg. The blood was collected in a vacuum tube with a culture medium of 1 per cent. glucose bouillon, to which had been added 2 per cent. sterile sheep's serum.

Post-mortem.—A streptococcus was found in the lungs and blood of one case, and a pneumococcus and staphylococcus in the lungs of another.

Fæces.—In the examination of the fæces of 8 cases a diplostreptococcus similar to that found in the pharynx was isolated in 4.

In August, previous to the outbreak of recognised cases of influenza, there had occurred at the Tuxedo Military Hospital 2 cases of pneumonia, followed by empyema. I now believe from a study of their history these cases to have been originally influenza. At the time a pure culture of streptococcus was obtained from the pus of both these cases. A small amount of vaccine was made from this culture, and four of the members of the laboratory staff were inoculated. Examination in two of those inoculated showed increased opsonic index for this streptococcus. This increased opsonic index persisted for four months in one case in which the examinations were continued.

The predominant micro-organism thus found has been a streptococcus or diplostreptococcus. This is a Gram-positive streptococcus appearing in either short or long chains. It is pleomorphic. The same micro-organism will appear at different intervals of cultivation as either a streptococcus or diplostreptococcus. No capsule was demonstrated. It is hæmolytic on first cultivation, but loses this power on subcultivation. Cultivated for some days in serum-glucose bouillon it assumes a lanceolate shape. It forms discrete colonies on hæmoglobin agar and confluent colonies on agar to which the blood had been added at 80° C. Grown in serum-glucose bouillon it forms a diffuse cloud. It coagulates litmus milk with acid formation in 72 hours and ferments lactose. It does not ferment inulin. The agglutination

reactions with Types I., II., and III. antipneumococcus serums were negative.

Preparation of the Vaccine.

For the use of members of the C.E.F. a vaccine was prepared as follows :—The strain of streptococcus obtained from an empyema that occurred in August was added to two strains of streptococci obtained from the naso-pharynx of soldiers who arrived from the East suffering from the disease on Oct. 1st, 1918. From time to time strains of streptococci were added ; these were taken from the naso-pharynx and one strain from blood culture and one from the lungs post mortem. One strain from the pharynx gave cultural characteristics of the *Streptococcus viridans.*

The streptococci were grown in 1 per cent. glucose bouillon to which 2 per cent. of laked sterile sheep's blood had been added. Strains of pneumococci were obtained from the naso-pharynx and sputum of the cases at the same time and grown in similar media. A strain corresponding to Type No. III. was not obtained. After 18 hours' incubation the cultures were centrifuged in deep tubes at high speed for half an hour. The supernatant fluid was poured off and the bacterial deposit of the tubes was diluted with normal saline and pooled. A dilution was made of the streptococci to give 1800 million per c.cm. and dilution of the pneumococci to give 900 million per c.cm. as by hæmocytometer count.

The influenza bacillus obtained from the naso-pharynx of the first cases to arrive was used ; it was grown in flasks of solid media. Hæmoglobin agar was made by adding 20 c.cm. of sterile sheep's blood to 1 litre of agar at a temperature of 80° C. This did not make a slightly medium, but the influenza bacillus grew freely on it. The flasks were incubated two days before using to test sterility. The culture was carried in Löffler's blood serum tubes to which had been added 2 c.cm. of serum glucose bouillon, the contents of one tube sufficed to seed a flask. Cultivation was carried out for 24 hours at 37·5° C. The growth was washed off with normal saline and filtered through sterile gauze. It was centrifuged and the bacterial deposit pooled and diluted with a normal saline solution, to give a count of 1200 million per c.cm. This was judged by the turbidity of a standard suspension. The saline suspensions of the streptococci, pneumococci, and influenza bacillus were mixed in equal parts, and 0·2 per cent. trikresol added. After bottling in rubber-capped, sterile bottles, the vaccine was sterilised for a half-hour at 60° C. Sterility was tested by inoculation of media and guinea-pigs.

The dose was 0·5 c.cm., containing approximately 300 million streptococci, 300 million influenza bacilli, and 150 million pneumococci. Preliminary inoculations were carried out on the staff of the laboratory to determine size and interval of doses.

Inoculations.

With the permission of Major-General Fotheringham, C.M.G., D.G.M.S., the soldiers of the district were inoculated under the direction of Colonel Webster, A.D.M:S. The inoculation was voluntary.

The first inoculations were given on Oct. 20th, 1918, and a second inoculation seven days later. There were some 7600 soldiers in the district at the time and 4842 were inoculated once ; about half of these were inoculated twice. In anticipation of an outbreak there had been established a special military hospital for the purpose of receiving such influenza cases as might develop. This hospital was under the charge of Captain D. A. Macdonald, C.A.M.C.

From Oct. 1st, 1918, to Feb. 28th, 1919, 520 soldiers were admitted to this hospital suffering from the disease.

Clinical Diagnosis.

The onset was, as a rule, sudden. The soldiers complained of general depression. In all the cases there was an initial chill or chilly sensations. Pains in the back and legs were common and more severe on the second day. Headache was a direct initial symptom, especially so in the latter stages of the epidemic. Sore-throat was a common complaint. The throat was dry and congested. A dusky appearance of the face and congestion of the conjunctiva were common. Some cases exhibited a coryza. A loose cough developed with the disease. Nose-bleed occurred in about one-third of the cases. In all cases the temperature rose rapidly to at least 101° F. The pulse-rate was from 90 to 120.

Cadham – The Lancet – May 29 1919 885-6

886   THE LANCET.]   MR. J. P. WILLIAMS: BLACKWATER FEVER.   [MAY 24, 1919

Statistics of the Hospital.

Of the 520 cases admitted, 282 had been inoculated with the vaccine and 238 were uninoculated. There was a total of 58 cases of pneumonia and 22 deaths. Among 282 inoculated 17 developed pneumonia and 5 died. Of the 5 that died 3 had received their first inoculation on the day they were admitted to the hospital. One developed the disease three days subsequent to the first inoculation and 1 ten days subsequent. The latter soldier was suffering from tubercular glands of the neck.

No soldier died who had been admitted subsequent to the second inoculation.

Among the 238 admitted who had not been inoculated with the vaccine there occurred 41 cases of pneumonia and 17 deaths.

TABLE I.—*Report of Military Hospital for Influenza.*

—	Admissions.	Pneumonia.	Deaths.
Inoculated	282	17 ... 6·05 %	5* ... 1·7 %
Uninoculated ...	238	41 ... 17·1 %	17 ... 7·1 %

* Of these 5, 3 received their first inoculation on day of admission.

Captain D. A. Macdonald states that the disease and complications were not so severe in the inoculated. The average stay in the hospital of a patient was twice as long for the uninoculated as for the inoculated.

The cases came from the troops in the district, except for 40 cases which were taken from troop trains passing through Winnipeg. The troops were quartered in barracks throughout the city, in military hospitals, and some at their homes. Cases developed in all quarters.

The inoculations were carried out two weeks previous to the peak of the epidemic in the city. The incidence of admissions into the hospital followed closely the curve of the epidemic in the city.

Conditions of exposure were practically the same in all the barracks, and were no different for the inoculated and the uninoculated, except in the 40 cases which developed the disease on troop trains. Both the inoculated and uninoculated were admitted to the hospital at all stages of the epidemic.

A quarantine was placed on the barracks following the placing of a ban on public gatherings in the city. As the business of the district required to be carried on absolute quarantine was not considered. Cases developed in all barracks and the military hospitals irrespective of the quarantine. The quarantine was lifted a week before Christmas and the men allowed leave. They scattered through all the infected districts of the city and province, with no increase in the incidence of influenza among them.

Inoculations in the Civilian Population.

Under the direction of Dr. Gordon Bell, chairman of the Manitoba Provincial Board of Health, there were prepared in the same laboratory 600,000 doses of vaccine for the use of civilian practitioners. This was supplemented by 100,000 doses prepared by Dr. Boyd, pathologist of the Winnipeg General Hospital. The vaccine was distributed to physicians of Winnipeg and throughout the West.

Approximately one-quarter of this vaccine was prepared as before stated; the balance contained strains of bacteria as obtained from Dr. E. C. Rosenow, of the Mayo Clinic, Rochester, Ill. The dose of this vaccine was 0·5 c.cm., containing approximately 300 million pneumococci, 200 million influenza bacilli, and 150 million streptococci. A second dose was advised.

Reports were received from 108 physicians at various points in Manitoba and Saskatchewan. These reports are summarised in Table II.

To the question, "Do attacks of influenza appear to be modified if contracted following one or more injections of the vaccine?" 101 physicians out of 108 reporting replied in the affirmative. There was no definite report of the vaccine being valuable in the treatment of influenza or pneumonia.

In reply to the question, "Since influenza and pneumonia have been fatal in such large percentage of pregnant women, has vaccine apparently afforded protection?" 32 out of 37 physicians answering this question answered in the affirmative.

TABLE II.—*Incidence of Disease and Mortality in Civilian Population.*

(A) Number of persons inoculated—once, 28,815; twice, 24,184. Total, 52,999.
(B) Number of uninoculated in clientele of physicians reporting, 85,941.

Incidence of—	(A) Inoculated.			(B) Uninoculated.
	After first inoculation.	After second inoculation.	Total.	
Influenza ...	2843, 9·7%	2360, 9·7%	5203, 9·8%	21,285, 24·8%
Pneumonia.	177, 0·65%	133, 0·60%	300, 0·57%	1869, 2·2%
Deaths ...	61, 0·21%	24, 0·09%	85, 0·16%	563, 0·66%

The majority of these inoculations were given in the earlier stages of the epidemic, but no attempt was made to keep accurate statistics on this point. The ages of those inoculated were not obtained. Due to the exigency of war the profession was depleted and all branches were forced to work under a great strain; also the people were nervous, so that it was difficult to obtain full statistics or to divide any portion of the population in two parts for the purpose of running controls.

These records, as indicated in Table II., show that the incidence of pneumonia was about four times as great, and the mortality rate was four times as great, in the uninoculated as in the inoculated.

Comment.

It is a difficult matter to estimate the value of prophylactic vaccine as used in this epidemic of so-called influenza. Bacteriological findings show that the kinds and strains of bacteria found complicating the disease vary in different districts, and even at different stages of the epidemic in the same district. The disease is known to vary in severity in localities not widely separated geographically and during different stages of the epidemic in the same localities, so that in estimating the value of a vaccine these facts should receive careful consideration.

I believe the vaccine used as a prophylactic for the military personnel of this district to have been of value. The incidence of pneumonia was less than one-half and the mortality rate less than one-third in the inoculated as compared with the uninoculated admitted to the Special Military Hospital under similar conditions. The mortality rate for the city for the period of time under consideration was 6·28 per 1000; 53·6 per cent. were males, and 75 per cent. of these were at the age known as military age. The mortality rate of the soldier in the city for the same period of time was 2·5 per 1000.

The statistics obtained from the physicians as to the use of the vaccine in civil practice appear favourable.

Winnipeg.

BLACKWATER FEVER.

BY J. P. WILLIAMS, M.R.C.S., L.R.C.P. LOND.

DURING the past four years ten cases of blackwater fever have been under my care in hospitals on the Gold Coast. The previous history of the cases showed without exception (1) that they had never taken quinine as a prophylactic according to any recognised system, although each had resided several months in an endemic area; and (2) that each of them had for some three to six months preceding the onset of blackwater fever suffered from repeated attacks of malaria, but had either "treated" themselves or neglected to carry out the instructions of their medical attendant.

Treatment.

The treatment I employed in these cases may be summed up as follows: (1) careful nursing; (2) drugs; (3) vigorous hydrotherapy; (4) precautions against heart failure, particularly during convalescence; (5) invaliding.

In addition to the ordinary four-hour temperature chart it is of great importance to keep a chart of the total volume of all fluids administered to and excreted by the patient. The urine in particular should be accurately measured and specimens of each portion passed put in a series of labelled test tubes kept where they are not visible to the patient. A blackwater case is invariably in a state of great mental anxiety, and every precaution should be taken to prevent

Leishman – The Lancet – Feb. 14 1920 366-8

366 THE LANCET,]   MAJ.-GEN. SIR W. LEISHMAN: INOCULATION AGAINST INFLUENZA.   [FEB. 14, 1920 3

Crile upheld the view that traumatic shock is due to exhaustion of brain cells by intense sensory excitation, and that such could be prevented by local anæsthesia which blocked the sensory nerves. By suitable anastomoses of blood-vessels he cross-circulated two dogs, so that the blood of each intermingled; only the animal submitted to traumatism showed the characteristic changes in the brain cells. These were produced then not by products of traumatism in the blood but by sensory excitation. Severe traumatism of the brain itself did not produce the changes in the brain cells. No shock was produced in spinal animals by traumatism of the body below the point of section of the spinal cord. Similar changes in the brain cells were produced by fear, exhaustion through excessive activity, prevention of sleep, great loss of blood.

The sub-committee of the Medical Research Committee on Shock has brought forward evidence which favours the view that shock can be brought about by absorption of a substance or substances from killed and dying tissues; thus amputation of a limb may relieve shock by putting an end to such absorption. So, too, in the case of extensive burns of the skin, shock is regarded as resulting from absorption of products of protein decomposition. Local trauma—a burn or the wheal of a cane—causes capillary flushing and œdema provoked by damaged tissue products. Noteworthy is the observation by Dale that an etherised cat can be put into the condition of shock by an injection of histamine, but not the normal cat nor one anæsthetised with nitrous oxide and oxygen. On the one hand there is the cumulative effect of two poisons, on the other the protective effect of oxygen. In the state of shock produced by the injection of histamine in the etherised cat the whole of the potentially available capillary channels become patent, the blood percolates into the network of channels as a sponge. 50 to 60 per cent. of the plasma may pass out. A constriction of the arterioles holds up the arterial pressure, but the venæ cavæ are flaccid, half empty, the portal vein flat, the filling of the heart in diastole wanes. The liver and spleen are moderately pale, but the bowels show a diffuse dusky congestion.

Shock due to Increased Imbibition.

It seems to me that shock is due to metabolic products opening up all the capillaries and increasing imbibition in all the cells of the body at the same time; such products can be evoked in the cells by violent nervous stimulation, by want of oxygen or by toxic substances in the blood. Waller finds in people of nervous temperament that the electrical resistance of the current passing between the back and palm of the hand is lowered by emotional changes of consciousness. This is probably an index of the change brought about in the imbibition forces of the cell by nervous shock. The concentration of ions on the cellular membranes and imbibition of fluid by the cells are so changed in shock, that a generalised passage of fluid into extracellular spaces and flaccidity result, with pooling of the blood in dependent parts; the consequent failure of the circulation and oxygen supply intensifies the evil.

The quick breathing set up in shock by cerebral anæmia and want of oxygen washes CO_2 out of such of the blood as continues to circulate and increases the alkalinity of the tissues which receive it—e.g., heart and brain—for the alkali, which was bound to CO_2 in the blood, is taken up by the tissues when set free. There is, then, an alkalosis and not an acidosis in shock, and the injection of sodium bicarbonate is contra-indicated. (B. Moore.) The alkalosis lessens the sensitivity of the respiratory centre, and thus air containing 2 per cent. of CO_2 acts as a stimulant and secures better oxygenation of the blood.

Injection of Bayliss's gum saline is required to fill up the blood-vessels; the colloid gum retains the necessary salts within the blood-vessels. At the same time the patient requires oxygen inhalation, which can be given most suitably in an oxygen chamber. I have constructed, and am now testing, a light, collapsible, and transportable oxygen chamber, large enough to take nurse and patient, to be used in conjunction with liquid oxygen containers, and ventilated so that no recirculation or purification of the air is required.

CONCLUSION.

In conclusion I ask you to consider not increased capillary pressure and filtration as the causes of œdema, but stagnation of flow with consequent oxygen want and increased imbibition. The result of such a shifting of ideas will, I believe, prove fruitful.

THE RESULTS OF
PROTECTIVE INOCULATION AGAINST
INFLUENZA
IN THE ARMY AT HOME, 1918-19.

BY MAJOR-GENERAL SIR WILLIAM B. LEISHMAN,
K.C.M.G., C.B., K.H.P., M.B., F.R.C.P., F.R.S.,
DIRECTOR OF PATHOLOGY, WAR OFFICE.

THE LANCET published on Oct. 26th, 1918, the proceedings of a Conference of bacteriologists, summoned by the Director-General of the Army Medical Service to consider the advisability of employing in the army a preventive vaccine against influenza. This Conference, of which I had the honour to be chairman, agreed that such a vaccine might be expected to be of service, and made recommendations as to its constitution and use. The vaccine recommended was accordingly prepared at the Royal Army Medical College, and, in certain commands, used on a considerable scale.

In view of the opinion, widely expressed in both medical and lay journals, that we are threatened with another epidemic wave of influenza, it is felt that the results obtained in the army commands at home last winter with the vaccine in question should be made known, not only because it is proposed to advocate its employment again in the army, if we should be so unfortunate as to find ourselves in the presence of a serious recrudescence of the disease, but also because the modified vaccine now in army use has, I understand, been adopted by the Ministry of Health for employment in the civil community.

The Original Formula.

The vaccine formula recommended by the Conference mentioned above was as follows:—

B. influenzæ	60 millions	
Streptococci	80 ,,	in 1 c.cm.
Pneumococci	200 ,,	

Several strains and types of each organism were used, all comparatively freshly isolated from cases of the disease. Two doses were recommended, the first 0·5 c.cm., and the second, given after 10 days' interval, 1 c.cm. The statistical results recorded below apply solely to the vaccine prepared in accordance with the above formula.

Leishman – The Lancet – Feb. 14 1920 366-8

THE LANCET,]   MAJ.-GEN. SIR W. LEISHMAN: INOCULATION AGAINST INFLUENZA.   [FEB. 14, 1920 367

As was naturally to be expected, in view of the divergent views held as to the bacteriology of the epidemic, the proposed constitution of the vaccine was subjected to a certain amount of criticism in subsequent issues of the medical press, and the points made in these communications, many of them most valuable and helpful, were duly noted. One of the principal criticisms was concerned with the dosage which had been agreed on as appropriate for the *B. influenzæ* moiety of the vaccine, it being urged that a considerably larger dose of this might be given with safety and with the prospect of an enhanced degree of immunity. In view of this, and also of the fact that, as the bacteriological experience of the epidemic extended, the ætiological rôle of Pfeiffer's bacillus came more and more into prominence, I consulted my colleagues of the original Conference afresh upon this point and found them all in agreement with an increased dose of Pfeiffer's bacillus, which I proposed should be raised from 60 millions to 400 millions in 1 c.cm., it being understood that the strains employed should not have been so cultivated or so recently derived from cases as to be unduly toxic in their action.

The Revised Formula.

The formula of the vaccine as thus revised, and as now employed in the army, is therefore :—

$$\left.\begin{array}{lr}\text{B. influenzæ} & \text{400 millions} \\ \text{Streptococci} & \text{80 ,,} \\ \text{Pneumococci} & \text{200 ,,}\end{array}\right\} \text{in 1 c.cm.}$$

From the first it was desired that every attempt should be made to secure clear statistical evidence of the results of the inoculations with the vaccine, and the necessary instructions to this effect were circulated by the War Office, returns in accordance with a simple *pro formâ* being called for at regular intervals. In theory such clear evidence should have been easy to collect through the workings of official machinery ; in practice it has been very difficult. Only those familiar with the strain thrown on the medical personnel by the addition of a severe and widespread epidemic to the already sufficiently arduous labours of those days of urgent and wholesale demobilisation can appreciate the difficulties of collecting and recording, in accurate detail, the information required for the returns. In spite of these difficulties, which, unfortunately, vitiated some of the returns, a considerable number of inoculations were carried out, and the records were received and analysed at the War Office.

Although it is very far from my intention to make any claim that the figures presented below are conclusive and free from all or even, in some cases, from possibly large fallacies, they serve, I think, to show at least the general trend of the inoculation results, and they have encouraged the hope that, with the larger dose of Pfeiffer's organism now employed, the vaccine, should it be needed, may prove a powerful reinforcement to other measures of protection.

Explanation of the Table.

A few words are called for in explanation of the table. The individual returns are shown under the name of the unit or the principal station in or near which the soldiers in question were located. The period covered by each return is shown in a separate column. The "strength" is the "average strength" of the unit or station ; no other method was possible in view of the fluctuations of the population. The "inoculated" include those inoculated before the period in question, as well as those done during it, while the "uninoculated" are arrived at by deducting the inoculated from the average strength. The number of cases, complications, and deaths are, of course, not averages, but actual figures derived from the hospital records. The recording of pulmonary complications is probably lacking in uniformity, since different medical officers may have taken different views as to the

TABLE OF RESULTS OF INFLUENZA INOCULATIONS IN THE HOME COMMANDS, 1918-19.

	Period covered by return.	Average strength during period. All ranks.	Number Inoculated.		Number of cases of influenza during period.		Incidence of attack per 1000.		Number of cases in which pulmonary complications occurred.		Deaths.	
			1 dose only.	2 doses.	Inoc.	Non-Inoc.	Inoc.	Non-inoc.	Inoc.	Non-inoc.	Inoc.	Non-inoc.
Northern Command.												
1. Cramlington ...	31/12/18-28/2/19	1000	20	230	4	40	16·0	53·5	—	—	—	—
2. Wallsend ...	1/11/18-30/11/18	2149	774	591	1	5	0·7	6·4	—	1	—	1
3. Forest Hall	1/11/18-30/11/18	841	30	57	—	17	0	22·5	—	1	—	2
4. Seaton Deleval ...	1/11/18-30/11/18	1100	109	94	5	24	14·7	26·7	—	—	—	—
5. York	1/2/19-30/4/19	3100	1450	50	9	240	6·0	150·0	1	65	—	25
6. Newcastle ...	1/11/18-30/11/18	2794	324	41	1	62	3·0	25·5	1	16	—	5
7. Catterick ...	1/3/19-30/4/19	3352	78	395	4	76	8·4	26·3	—	—	—	—
8. Ripon (Reserve Centre)	1/4/19-30/4/19	1824	71	1174	1	5	0·8	5·1	—	—	—	—
9. Ripon ...	1/11/18-30/11/18	5246	365	408	4	81	5·1	18·0	1	12	1	3
10. Alnwick ...	1/11/18-30/11/18	668	25	175	—	20	0	30·0	—	—	—	—
11. Bradford ...	1/11/18-30/11/18	643	31	170	—	5	0	11·5	—	—	—	5
12. Tyne Garrison ...	1/11/18-30/11/18	5270	1048	765	6	79	3·3	22·8	—	2	—	5
13. 3rd Cheshires ...	1/11/18-30/11/18	2180	222	412	12	48	19·0	31·0	—	25	—	3
14. West Hartlepool ...	1/11/18-30/11/18	670	127	60	—	30	0	62·0	—	5	—	4
15. Clipstone ...	1/11/18-30/11/18	11,509	525	1734	38	228	16·8	24·6	—	2	—	2
16. Bagthorpe ...	1/11/18-30/11/18	800	121	31	14	6	92·0	9·4	4	2	—	—
Eastern Command.												
17. Maidstone ...	9/11/18-30/4/19	4197	80	410	1	504	2·0	135·9	—	403	—	41
Irish Command.												
18. Finner ...	1/11/18-30/11/18	760	79	559	55	36	86·0	295·0	7	11	1	2
19. Charles Fort ...	1/11/18-30/11/18	1453	380	191	4	7	7·0	7·6	--	—	—	—
20. Cahir ...	1/11/18-30/11/18	526	58	318	4	16	11·2	94·1	—	—	—	—
21. Buttevant ...	1/11/18-30/11/18	855	126	428	—	7	0	24·8	—	1	—	3
Western Command.												
22. Prescot ...	1/11/18-30/11/18	4151	483	100	1	31	1·7	5·1	—	—	—	—
Scottish Command.												
23. 4th Seaforths ...	1/11/18-30/11/18	2326	500	—	—	102	0	55·0	—	2	—	—
London District.												
24. Battersea ...	1/11/18-30/4/19	1750	—	221	59	402	267·0	263·0	12	35	—	—
—	Totals ...	59,144	7010 / 8614 (15,624)		221	2059	—	—	36	583	2	98

1 dose only.

Leishman – The Lancet – Feb. 14 1920 366-8

Summary of Table.

	Strength.	Ratios per 1000.		
		Incidence of attack.	Incidence of pulmonary complications.	Deaths.
Inoculated ...	15,624	14·1	1·6	0·12
Non-inoculated ...	43,520	47·3	13·3	2·35

degree of bronchial or pulmonary involvement which should be taken as a complication.

The returns, all of which lie within the period between November, 1918, and April, 1919, comprise all those relating to this period which conformed to the following requirements:—

1. That the vaccine used was that prepared at the Royal Army Medical College, according to the original formula.

2. That influenza should have been present in the unit during the period under review. In many stations where inoculation has been largely carried out there was a rapid cessation of the epidemic. Such returns would have swelled the total of the inoculations without throwing any light on their protective effects.

3. That only such returns are included as showed that at least one-tenth of the average strength had been inoculated, whether with one dose or two.

Information was asked for as to the interval occurring between inoculation and a subsequent attack of influenza, but the figures in response to this are too few to be worth analysing; it need only be said that they furnish little or no evidence of any increased susceptibility in the days immediately following inoculation, and that they throw no light of any value on the duration of the immunity conferred by the inoculations. The figures bearing on the latter point would, in any case, have been exposed to the fallacy that the epidemic was rapidly declining throughout the country, and that the inoculated population was drifting, with increasing rapidity, out of our control into civil life.

No bad effects were reported from the inoculations, and the reactions, in the overwhelming majority, were trivial or non-existent.

It will be noted from the table that nearly one-half of the inoculated had received only the first dose of the vaccine—i.e., one-third of the amount which we considered essential to effective protection. It is reasonable to assume that, had all received the full dosage, the protective results would have been still more evident. No statistical evidence bearing upon this point is, however, available.

The table had best be left to speak for itself, but it will, I think, be admitted that in general the results are encouraging and that they tend to confirm, and even strengthen, our original anticipations, which were, briefly, that at least a moderate degree of protection against infection might be expected, while more decidedly beneficial effects might be hoped for in a diminution of both the frequency and the gravity of the pulmonary complications.

Periodic returns have continued to be received since the period dealt with in the table, but these have been either negative altogether, as regards incidence of the disease, or show so few cases of influenza in either group as to be valueless from a statistical standpoint.

BRISTOL HOSPITAL SUNDAY FUND.—The Lord Mayor of Bristol has expressed his delight at the satisfactory progress of his Sunday Fund, which bids fair to show a substantial increase on last year's record total of over £5000. Collections to hand so far are bigger by 25 per cent. than the corresponding figures of last year. It is interesting to note that the movement towards coöperation between the hospitals receives such tangible support from the Bristol public, who, by means of this fund and the collections made by the various firms, show a certain approval of the principle of hospital union which has for some time past been under discussion in Bristol.

COMPLEMENT-FIXATION EXPERIMENTS IN INFLUENZA.

BY H. J. B. FRY, M.D. OXON.,
CAPTAIN, R.A.M.C.(T.),
AND
C. LUNDIE, M.D. GLASG.,
CAPTAIN, R.A.M.C.(T.C.)

IN the first part of a previous note [1] by one of us (H. J. B. F.) an organism isolated from cases of influenza was described and its morphological and cultural characters given. It was there stated that the serum of a patient from whose blood the organism had been isolated had shown definite complement-fixation with an antigen prepared from the organism. This result encouraged us to try a similar experiment with sera obtained from other cases of influenza, which had been investigated (H. J. B. F.) during the two previous waves of the epidemic. The sera from these cases were old at the time of this experiment. Although preserved in sealed glass capsules, and, as far as possible, kept on ice, some deterioration was to be expected. Owing to the decline of the influenza epidemic cases of recent influenza being infrequent, but the sera from a few definite cases of a mild type have been examined together with other sera as controls. One of us (C. L.), as the pathologist in charge of the serological work of No. — General Hospital (Venereal), had very favourable opportunities for examining sera from syphilitic and other patients as controls. The complement-fixation experiments described below were carried out by him, and in order to render the test more rigid he was ignorant of the nature of the cases from which the sera were derived.

Experiments.

The experiments group themselves under the following headings:—

1. Old sera obtained from cases of influenza at the height of the epidemic 1918–19.

2. Fresh sera and cerebro-spinal fluids from recent cases of influenza.

3. Control sera (a) from normal individuals; (b) from syphilitic patients who have never had influenza; (c) from patients with no recent history of influenza; and (d) sera from patients suffering from other pyrexial diseases, typhoid fever, malaria, tuberculosis, &c.

The total number of influenza sera examined is 15, which includes: Influenza old sera, 5; influenza fresh sera, 8; and influenza cerebro-spinal fluids, 2.

Control Cases (32).

(a) Normal	Sera 3	with no history of influenza .. 4
	Cerebro-spinal fluid 1	
(b) Syphilitic sera with no history of influenza	...	10
(c) Syphilitic sera with histories of influenza not later than one year		6
(d) Sera from specific diseases	Typhoid	1
	Malaria	5
	Tuberculosis	3
(e) Sera from non-specific diseases		3

Serological Technique (C.L.).

(a) *Hæmolytic system.*—Sheeps' corpuscles were used in a 5 per cent. suspension after washing six times with saline. The corpuscular suspension was sensitised with 5 M.H.D. of rabbit anti-sheep serum (Burroughs and Wellcome) titre 1 in 2000-3000. Complement was guinea-pig's serum used fresh on the same day, and

Ely etal – JAMA – Jan. 4 1919 24-28

24   INFLUENZA—ELY ET AL.   Jour. A. M. A.
                                                              Jan. 4, 1919

MISPLACED KIDNEY: REPORT OF A CASE

Allen H. Bunce, M.D., Base Hospital No. 43
Captain, M. C., U. S. Army, A. E. F., France

In a necropsy on the body of G. W., a well developed adult male negro, height 5 feet, 11 inches, weight, 170 pounds, who had died of lobar pneumonia, an anomaly in the location, shape and blood supply of the left kidney was observed. The kidney could not be found by feeling in the left renal fossa. After careful dissection the left suprarenal gland, somewhat larger than normal, was located in the usual position. The right kidney and suprarenal gland were in the normal position and had a normal blood supply. The gastro-intestinal tract was removed and the left kidney found inside

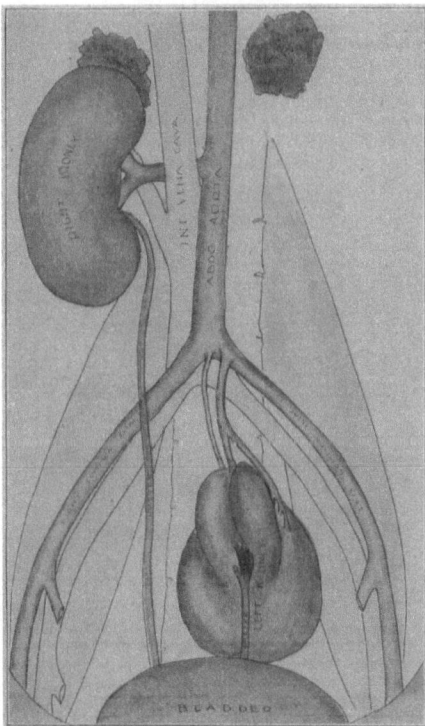

Location, shape and blood supply (diagrammatic) of misplaced kidney.

the bony pelvis slightly to the left side. It was retroperitoneal, as would be expected. The kidney was somewhat pear-shaped, with the small end pointing upward. Its blood supply consisted of a main artery branching from the left common iliac and a smaller branch from the bifurcation of the abdominal aorta. Both arteries entered the anterior surface near the upper end. The veins, two in number, left the kidney on the posterior surface at the upper and lower ends, respectively, and emptied into the left iliac vein. The ureter, which was 9 cm. in length, left the anterior surface of the kidney and passed behind the peritoneum into the bladder in the usual location. The bladder, when distended, partially covered the kidney. The two kidneys, the ureters, the aorta and the bladder were dissected out and removed together. The diagrammatic drawing illustrates the condition clearly.

Military Medicine and Surgery

INFLUENZA AS SEEN AT THE PUGET SOUND NAVY YARD

C. F. ELY, M.D.
Commander, M. C., U. S. N.

B. J. LLOYD, M.D. (Seattle)
Surgeon, U. S. Public Health Service

C. D. HITCHCOCK, M.D.
Lieutenant, M. C., U. S. N. R. F.

AND

D. H. NICKSON, M.D. (Seattle)
Lieutenant, Junior Grade, M. C., U. S. N. R. F.

NAVY YARD, PUGET SOUND, WASH.

In the present state of our knowledge of this disease, one is tempted to ask, "When is influenza not influenza, and why?" Are we dealing with a definite disease caused by a specific micro-organism? If so, is that organism the influenza bacillus? Is it a hemolytic streptococcus? Is it an aberrant form of the pneumococcus (streptopneumocòccus)? Is it a combination of two or more of these, and if so, is infection with the different organisms simultaneous or does the streptococcus follow the influenza bacillus as a secondary invader? May still other organisms than these cause the disease? Are there two or more separate diseases that are being confused both clinically and bacteriologically, and may they coexist in the same patient? May a group of human beings (camp, city or community) be attacked by this epidemic disease and some of them suffer from one infecting organism and some from another and still others from combinations? Are the pathogenic streptococci really a large family that can change form and affinity (for human tissues) and run up and down the scale of virulence ad lib.?

One of us (Lloyd) observed in 1915, 1916 and 1917 that hemolytic streptococci, fatal to rabbits in pure culture (intravenously), could usually be found in certain types of influenza. In one instance he obtained such an organism from the blood (before death) of a patient who had severe cholecystitis, for which operation was performed. The patient recovered, returned home, and became suddenly ill with fever, collapse, signs of pulmonary edema, and intense jaundice. The patient died twenty-one days after operation, and forty-eight hours after the last illness began. It is interesting to note in this connection that in some of the fatal cases of influenza at this station there was marked jaundice.

Nickson also found hemolytic streptococci in the blood of two persons suffering from influenza (bronchopneumonia) previous to his assignment to this station.

Based on previous observations, Lloyd suggested that we would probably find a hemolytic streptococcus the cause of this disease should influenza present itself among our personnel in epidemic form, and also expressed the opinion that a vaccine made from such an organism might be useful as a prophylactic. All of us felt that the influenza bacillus should be added if found. To Drs. Hitchcock and Nickson were assigned the tasks of making the pathologic and bac-

Ely etal – JAMA – Jan. 4 1919 24-28

VOLUME 72
NUMBER 1
INFLUENZA—ELY ET AL.   25

teriologic.studies, following out a more or less definite plan on which all were agreed.

In boldly announcing the fact that this work was undertaken with what might be termed "preconceived ideas" on the part of at least two of us, it might be argued that we were looking for a streptococcus infection. We were; but we were also looking for anything else we could find. Nothing else was found in the blood, nor did we find anything else in the tissues at the necropsies; and a reasonable, though not a persistent, effort was made to obtain the influenza bacillus from the sputum without success. Never did blood cultures show anything but diplococcal or streptococcal forms; only once did tissue cultures show anything else, and that was when they were contaminated by the colon bacillus. Lieutenant Henry reports that in a few cases studied by him at the Seattle training camp he obtained only diplococcal forms, which he regards as pneumococci.

CLINICAL DATA

The onset is sudden. The patient usually has a chill or chilly sensations. There may be headache, and pain in the back; and there is a tendency for the knees to give way. There may be nosebleed. The temperature rises rapidly and may reach 104 or 105. In two fatal cases a temperature of 108 was recorded. The pulse is from 100 to 120, and higher in severe cases. Lung symptoms soon make their appearance with pain over the lungs, usually the lower border. Constipation is the rule, and the patient frequently complains of pain over the upper abdomen.

Examination of the lungs in moderately severe cases shows fine and coarse râles and areas of dulness. The liver and spleen are enlarged and tender. The respiratory rate averages from 28 to 30 and, though higher in very severe cases, there is not the rapid rate seen in ordinary lobar pneumonia. The cough is usually loose, and an abundant frothy, greenish fluid, pink with blood, is brought up. The contrast between this material and that usually seen in lobar pneumonia is quite marked. In severe and fatal cases delirium is present, the facial expression is anxious, and there is often marked cyanosis. In many fatal cases the respiration continued for some time after the heart had stopped.

CLINICAL PATHOLOGY AND PATHOLOGIC ANATOMY

Of sixty-two urinary examinations made fairly early, twenty-six showed albumin and hyaline and granular casts; seven showed albumin only, and twenty-nine were normal.

Of seventy-five blood examinations, twenty-five gave a leukocyte count of 5,000 or less, thirty-four gave a count of between 5,000 and 10,000 and sixteen a count of more than 10,000. Several cases gave a count of from 30,000 to 56,000; but in these cases there was some complication, usually cerebrospinal. In convalescent cases the leukocyte count tends to rise.

Necropsies were performed in thirty-nine cases, only six of which showed varying degrees of consolidation, sometimes complete for some portion of the lung. There was marked engorgement of the lung tissue with a large amount of bloody fluid exuding from the cut surface; not infrequently the cut surface of certain areas showed small amounts of pus in the smaller bronchi. Pleural effusions, varying in amount, usually right sided, serofibrinous, and occasionally purulent, were

fairly constant. The heart was slightly enlarged and the right auricle dilated. The kidneys were enlarged and congested, an edematous condition frequently being found about the suprarenals. The spleen was large and soft, the cut surface exuding bloody fluid.

BACTERIOLOGIC FINDINGS

Sputum examinations were made in forty-nine early cases and twenty-five late cases with these results: Smears were made from selected portions. Gram positive cocci were found in pairs and chains, streptococci predominating throughout all examinations. Portions of sputum washed, plated on blood agar and incubated for twenty-four hours showed large numbers of hemolyzing colonies composed (microscopically) of chain-forming cocci (sometimes paired). Subcultures of these in bouillon, with one exception, showed chain formations. Two rabbits were injected intravenously with small amounts of washed sputum, suspended in broth. These animals died after thirty-six and seventy-two hours. Pure cultures of hemolytic chain-forming

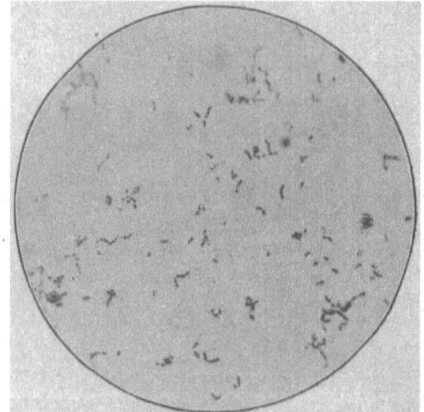

Fig. 1.—Smear direct from pus from joint of rabbit inoculated from washed sputum, × 1,000, showing streptococci.

cocci were obtained from the heart's blood and from the pus from the joints, in both animals.[1]

Cultures made postmortem in twenty cases gave hemolytic streptococci from the heart's blood 17 times; from the pericardium, 12 times; from the liver, 13 times; lung, 14 times; spleen, 5 times; kidney, 17 times; bile, twice. In only one case the cultures were entirely negative. It is believed that this was due to an error in technic. In one case, cultures were contaminated with the colon bacillus.

A total of fifty-two attempts at blood culture on living patients gave twenty-four positive results, all streptococci except one, which gave only a diplococcus, which would not chain. This patient had the physical signs of lobar pneumonia and was clinically fairly typical of that disease; but five members of his family had "influenza" at the same time that he had "pneumonia," all being in the emergency hospital together (civilians). Two patients yielded blood cultures

1. Since this was written, one rabbit was killed three weeks after inoculation. It was greatly emaciated; pus from joints was somewhat caseated but showed streptococci.

Ely etal – JAMA – Jan. 4 1919 24-28

eighteen hours after onset, eight within three days and one after three weeks' illness.

The technic of blood cultures was as follows: Three c.c. of blood were drawn under aseptic precautions and placed in an Erlenmeyer flask containing 30 c.c. of

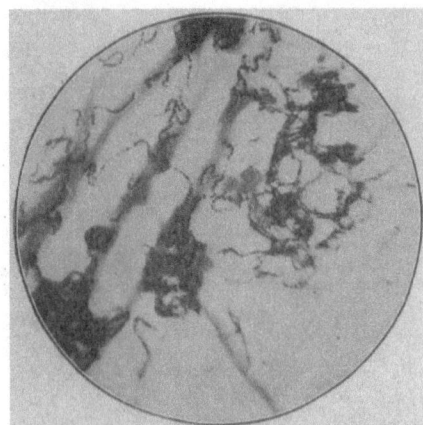

Fig. 2.—Marked chain formation in bouillon culture (twenty-four hours) made direct from human blood from patient who recovered; × 1,000.

1 per cent. glucose broth plus 1 per cent. of sheep serum. After incubating for twenty-four hours there was usually an abundant growth.

CULTURAL AND STAINING CHARACTERISTICS, AND REACTIONS

On tubed solid mediums the organism we are describing grows in small, discrete colonies. On blood agar plates the colonies are usually larger, and when recently from the human body are surrounded by a well marked hemolytic zone. Hemolytic properties are quickly lost in subcultures, but may be restored by passage through rabbits or white mice. The microscopic appearance in smears from human and animal tissues is that of a coccus, occurring in short or long chains; once a diplococcus only was obtained from a blood culture. In the mouse the organism may show as mixed diplococci and streptococci. On agar the growth may also show mixed diplococci and streptococci, or there may be chains of diplococci, and after a few generations bouillon cultures may show diplococci predominating and even groups suggesting staphylococci, though when grown in bouillon direct from human and animal tissues, chain formation is the rule, the units in the chains varying in number from four to twenty. Some strains retained their chain-forming properties much more persistently than others. The size of the organisms varied from 0.3 to 1 micron; they were usually true spheres, but occasionally were somewhat elongated. The development of the organism in broth produces diffuse cloudiness accompanied by varying amounts of sediment. Acid was produced in glucose and lactose 4.6 and 2.1 degrees respectively (phenolphthalein). No gas was produced. The organism is gram-positive and stains readily with the ordinary anilin dyes. A capsule was demonstrated in only one strain from the peritoneal cavity of a

mouse. In addition to the hemolytic property noted on blood agar plates, it was found that when 0.5 c.c. of a twenty-four-hour broth culture was mixed with the same amount of a 5 per cent. suspension of red blood cells (rabbit) in physiologic sodium chlorid solution and incubated at 37 C. for one hour, the cells were completely hemolyzed. This was also true of a strain that grew as a diplococcus.

BILE SOLUBILITY

A twenty-four-hour broth culture was filtered through gauze and cotton to remove sediment and large clumps. The filtrate was then centrifuged in Hopkins tubes, the liquid pipetted off and just enough salt solution added to the precipitated organisms to make a distinctly cloudy suspension. Two-tenths c.c. of fresh sterile ox bile was added to 1 c.c. of this suspension and incubated at 37 C. for one hour. Solution of the organisms did not occur. It will be recalled that the organism was obtained direct from the bile at two necropsies.

AGGLUTINATION AND PRECIPITIN REACTIONS

The organism did not agglutinate in Types I, II and III antipneumococcic serum nor in serum from convalescent patients.

A precipitin reaction was obtained in a 1 : 25 dilution in Type I serum and in a 1 : 50 dilution in Type III serum. Similar reactions were thus obtained in serums of persons ill of the disease: 1 : 25, one; 1 : 50, two; 1 : 800, one. No others were tried.

PATHOGENICITY FOR MICE AND RABBITS

Injections of 1 c.c. of a twenty-four-hour broth culture into the ear veins of rabbits invariably killed the animals in from eighteen to seventy-two hours. A marked and constant lesion in these animals was a

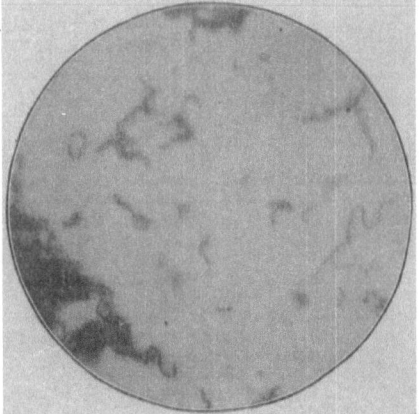

Fig. 3.—Marked chain formation in subculture from bouillon on blood agar plate; × 1,200.

purulent arthritis affecting the larger joints particularly the midjoints of the limbs (corresponding to the elbows and knees). The organism could be demonstrated in great numbers in the tissues and particularly in the pus from the joints, always in chains. Five-tenths c.c. of a twenty-four-hour broth culture invaria-

Ely etal – JAMA – Jan. 4 1919 24-28

VOLUME 72
NUMBER 1   INFLUENZA—ELY ET AL.   27

bly proved fatal when injected intraperitoneally into white mice, death occurring in from twelve to twenty-four hours. Smears from the peritoneal fluid showed usually chains, occasionally pairs only, and sometimes both. Cultures made from this fluid, in bouillon, rarely failed to show marked chain formation, even though smears from the fluid showed only diplococci.

TECHNIC OF PREPARATION OF VACCINE

(*a*) Mixed virulent strains of hemolytic streptococci obtained as related are grown for twenty-four hours in 1 per cent. glucose broth plus 1 per cent. sheep serum.

(*b*) At the end of twenty-four hours the supernatant liquid is poured off from the sediment.

(*c*) The organisms from the supernatant fluid are thrown down in a centrifuge.

(*d*) The sediment left in the culture flasks is filtered through gauze and cotton and centrifuged.

(*e*) The two portions of solid micro-organisms are mixed, enough 0.8 per cent. salt solution plus 0.25 per cent. phenol being added to make a heavy suspension. Care should be taken not to add too much salt solution at this stage.

(*f*) The suspension is placed in a sterile bottle with beads and it is shaken to break the clumps.

(*g*) It is filtered again through gauze and cotton.

(*h*) It is filtered again through an alendem filter crucible at 15 pounds pressure; this does not remove the organisms.

(*i*) A small quantity of the filtrate is taken as it comes from the alendem crucible, and by means of a Hopkins tube the number of organisms per cubic centimeter is estimated.

(*j*) Salt solution (plus phenol) is added to make a dilution of 250 million organisms per cubic centimeter.

(*k*) This is tubed, capped and immersed in a water bath for one hour at 56 C.

(*l*) Each tube is tested by planting 3 or 4 drops on blood agar and incubating for twenty-four hours.

The dose used here is 0.25, 0.5 and 1 c.c., given at forty-eight-hour intervals.

INCIDENCE IN VACCINATED AND UNVACCINATED PERSONNEL

Influenza was introduced at the Puget Sound Navy Yard by a draft of men (987 in number) from Philadelphia, many of whom arrived ill or came down within a few hours after reaching this station. A tabulated statement of cases and deaths in the different units is given herewith.

It is fair to say that no unit was divided into two parts for the purpose of running experimental subjects and controls side by side. Circumstances were such that this could not well be done. It is also fair to say that in our largest unit (seamen's barracks) many cases had already occurred before vaccination could be done; we do not know how many. This is also true of the Philadelphia unit. It is not true of the rest of the command.

Conditions of exposure were not materially different in the different units. Conditions of housing differed in that some men were in barracks and some in tents; but this seemed to make no difference with regard to incidence. All of the marines were in barracks, rather closely quartered. All of the Seattle training camp men were in tents, two men to a tent (8 by 10).

The following facts stand out prominently:

Of 4,212 men who were vaccinated, not one man died. Among 111 Filipinos isolated and vaccinated early and later exposed, there occurred only two cases, both the patients recovered. Among 361 marines vaccinated early with no attempt to control exposure,

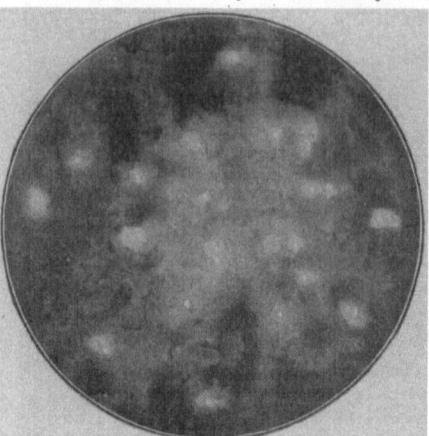

Fig. 4.—Drawing from blood agar plate to show hemolysis (not a very satisfactory picture of the plate).

there occurred two cases, both patients coming down after the first injection; both recovered. Among sixty-two marines at the ammunition depot who were vaccinated early, there occurred three cases; two after the first injection and one after the third; there were

INCIDENCE AND FATALITY IN VACCINATED AND UNVACCINATED PERSONNEL

	Complement		Cases		Per Cent. Attacked		Deaths		Case Fatality Percentage	
	Vaccinated	Unvaccinated	Vaccinated	Unvaccinated	Vaccinated	Unvaccinated	Vaccinated	Unvaccinated	Vaccinated	Unvaccinated
Philadelphia Unit......	131	855	37*	168	28.2	19.6	0	21	0	12.5
Seattle Training Camp No. 1...............	....	4,159	....	813	....	19.5	..	33	..	4+
Seattle Training Camp No. 2...............	662	....	11	...	1.60	....	0	..	0	
Seamen's Barracks, Puget Sound......	2,800	3,472	57†	428	2.03	12.3	0	42	0	9.8
Marines, Puget Sound Navy Yard and Ammunition Depot.......	425	....	5	...	1.2	....	0	..	0	
Filipino Unit.............	111	....	2	...	1.8	....	0	..	0	
Aviation Unit...........	83	....	32‡	...	38.5	....	0	..	0	

* Twenty-six of the thirty-seven vaccinated came down before vaccination was completed.
† Fifty-five of the fifty-seven came down after one injection and did not complete the process.
‡ Thirty-one of the thirty-two came down after the first injection.

no deaths. Among 662 bluejackets at the Seattle training camp, three men developed the disease after the first injection, one after the second injection and seven after the third; there were no deaths. Among eighty-three of the Aviation Corps there occurred thirty-two cases, thirty-one of the patients coming down within a few hours after the first injection and

Ely etal – JAMA – Jan. 4 1919 24-28

one after the third injection; there were no deaths. Altogether there were 1,279 men who were vaccinated either before exposure or about the time they were exposed, and of these ninety-four developed the disease before vaccination was completed and eleven afterward. All recovered. Some of the cases in the vaccinated were fairly severe and from the blood of one of these patients a streptococcus was recovered.

The period of observation was from September 17 to Oct. 21, 1918. Up to November 3 there had occurred but forty additional cases at the Seattle training camp and sixteen at the Puget Sound Navy Yard, facts which seem to indicate that the epidemic was practically over at the time these data were obtained. There have been several deaths since October 21, but so far none among those who were vaccinated (November 9).

CONCLUSIONS

We believe that the disease called influenza at the Puget Sound Navy Yard was due to the organism described above, and that despite variations it should be classed as a hemolytic streptococcus, at least until such time as the relationship between diplococci and streptococci is more accurately established. Our findings failed to show that the influenza bacillus was in any way connected with the production of the disease at the Puget Sound Navy Yard.

We believe that the use of killed cultures as described prevented the development of the disease in many of our personnel and modified its course favorably in others. We at first used a single strain, but later mixed two or more strains. We do not know that the latter is advantageous.

Attention is invited to the fact that a vaccine made from streptococci apparently protected 662 blue jackets in a camp where Henry found what he considered pneumococci only.

We suspect that there may be different strains of the organism causing influenza (call it what you please), and recommend for vaccines cultures recently from human tissues, preferably from cases in the same community where the disease is prevalent; such cultures must kill rabbits promptly when given intravenously. One should not forget to add a little serum to the culture medium.

We offer no suggestion with regard to the duration of the immunity produced, and in our experience vaccination may be repeated without inconvenience.

We further suggest that the vaccine be tried out in smaller doses as a therapeutic agent in cases in which there is delayed convalescence, unless there is empyema or other evidence of localized suppuration.

Flatulence and Sleep.—Take the earliest example—the infant "muling and puking in its nurse's arms"—keeping its careworn parents awake half the night. Why does the rocking the cradle or "dandling" in the arms so often soothe and produce sleep? Because, owing to the constantly changing axes of the loops of intestines, the bubbles of wind are enabled to pass on. "The hand that rocks the cradle moves the wind." Far better than "ruling the world"! For just the same reason the sleepless adult tosses on his bed from side to side. By doing so he involuntarily coaxes the flatulence to move on from the loops of intestine where it has been accumulating and sending those disturbing messages to the higher centers. And hence many a patient will sleep better after a dose of calomel or blue pill than after one of the recognized hypnotics.—G. King Martyn, M.D., *Medical Press and Circular.*

DEPRESSED FRACTURE OF THE MALAR BONE

A. E. ROCKEY, M.D. (PORTLAND, ORE.)
Major, M. C., U. S. Army
CAMP LEWIS, AMERICAN LAKE, WASH.

Preparation for the activities of war has made this lesion more frequent than was usual in civil life. It is caused by direct violence of a fall or blow. Automobile or motorcycle mishaps, bayonet and trench drill, mule kicks, and blows in boxing and baseball have been factors in cases brought to our hospital. The extent of the depression, the location of the fracture line, and complicating fractures of other bones differ with the force and direction of the trauma.

In construction, the malar bone itself is more rugged than the maxilla in the immediate vicinity of its articulations. The occasional occurrence of complete or

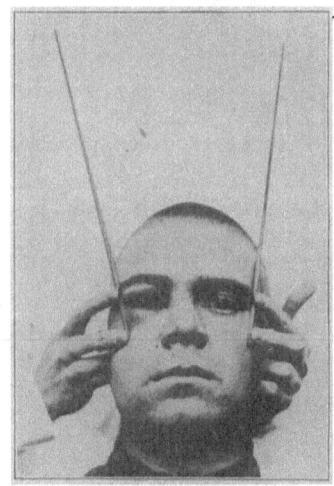

Fig. 1.—Method of diagnosis in depressed fracture of the malar bone.

partial anesthesia of the area of distribution of the infra-orbital nerve demonstrates definitely that the fracture line runs through its foramen of exit. The orbital plate is also involved. The temporal process may or may not be broken. Emphysema was present in one case. When depression is slight, the external aspect may be speedily covered by the resulting swelling. It is consequently not discovered until the swelling subsides and the deformity becomes manifest.

We have devised a method of diagnosis, illustrated in Figure 1, which definitely determines even a slight depression. Two straight wooden applicators are placed, vertically at the outer edge of the orbit from the prominence of the cheek bone upward, as shown. If depression exists, the difference in angle is obvious. The swelling may be pushed out with the finger tip and the end of the applicator given firm rest on the bone.

The bone may usually be easily raised into position by grasping it through the skin with heavy tenaculum forceps. The ordinary towel clips at hand in every

Watters – Bost.Med. & Surg. J – Dec. 25 1919 727-731

TABLE OF CONTENTS

December 25, 1919

Original Articles.

VACCINES IN INFLUENZA.

BY W. H. WATTERS, M.D., BOSTON,

Pathologist, Massachusetts Homeopathic Hospital.

EARLY in September, 1918, the epidemic of influenza that had been raging in certain parts of Europe made its expected appearance in America. The first outbreak occurred in the Boston district and from here to a large extent it spread over the entire country. At this time comparatively little was known about it by the American medical world, although its arrival had been clearly foreseen by many. Since then all of the many phases have been studied by most competent men from the Atlantic to the Pacific; and, literally, volumes have been written concerning it.

It is not, therefore, with the expectation of adding anything new to these accumulated data that the writer has prepared this article, but merely with the desire to add the results of a somewhat extensive personal experience of one who happened to have a very early opportunity to study the cases at first hand.

Starting in the Chelsea Naval Hospital, the number of cases almost immediately exceeded all accommodations. The Haynes Memorial for Contagious Diseases, a department of the Massachusetts Homeopathic Hospital, was offered to the Government and was accepted, the personnel of the institution and its directors being continued as before. Here and later in the main hospital many hundreds of cases of influenza and its complications were treated during the next two months. Other phases than attempts at immunization will at this time be entirely eliminated on account of space limitations.

Prior to this time, Dr. Timothy Leary of Tufts Medical School, and the writer had discussed the possibilities of vaccines in this disease and had agreed that their administration was at least logical from the prophylactic standpoint.

Immediately upon the arrival of these cases at the Haynes Memorial, Dr. Leary made a large number of cultures and from these obtained his first vaccine. To Dr. Leary, therefore, belongs the credit of first applying vaccines as a prophylactic measure. The writer also obtained cultures, prepared vaccines, and administered them. Neither was able to isolate or then discover the so-called influenza bacillus, the organism predominating being a diplococcus, doubtless of the group of the *Micrococcus catarrhalis*. Very shortly, however,

Watters – Bost.Med. & Surg. J – Dec. 25 1919 727-731

post-mortem examinations of fatal cases revealed the influenza bacilli in the lungs and pure cultures were obtained. From this time onward the two investigators varied. One, Dr. Leary, decided to prepare his vaccine from various strains of influenza bacilli alone; the other, the writer, assuming that a mixed infection was active in various phases of the disease, prepared a vaccine with various bacteria included. The following is a report of the latter study:

From the lungs at post-mortem examinations a number of organisms were isolated and from these a mixed vaccine was prepared as follows:

```
Micrococcus catarrhalis ..........400 million
Pneumococcus ....................400    "
Streptococcus hemolyticus .......400    "
Bacillus influenzae .............100    "
```

Of this, the recommended dosage was .2 c.c., .3 c.c., and .4 c.c., administered at 3-day intervals. It was stated that the procedure was experimental, was theoretically logical, and was relatively harmless, and the duration of its efficiency would probably be about four weeks. Public clinics were opened where it could be obtained by any one, free of charge, and large amounts were distributed to physicians and boards of health without charge, the only proviso being that it should be similarly freely administered. In all a sufficient supply was sent out for about fifty thousand doses. A request accompanied each lot that records of results be kept and returned. As might be expected, however, in the most unusual stress of sickness and death, a large number of such records were either lost or not made. From one state department of health, in particular, to which thousands of doses were sent, no adequate report was ever obtainable. Many reports did come in, however, frequently accompanied by comments from the one submitting them. These coming as they did, from trained observers entirely unbiased either for or against the method, seem to be of sufficient value to justify placing them on record.

The first immunizations were upon the laboratory staff itself. Here, of the total fourteen, ten received inoculations. None of these contracted the disease. Of the four others, two had influenza rather severely. This seemed rather suggestive because all were in close and intimate contact with a great many cases continually. Among the nurses inoculations were

offered as optional and were begun practically as soon as the epidemic appeared. For the combined senior and intermediate classes the statistics have been collected, but, unfortunately, those for the lower classes were lost in the stress of active work.

For the two upper classes the results are as follows:

		SICK	PER CENT. SICK
Not vaccinated	41	33	80
Vaccinated once	27	9	33
Vaccinated twice	9	3	33
Vaccinated three times	6	2	33

The high disease incidence here was undoubtedly due to the fact that all these nurses were constantly and continually exposed to the infection in caring for the hundreds of cases in their wards and were exposed under conditions of physical and mental fatigue that were almost ideally favorable to the contagion.

In the catgut factory of W. D. Young & Co., in one room where the raw gut was manufactured, nineteen employees were inoculated and one refused. Within a week, the only case of the disease that had occurred was the one uninoculated individual.

Among the commercial firms of the city, many desired or requested the treatment. Perhaps the most carefully controlled study was here made among the employees of the H. P. Hood Milk Co., with the very efficient coöperation of the medical supervisor, Dr. N. R. Davis, who superintended the entire work. Upon the first appearance of the epidemic, Dr. Davis foresaw the coming storm and recommended that all of the employees be immunized. At this time an occasional worker was sick but the number was very insignificant. Injections were immediately begun and vigorously carried forward. Following the subsidence of the epidemic wave, Dr. Davis carefully collected statistics comparing the results among those immunized and those not immunized. These, he reports as follows:

	NON- VACCINATED	VACCINATED
No. persons under observation	300	247*
No. cases of influenza	93	17*
No. cases of pneumonia	5	2†
Percentage of influenza	81	6.8
Percentage influenza mortality	4.3	0

Dr. Davis states "that the majority of these people were route salesmen whose duties took them in all kinds of homes during this epi-

* This includes six with only one inoculation and five with two inoculations.
† These each received but one inoculation.

Watters – Bost.Med. & Surg. J – Dec. 25 1919 727-731

Vol. CLXXXI, No. 26]   BOSTON MEDICAL AND SURGICAL JOURNAL   729

demic. They were out in all kinds of weather and some of them had to take the pocketbook from underneath the mattress of people who were ill, to get their money. The other people were men and women in the office. A great many of our force were ill with influenza who did not care to be vaccinated. These employees were equally exposed."

At the same time a similar study was being conducted at the Boston Confectionery Co. The results may be thus summarized:

	Not Vaccinated	Vaccinated
Boston Confectionery Co.		
No. persons under observation	200	250
No. cases of influenza	75	3
No. cases of pneumonia	4	0
Percentage of influenza	30	0.8
Percentage influenza mortality	2.7	0
F. H. Roberts Co.		
No. persons under observation	339	329
No. cases of influenza	9	3
No. cases of pneumonia	1	0
Percentage of influenza	2.7	0.9
Percentage influenza mortality	11	0
Miller Candy Co.		
No. persons under observation	25	90
No. cases of influenza	18	5
No. cases of pneumonia	1	0
Percentage of influenza	72	5.5
Lovell & Covell Co.		
No. persons under observation	100	185
No. cases of influenza	90*	0
No. cases of pneumonia	?	0
Percentage of influenza	90	0

* The majority of these cases contracted the disease prior to the time when their associates were vaccinated. Therefore comparative deductions must be made with caution.

A little later word came that the epidemic had appeared in the male wards of the Allentown State Hospital in Pennsylvania. A supply of vaccine was immediately sent to Dr. L. B. Pierce, from whose report the following facts are taken. The outbreak started and spread rapidly among the buildings for males and when the vaccine was received had practically not appeared in the buildings for females. Immunization attempts were therefore largely directed to the uninvolved departments, although a few in the other parts were treated. The report includes accordingly largely a comparison of disease incidence morbidity and mortality between a non-immunized department and an immunized one, both presumably equally exposed to infection. The results are interesting:

	Not Vaccinated	Vaccinated
Allentown State Hospital.		
No. of cases under observation	575	722
No. of cases of influenza	186	61*
No. cases of pneumonia	77	11†
Percentage of influenza	32.4	8.4
Percentage influenza mortality	17.7	13.1

* Of these, 18 had received but one, and eight, two inoculations.
† Of these, three had received but one, and two, two inoculations.

Of the 61 cases vaccinated 22 showed the disease in less than one week, three from the first to the fourth week, 18 after the fifth week, 17 after the fifth. This suggests the onset of the immunity to be about one week, the persistence of its highest efficiency about three or four weeks, and its gradual disappearance thereafter. Dr. Pierce states that "the epidemic among the women came later, after the inoculations were completed, and was much less severe in character, those who had the disease exhibiting it in a much milder form. It would look as if the vaccine must have been atleast a factor in this result."

The writer in person in association with the Bridgeport Board of Health, organized the immunizing staff of the Remington Arms Company and the Bullard Machine Works. On account of the relatively light course of the epidemic here and the sudden disarticulation of lines of work in these industries subsequent to the armistice, full reports were not obtainable. From the report of the Board of Health, however, the following is abstracted:

	No. Receiving 1 Inoculation	No. Receiving 2 Inoculations	No. Receiving 3 Inoculations
Remington Arms	1079	905	660
Bullard Machine	1099	707	409
Bridgeport Brass	846	576	400
Total	3024	2188	1469
Grand Total of Inoculations			6681

Results:

It was impossible to follow up closely all of the cases that were vaccinated. Except in a general way there is nothing that can be said of cases in the Remington Arms and Bridgeport Brass Co. The physicians at these factories report that the cases of influenza materially decreased, that there were no severe cases after the vaccinations and that only a few men reported to them with any of the symptoms. However, this does not apply particularly to the vaccinated group, but to the entire factory. It may have been due to the fact that the epidemic has reached its height at about this time and that the decrease of cases would have followed even if there had been no inoculations.

In one case, the arm was swollen and became very painful after the first inoculation and continued in this condition for two or three days. In another case, a very severe headache resulted and there was a general reaction

Watters – Bost.Med. & Surg. J – Dec. 25 1919 727-731

730   BOSTON MEDICAL AND SURGICAL JOURNAL   [DECEMBER 25, 1919

which lasted for two or three days. The other two cases did not seem to be important. One man tried to faint as the vaccine had been given, claiming that his head and arm hurt. Another case reported a stiff arm the next day.

There were three cases and one death among the men vaccinated at the Bullard factory. Two of these cases, including one that died, had received only one inoculation and probably had the infection before he was vaccinated. It was also reported by the physician that the patient who died had other serious complications which contributed to his death. The third case had had two inoculations before the onset of the disease, but his illness was not severe. Several cases, with no deaths, were reported at this factory among the unvaccinated employees. There was no practical way in which records could be obtained on the unvaccinated group so that the actual number of cases is not known."

From various other boards of health, the reports are either entirely missing or are so sketchy as to be practically valueless. To practicing physicians the vaccine was sent in abundance. The reports that were submitted may be summarized as follows:

Doctor	No. Inocu-lated	No. Contract-ing Diseases	Pneumonia Cases	Deaths
Barney	47	None	None	None
Bell	25	"	"	"
Bowen	200	1	"	"
Cahill	40	None	"	"
Coffin	13	"	"	"
Cross	48	2	"	"
Emerson	39	"	"	"
Gould	30	1	1	"
Hanson	30	None	None	None
Johnson	6	"	"	"
Jones	123	5	"	"
Kirkland	160	2	"	"
Leard	100	3	"	"
Leeds	2	None	"	"
Phillips	105	....	....	....
Piper	31	None	None	None
Rice	98	"	"	"
Ring	26	5	"	"
Southwick	125	None	"	"
Sylvester	88	2	1	"
Ventrone	60	None	None	"
Weston	2	"	"	"
Wooldridge	75	"	....	....

Dr. Barney: There is no comparison in my cases, as everyone inoculated has escaped the disease with possibly one exception. I am not quite sure of the diagnosis yet. Some of the patients inoculated were intimately and continuously exposed, three of them being nurses. They escaped. In three other instances all members of the family had influenza except the one inoculated, who was intimately associated with the other members. I am very enthusiastic in regard to the influenza prophylactic vaccine.

Dr. Bell: Prophylactic measure seemed of value.

Dr. Bowen: I used the prophylactic vaccine in a great many cases all the way from six months to 60 years, and while I do not wish to be over enthusiastic will say that I am confident it does not do to neglect it as one of the prophylactic measures.

Dr. Cahill: It seemed in general that I found the disease in 70% of the same number of uninoculated persons under same conditions and in same length of time.

Dr. Emerson: I see absolutely no objections to the method and so far as I know no one to whom I gave the vaccine has had the "Flu."

Dr. Gould: I am sure it must have been of much service.

Dr. Jones: Personally I feel that this method of inoculation is very valuable in preventing and modifying the severity of influenza and pneumonia.

Dr. Leard: The doctor states under date of December 1st, two months after inoculations, that since filling out the above record he has had several cases ranging from light to severe.

Dr. Phillips: During the first three weeks of the epidemic and following the inoculations, not a case occurred among our nurses, while in the other hospitals here nurses by the dozens were attacked, and many died. In the fourth week, however, one after another of the ten came down. I think the explanation is that their immunity was short lived, and only partial, and that we would have done much better had we continued the vaccine until reaction ceased to fairly large doses. Only one patient outside the hospital who was inoculated came down with the infection.

Dr. Piper: In several cases, four at least, I gave prophylactic vaccine to persons who were much exposed to patients ill with influenza and in no instance did persons so treated contract the disease. I am confident the vaccine is a helpful measure.

Dr. Rice: Not quite fair in my case because the disease was rather on the wane when inoculation began.

Dr. Southwick: I have great confidence in the prophylactic value of the influenza vaccine prepared by Prof. Watters. I used in most of the cases one-third larger dose than the amount originally recommended.

Dr. Sylvester: I found that 75% of household contracted it if not inoculated, while only two out of all treated contracted same. I feel it was a decided benefit.

Dr. Ventrone: Those inoculated, according to my experience, were immune.

Dr. Wooldridge: Personally we inoculated about seventy-five cases and as far as we know not one case developed influenza. We inocu-

Watters – Bost.Med. & Surg. J – Dec. 25 1919 727-731

Vol. CLXXXI, No. 26]   · BOSTON MEDICAL AND SURGICAL JOURNAL   731

lated one prospective confinement case after she had been exposed to influenza and she developed a severe attack of pneumonia, but recovered without having a miscarriage.

It will· be seen that there is practically a unanimity of opinion in favor of the idea that active immunization by the use of vaccines may be obtained, a fact which while not, of course, to be considered as scientific proof, still should be considered to have distinct value. Another interesting note is found in the comment upon reactions. These, while infrequent, were almost always mistaken for the beginning of influenza, being characterized by sudden chill, fever, headache and prostration, persisting for a few hours and subsiding gradually.

It may be of further value to note in combining the above figures, excluding the Bridge-, port Board of Health and the Lovell & Covell Company, where comparisons are indefinite, that there was disease incidence among those inoculated of approximately 3.5%, while at the same time among others not inoculated the disease incidence amounted to 28% and under similar surroundings. Among those immunized the incidence of pneumonia was very low, there being only fifteen cases definitely reported. The total of eight deaths has been reported, these all coming from the Allentown State Hospital where three of the patients had received but one inoculation and three, two inoculations. Apart from this the mortality records are clear.

In preparing this paper, the writer fully realizes the fact that epidemics afflict first those most susceptible and that measures for immunization employed later upon those not yet infected may consist of administering them to persons already naturally immune. As such, it is obviously unfair to compare early morbidity among a non-immunized community and later morbidity among a hopefully partially immunized one after the most susceptible have already become diseased.

In the Allentown report, however, this possibility seems to be successfully met when it is noted that of those vaccinated persons contracting the disease 36% did so within one week of the first inoculation when the immunity should ·be theoretically only beginning and 57% did so after the fourth week when the immunity was decreasing. It would suggest that for a period of three or four weeks, a distinct degree of resistance to infection might be produced.

Again, in the report of Dr. Phillips, no inoculated nurses in the hospital with which he is associated contracted the disease until after three weeks subsequent to inoculation, even though constantly exposed.

Dr. Leard also reports occurrence of the disease in vaccinated cases later than four weeks after inoculation.

These notes seem strongly to suggest that there is a period of three to five weeks subsequent to inoculation during which a distinct degree of immunity exists.

With these facts in mind and even with the incomplete returns necessarily incident to an almost unprecedented epidemic at a time when the medical profession of the country was seriously depleted by war, it has seemed that the results reported in this article deserve to be thus recorded.

PRIMARY SARCOMA OF THE STOMACH. REVIEW OF THE CASE SIX YEARS AFTER OPERATION.

By A. R. Kimpton, M.D., F.A.C.S., Boston.

In June, 1914, in this Journal,[1] the case of round celled sarcoma of the stomach which is here to be reviewed was reported. Coincidently Frazier[2] published an article on gastric sarcoma in which he states that of 12 cases of sarcoma of the stomach the longest period of survival after operation was 14 years, while the remaining cases survived "2 two years, 1 one year, 1 had recurrence in three years, and 8 were reported as well from two to eleven months after operation."

The following case is of particular interest in that the patient is ·alive and perfectly well, with no evidence of return of the sarcoma five years and ten months after an extensive resection of the stomach for a very rapidly growing sarcoma of the round celled type. She is able to drive, oil and grease, and even change the tires of her own car.

(Quotation from Journal of June 11, 1914.)[1]

"The following case is of interest, not only because of the comparative rarity of gastric sarcoma, but also because of the fact that the patient was known to have had an abdominal tumor for years. Yet at the time of operation she was not anemic or emaciated, nor did she have any gastric symptoms other than indigestion (apparently hyperacidity).

Rosenow-Sturdivant – JAMA – Aug. 9 1919 396-401

than on digital exploration. This is very good so far as it goes, but it seems to be a confession that the exploration cannot be made completely. I would not feel satisfied to close the abdomen without feeling the gallbladder, kidneys, pancreas and other viscera. You cannot make a satisfactory exploration of the abdomen without using the sense of touch. In anesthetizing the peritoneum near the abdominal incision, one of the best bits of technic is, as soon as a small opening is made through the peritoneum, to slip one finger on the inside of the peritoneum about 2 inches back from the margin of the wound and by placing the hypodermic needle directly through the rectus muscles the point of the needle touches the finger; the opening in the needle is exactly in the right 'position to infiltrate the subperitoneal tissue at the site of the most sensitive nerves. By doing that up and down both sides of the incision you secure the best sort of anesthesia of the abdominal peritoneum in the neighborhood of the wound. One part of abdominal work which cannot be done with local anesthesia without pain is in conditions in which you have to make traction on the mesentery. As soon as you pull on the meso-appendix in appendix operations, pain is produced. In ovarian cyst found during pregnancy, when you fear to give a general anesthetic we get magnificent results from local anesthesia. I have used it in diffuse peritonitis where the patient had double pneumonia and yet I did not dare let the peritonitis go without drainage and had equally good results. I have also used it in gastrectomy and conditions of that kind.

Dr. Robert E. Farr, Minneapolis: I am not much of a golf player and do not believe in making all shots with one stick. However, when I do shoot I generally use my best stick. To my mind, the best stick in anesthesia up to date is local anesthesia, providing it can be used successfully. We see the same difficulty today with local anesthesia that we usually see when a man reads a paper on this subject. He is like the Christian scientists: he will not argue. These papers are discussed by local anesthesia enthusiasts who spend their time picking out a few of the known shortcomings of the method. Dr. Scott says: "You can not explore the abdomen." I say I can. If he cannot, I can not help that. Dr. Ruben says: "We have necrosis of the skin." I say we do not. We never have necrosis of the skin. If we keep the epinephrin below five drops to the ounce and put procain up in Ringer's solution, and make subdermal instead of intradermal infiltration, we do not have necrosis. Local anesthesia should not be blamed for the shortcomings of those who use it. I have been trying to make the use of local anesthesia simple. This can be done by the method I described and by the use of the apparatus shown. If by this method we can get anesthesia in approximately 100 per cent. of cases, why should we introduce double the amount of anesthetic surrounding the field of incision instead of infiltrating directly into it? Nerve blocking has its place and is an excellent method, but it requires an expert to spear for nerves, and this method will never become common. The method should be simple and easy for all to learn. I am not in sympathy with the idea of reserving local anesthesia for extreme cases. If this is a good thing for bad cases it should be a good thing for good cases. I believe that it is a good thing for all cases in which it can be used.

Virginia Antituberculosis Work.—The work is done county by county. One of the workers gets permission to appear before the council or board of supervisors, outlines the nature of the work and asks to be allowed to make certain investigations, saying that no obligation is attached to this, but that when the work is completed, certain reports and resolutions will be made which can be acted on at the discretion of the governing bodies. A few interested people are interviewed, the field nurse is introduced, and she does the rest, such as get in touch with families and with the doctors of the community, and offers her services for instructive care and beside nursing when necessary. She will send patients to sanatoriums, arrange for free clinics, and health talks in the churches and at public meetings.—*Journal of Outdoor Life.*

STUDIES IN INFLUENZA AND PNEUMONIA

IV. FURTHER RESULTS OF PROPHYLACTIC INOCULATIONS *

E. C. ROSENOW, M.D.

AND

B. F. STURDIVANT, M.D.

ROCHESTER, MINN.

To determine the value of vaccination against disease, it is essential that the disease shall be one which a relatively large number of persons will develop unless protected, and that it be accompanied by serious consequences. These conditions were amply fulfilled during the pandemic of influenza. Moreover, the vaccine should contain the killed bacteria that produce symptoms and which are at least contributory to the cause of death. We have attempted, so far as possible, to fulfil this requirement by making a careful bacteriologic study of the disease, and by incorporating into the vaccine the important bacteria isolated. The epidemic was severe, and the need and the demand for vaccination were great; a large number of cases were available for bacteriologic study and to supply the proper strains for the vaccine. Vaccinations in large numbers during the past ten years with bacteria belonging to the group found in influenza have at least proved harmless, and in the case of pneumonia, prophylactic vaccinations have been successfully carried out by Wright,[1] Lister,[2] and Cecil and Austin.[3] A splendid opportunity to study the effect of prophylactic inoculation was at hand. Owing to the foresight of the founders of the Mayo Foundation, necessary funds to meet the emergency were available. A large amount of the vaccine has been prepared and sent gratis on request to numerous physicians on condition that reports of the results be returned.

In a previous report,[4] the reasons for the use of a mixed vaccine containing, as far as possible, freshly isolated strains were discussed. It was pointed out that the streptococci, especially green-producing streptococci from influenza, have certain peculiar properties. The preliminary results, as reported from the use of this vaccine, indicate that considerable protection is afforded against influenza and especially against the accompanying pneumonia. Vaccinations were begun soon after the onset of the epidemic. The period of observation was six weeks. It is our purpose in this paper to emphasize essential points in the preparation of the vaccine, to present further results from its use, and to record certain immunologic experiments.

* From the Division of Experimental Bacteriology, Mayo Foundation.

* This paper and that of Dr. G. W. McCoy which follows are part of a symposium on "Influenza." The remaining papers and the discussion will appear next week.

* Read before the joint meeting of the Section on Pharmacology and Therapeutics, the Section on Pathology and Physiology and the Section on Preventive Medicine and Public Health at the Seventieth Annual Session of the American Medical Association, Atlantic City, N. J., June, 1919.

1. Wright, A. E.; Morgan, W. P., et al.: Observations on Prophylactic Inoculation Against Pneumococcus Infections and on the Results Which Have Been Achieved by It, Lancet 1: 1-10 (Jan. 3) 1914.

2. Lister, F. S.: Prophylactic Inoculation of Man Against Pneumococcal Infections and More Particularly Against Lobar Pneumonia; Including a Report on the Results of the Experimental Inoculation, with a Specific Group Vaccine, of the Native Mine Laborers Employed on the Premier (Diamond) Mine and the Crown (Gold) Mines in the Transvaal and the De Beers (Diamond) Mines at Kimberley—Covering the Period from Nov. 1, 1916, to Oct. 31, 1917, Publications of the South African Institute for Medical Research, Johannesburg, South Africa, W. E. Hortor and Company, Ltd., 1917, pp. 1-30.

3. Cecil, R. L., and Austin, J. H.: Prophylactic Inoculation Against Pneumococcus, J. Exper. Med. 28: 19-41 (July 18) 1918.

4. Rosenow, E. C.: Prophylactic Inoculation Against Respiratory Infections: Preliminary Report, J. A. M. A. 72: 31-34 (Jan. 4) 1919.

Rosenow-Sturdivant – JAMA – Aug. 9 1919 396-401

COMPOSITION AND PREPARATION OF THE VACCINE

Influenza bacilli were isolated in large numbers at the outset of the epidemic, but they were rarely found later in the epidemic. The small fraction of influenza bacilli included in the first few batches of vaccine were therefore omitted, and the vaccine was made to contain a proportionately higher percentage of the green-producing streptococci. In other respects, the original formula has been adhered to. The formula as used in almost all cases covered by the present report is given in Table 1.

TABLE 1.—FORMULA OF VACCINE

Pneumococci, Types I (10 per cent.), II (14 per cent.), and III (6 per cent.)	30 per cent.
Pneumococci Group IV and the allied green-producing diplostreptococci described	40 per cent.
Hemolytic streptococci	20 per cent.
Staphylococcus aureus	10 per cent.

The preparation of the medium, the method of cultivating and collecting the bacteria, and the procedure of standardizing the dose and killing the bacteria are described in the preliminary report.[4] The vaccine, it will be remembered, was made to contain approximately 5 billion bacteria for 1 c.c. Later, the concentration was made twice as great, and the quantity of liquid was reduced to one-half. The injections were given subcutaneously one week apart. The first dose of the concentrated vaccine (0.25 c.c.) contained 2.5 billion, the second (0.5 c.c.) 5 billion, and the third (0.75 c.c.) 7.5 billion bacteria. Considering the large size of these doses and the reactions obtained, the injections should not be given oftener than once a week in order not to overstimulate the mechanism of immunity.

The tendency of streptococci to undergo changes and to lose specific properties has been repeatedly emphasized by one of us. It was thought important that freshly isolated strains should be included in the vaccine. In Table 2 are given the culture generations of all the strains that have been used throughout the epidemic. The fermentation power was tested of fifty-seven strains of the green-producing streptococci included in the vaccine; only twenty-seven fermented inulin, and only eight were bile soluble.

The advantages which should come from the use of a lipovaccine, particularly when a series of strains needs to be included, have already been pointed out,

and a simple method for the preparation in oil of a vaccine of the formula given in Table 1 has been developed and submitted for publication. A further study of the sputum and other material shows that of all the bacteria isolated, the somewhat peculiar green-producing streptococcus or diplostreptococcus is the most important. This organism is present in large numbers at the very outset of symptoms of influenza and of the accompanying pneumonia; it is commonly present after death. If the sputum or mass cultures are injected intraperitoneally into animals, they die, usually from invasion of the green-producing streptococci or pneumococci. If injected intratracheally in guinea-pigs the picture of influenzal pneumonia is closely simulated. Immunologic experiments with the serum from a horse injected with one strain indicate that most of the strains are immunologically alike. The serum of cases of influenza develops agglutinating power over these strains.

AGGLUTINATING POWER

In Table 3 it is shown that the vaccine used possessed well marked antigenic powers. The strains S 1, S 3, 2598².2, 2604.2, 3048.3, and 2874².3 were green-producing streptococci or diplostreptococci; 2575.2, a hemolytic streptococcus, and 2608².2, a staphylococcus from cases of influenza. It will be noted that agglutinins appear in the serum on the tenth day and persist for six weeks. Table 3 shows, moreover, that

TABLE 2.—CULTURE GENERATION OF BACTERIA FROM INFLUENZA AS USED IN THE VACCINE

Cultures	Green-Pro-ducing Strep-tococcus	Hemolytic Strepto-coccus	Staphylo-coccus
Third generation or below	58	18	18
Fourth to tenth generation	95	20	8
Eleventh to twentieth generation	21	0	0
Total	174	38	26

the bacteria in the vaccine (492) used as the antigen in the first column were susceptible to agglutination. This vaccine was prepared three months previously and was kept in the ice chest. Most of the strains used as antigen in the experiment recorded in this table were not included in the vaccine used to immunize the persons whose serums were tested. All the green-producing streptococci were agglutinated, however, by the monovalent horse serum.

TABLE 3.—AGGLUTINATING POWER OF THE SERUM OF PERSONS INOCULATED WITH SALINE VACCINE

Serums (Dilutions 1:20)	Strains								
	492	S 1	S 3	2,598².2	2,604.2	3,048.3	2,874².3	2,575.2	2,608².2
2,542 24 hours before third dose saline vaccine	0	0	0	0	0	+	0	0	0
2,542 24 hours after third dose saline vaccine	0	0	0	0	0	+	+	0	0.
2,542 48 hours after third dose saline vaccine	0	0	0	0	++	++	++	0	0
2,542 10 days after third dose saline vaccine	+	++	+	0	++	++	+++	++	0
2,542 6 weeks after third dose saline vaccine	+	++		..	++				0
2,543 24 hours before third dose saline vaccine	0	0	0	0	+	0	0	0	0
2,543 24 hours after third dose saline vaccine	0	0	0	0	+	0	0	0	0
2,543 48 hours after third dose saline vaccine	+	0	0	0	++	0	++	0	0
2,543 10 days after third dose saline vaccine	++	+	0	0	++	++	+++	+	+
2,543 6 weeks after third dose saline vaccine	++	0	0	0	++	++	++	+	0
2,545 24 hours before third dose saline vaccine	0	0	0	0	0	0	0	0	0
2,545 24 hours after third dose saline vaccine	0	0	0	0	0	0	0	0	0
2,545 48 hours after third dose saline vaccine	0	0	0	0	+	0	0	0	0
2,545 10 days after third dose saline vaccine	++	0	0	0	++	++	++	++	++
2,545 6 weeks after third dose saline vaccine	++	0	0	+	++	++	++	++	++
2,547 24 hours before third dose saline vaccine	0	0	0	0	0	0	0	0	0
2,547 24 hours after third dose saline vaccine	0	0	0	0	0	0	0	0	0
2,547 48 hours after third dose saline vaccine	0	0	0	0	+	+	+++	0	0
2,547 10 days after third dose saline vaccine	++	0	+	+	++	++	++	0	0
2,547 6 weeks after third dose saline vaccine	++	0	+	+	++	++	+	0	++
8,075 normal	0	0	0	0	0	0	0	0	0
8,076 normal	0	0	0	0	0	0	0.	0	0
NaCl	0	0	0	0	0	0	0	0	0

Rosenow-Sturdivant – JAMA – Aug. 9 1919 396-401

In Table 4 are given the results following the injection of a single dose of the lipovaccine (from 25 to 75 billions) in three persons. It may be noted that the amount of agglutination is greater than that following the injection of the saline vaccine, but here, as in the case following the injection of the saline vaccine, not all strains are equally susceptible to agglutination, and some are not agglutinated at all.

TABLE 4.—AGGLUTINATING POWER OF THE SERUM OF PERSONS INOCULATED WITH LIPOVACCINE

Serums (Dilutions 1:20)	3,271².3	3,296².2	3,331	3,332.2	3,334.2	3,334.2	3,342
						Strains	
3,074 normal.................	0	++	+	+	0	++	0
3,074 4 days after lipo-vaccine.............	+	+++	++	++	+	++	0
3,074 10 days after lipo-vaccine.............	+++	++++	+++	++	++	+++	0
3,074 6 weeks after lipo-vaccine.............	++	+++	++	+	+	++	0
3,075 normal.............	0	++	0	0	+	0	0
3,075 4 days after lipo-vaccine.............	++	+	0	0	+	++	0
3,075 10 days after lipo-vaccine.............	+	++++	+	+	++	++	0
3,076 normal.............	0	++	+	0	0	++	0
3,076 4 days after lipo-vaccine.............	+	+++	+	0	+	0	0
3,076 10 days after lipo-vaccine.............	++	+++	++	0	+	0	0
3,076 6 weeks after lipo-vaccine.............	+++	++++	+	0	++	0	0
NaCl..................	0	0	0	0	0	0	0

Table 5 shows the agglutinating power of various immune horse serums over strains of green-producing streptococci from influenza, strains included in the vaccine. The serum from Horse 15, immunized with one strain from the blood of a patient who died, has marked agglutinating power over most of the strains. Of the thirty-three strains tested in this manner, twenty-five were agglutinated specifically by this serum. The results indicate clearly that among the green-producing streptococci, including Group IV pneumococci in influenza, there are strains which have a specific

reacted severely to all three inoculations, others only to one or two. Persons coming down with a cold or with symptoms of influenza are often hypersensitive. Marked diffuse redness resembling erysipelas about the site of inoculation, with swelling and, later, marked induration, has occurred occasionally. In no instance were the symptoms alarming. The number of severe reactions is sufficiently large, however, to prevent general vaccination except at the time of an acute emergency. This is in accord with the experience of Cecil and Austin,[3] noted during prophylactic inoculations with pneumococci. An outline for records of persons vaccinated was sent with each batch of vaccine and later a questionnaire. The questionnaire asked for the date of the onset of the epidemic, the date when the vaccine was first used, the week of the height of the epidemic, the week in which the greatest number of vaccinations were given, and the duration of the epidemic. The number of cases of influenza from the time the vaccinations were begun until the end of the epidemic, or up to May 1, and the number of deaths which occurred among the vaccinated and unvaccinated in the same period, in the practices of the physicians supplied with the vaccine, were asked. The reports of the use of the vaccine after the epidemic had disappeared were excluded. The period of observation in most instances was from four to five months.

In determining a safe criterion as to the value of the vaccine, we have purposely been unfair to the vaccinated group. The protection afforded among the vaccinated patients was measured from the day of the first vaccination, whereas, judging by the agglutination experiments, it should be calculated from about one week after the third injection.

There is another reason why we have arbitrarily decided to make our calculations from the day of the first vaccination. A procedure, calculated to protect against an epidemic disease, such as influenza, should

TABLE 5.—AGGLUTINATING POWER OF VARIOUS IMMUNE HORSE SERUMS OVER STREPTOCOCCI INCLUDED IN THE VACCINE

Serums (Dilutions 1:20)	2,347.19	2,349.13	2,350.16	2,531.14	2,532.4	2,534.11	2,557.2	2,604.2	2,618².2	2,684.16	2,698².3	2,719²	2,769	2,800².2	2,825
								Strains							
Pneumococcus Type I....	0	·	0	+	0	0	0	0	0	0	0	0	0	0	0
Pneumococcus Type II...	++	0	0	+	0	+	0	0	0	++	0	0	0	0	0
Pneumococcus Type III..	0	0	0	+	0	0	0	0	0	0	0	0	0	0	0
Horse 9..................	++	++	0	+	0	++	0	0	0	0	0	+++	0.	0	++
Horse 15.................	+++	+++	+++	++++	+++	+++	0	+++	++++	++	++++	++	0	++	+++
Normal horse............	0	0	0	0	0	+	0	0	0	0	0	0	0	0	0
NaCl....................	0	0	0	0	0	0	0	0	0	0	0	0	0	0	0

TABLE 6.—RESULTS AS REPORTED IN QUESTIONNAIRES FROM ALL SOURCES

Groups	Total Number	Disease				Incidence for 1,000 Persons			Deaths				
		Influenza	Acute Edema of Lungs	Pneumonia	Empyema	Acute Edema of Lungs	Pneumonia	Empyema	Meningitis	Encephalitis	Total Deaths
Vaccinated once...	26,936	118.2	3.1	8.7	0.29	0.14	2.6	0.07	0.18	....	3.0
Vaccinated twice...	23,348	97.0	0.77	3.04	0.17	0.47	1.9	0.04	0.21	....	2.62
Vaccinated 3 times	93,476	87.9	0.8	4.4	0.18	0.18	1.2	0	0.05	....	1.43
Not vaccinated....	346,183	281.8	4.4	21.0	0.83	1.7	2.37	0.07	0.15	0.03	8.55

relationship, and that we were fortunate in successfully separating them from the ordinary *Streptococcus viridans* and including them in the vaccine long before the results of immunologic experiments were available.

The apparent protection against attacks of influenza noted in the preliminary report, difficult to understand at that time, now becomes rational.

METHOD OF SECURING DATA

In most instances the reactions were mild, about one person in each 100 reacted more severely. Some

have sufficient protective value when given after the onset of the epidemic to be measurable, for it is practically impossible to anticipate these epidemics and, moreover, persons will not present themselves for vaccination until the epidemic is at hand.

The questionnaire was arranged so as to yield information regarding the incidence of influenza, acute edema of the lungs, pneumonia and empyema, and the deaths from acute edema of the lungs, pneumonia, empyema, meningitis, and encephalitis among the vaccinated and the unvaccinated. Separate reports includ-

Rosenow-Sturdivant – JAMA – Aug. 9 1919 396-401

ing the foregoing points were asked for from institutions and in the cases of pregnant women. The impressions gained from the use of the vaccine regarding the severity of the disease if contracted following vaccination, and the effect, if any, which the vaccine had on certain chronic infections, such as bronchitis, sinusitis, myositis, and arthritis were asked for.

Many physicians were so overwhelmed during the height of the epidemic that accurate records could not be kept, and accordingly the reports containing accurate data are proportionately few. The reports of 530 physicians were fairly complete, however, and these are summarized in Table 6. It is realized that there must necessarily be errors in the morbidity figures as reported to us, just as in the case of reports to boards of health. It is generally agreed that as influenza became more prevalent and less severe, a proportionately smaller number of cases were reported, and that all morbidity figures reported are well below the actual figures. The error, however, among the vaccinated and unvaccinated groups in the reports to us, should be approximately the same, and hence the figures should be comparable. Mortality figures, on the other hand, may be considered as fairly accurate.

mer in these three decades were 23, 19, and 21, of the latter 13, 29, and 23, respectively. Through the cooperation of the Board of Health of Minnesota we were able to check the results as reported to us with the morbidity and mortality figures as reported to them. Reports on a considerable number of vaccinations were received from Brown, Chippewa, Clay, Dodge, Fillmore, Goodhue, Houston, Itasca, Lesueur, Lyon, Mower, Olmsted, Rice, Stearne, Steele, Wabasha, Waseca, Watonwan, and Winona counties. The total estimated population of these counties is 472,584. The total number of cases of influenza in these counties reported to the board of health during the epidemic until May 1 is 30,763, or sixty-five for each thousand. This is admittedly a low figure. The total mortality rate as reported to the board of health during this time is 4.2. The mortality rate, excluding the deaths which occurred in the respective counties prior to the date of the first vaccinations, is 3.2 (Table 7). The figures in the table indicating the cases and the deaths as reported to us are believed to be more accurate. The mortality rate, exclusive of that of the Mayo Clinic, in the 17,532 persons vaccinated three times is only one fourth of that reported to the

TABLE 7.—RESULTS AS REPORTED IN QUESTIONNAIRES FROM NINETEEN COUNTIES IN MINNESOTA EXCLUSIVE OF THE MAYO CLINIC

Groups	Total Number	Influenza	Acute Edema of Lungs	Pneumonia	Empyema	Acute Edema of Lungs	Pneumonia	Empyema	Meningitis	Encephalitis	Total Deaths
Vaccinated once...	4,828	115.1	0.4	8.28	0	0.4	0.2	0	0	0	0.2
Vaccinated twice..	4,029	88.3	0.74	3.7	0.47	0.47	1.9	0	0.47	....	3.2
Vaccinated 3 times	17,532	102.8	0.17	4.2	0.22	...	0.02	....	....	....	0.8
Not vaccinated....	36,100	373.5	1.35	20.4	0.6	1.4	4.0	0.13	0.16	0.02	6.35
As reported to State Board of Health..........	472,584	65.3	....	....	....	....	....	....	....	....	3.2*
(Estimated population)											

* Exclusive of deaths which occurred prior to the use of the vaccine and exclusive of the Mayo Clinic cases.

TABLE 8.—RESULTS IN OLMSTED COUNTY EXCLUSIVE OF MAYO CLINIC AND STATE HOSPITAL FOR INSANE

Groups	Total Number	Influenza	Acute Edema of Lungs	Pneumonia	Empyema	Acute Edema of Lungs	Pneumonia	Empyema	Meningitis	Encephalitis	Total Deaths
Vaccinated once...	2,424	100.2	0	6.1	0	0.41	2.8	0	0	0	3.2
Vaccinated twice..	1,021	221.8	2.9	0	1.9	...	4.8	0	1.9	....	6.7
Vaccinated 3 times	9,300	41.0	0.18	3.9	0.43	...	0.43	0.21	....	....	0.64
Not vaccinated....	8,700	246.0	3.2	13.1	0.45	0.9	2.6	0.46	0.12	....	4.0

RESULTS OF INOCULATION

The total number of unvaccinated persons recorded in Table 6 represents the sum of the estimated clienteles of the various physicians reporting the cases, and averages about 1,200 for each. It will be noted that the incidence of influenza, of acute edema of the lungs, of pneumonia following influenza, and the number of deaths from all causes among the vaccinated are consistently lower than that among the unvaccinated. Moreover, the incidence of disease and deaths is lowest in the group of 93,476 persons who were vaccinated three times. The reports included in this table were from many states, but the largest number came from Iowa, Minnesota, and Wisconsin. Thirteen thousand, six hundred and fifty persons inoculated and 2,083 who died were grouped according to age by decades. The curves indicating the percentage in each run roughly parallel.

The largest number of inoculations were given and the largest number of deaths occurred between the ages of 11 and 40 years. The percentages of the for-

board of health. Moreover, the total number of deaths among the vaccinated, including the persons inoculated only once and twice, is 1.6 for 1,000, or half the mortality rate as reported to the board of health during the same period of time. When we consider the fact that the deaths in each group were counted from the time the first vaccinations were given, which is really unfair to the vaccine, and the fact that our figures include all pneumonias, while those of the board of health include only the influenzal pneumonias, there seems little doubt that the difference must be due to the protection afforded by the vaccine. The figures given in Table 8 for Olmsted County, where about one third of the population was vaccinated, exclusive of the Mayo Clinic and the state hospital, are similar to those obtained elsewhere. The incidence of disease and the death rate among those vaccinated three times are well below that of those not vaccinated.

The results obtained in institutions in which the conditions among the vaccinated and the unvaccinated

Rosenow-Sturdivant – JAMA – Aug. 9 1919 396-401

were comparable are summarized and given in Table 9 in order still further to check the figures. The number of persons in most of the institutions included (fifty-three in all) was small. The opportunity for accurate observation was, therefore, favorable. The institutions included factories, personnel of hospitals, schools, and offices. The proportion of the vaccinated and unvaccinated varied between wide limits. The period of observation in the two groups was the same. The

TABLE 9.—RESULTS OF PROPHYLACTIC INOCULATION IN INSTITUTIONS WHERE THE CONDITIONS AMONG THE VACCINATED AND UNVACCINATED WERE COMPARABLE

		Incidence for 1,000 Persons					
		Disease			Deaths		
			Acute			Acute	
Groups	Total Number	Influenza	Edema of Lungs	Pneumonia	Empyema	Edema of Lungs	Pneumonia
Vaccinated 3 times	8,306	31	0.1	1.0	0.2	0	0.5
Not vaccinated....	9,388	200	0.5	12.0	0.8	0.4	5.5

incidence of disease and the number of deaths in almost all instances were lower in the vaccinated than in the unvaccinated group. The total average, as given in Table 9, compares favorably with that of the others. The death rate among the vaccinated is decidedly lower than among the unvaccinated.

The results given in the tables are in agreement with the numerous reports received by which it appeared that the vaccine had afforded striking instances of pro-

10. The incidence of disease and that of miscarriages and the mortality rate are consistently lower among those vaccinated than among those not vaccinated. The mortality (20 per cent.) of the unvaccinated pregnant women who developed influenza is somewhat lower than that reported from similar statistical studies by Bland[5] and by Harris.[6] They report a mortality of 37.7 per cent. and 27 per cent., respectively. The mortality of 12 per cent. in the 997 pregnant women inoculated in our series is in sharp contrast and calls for a further trial of this measure.

Almost from the beginning of the epidemic of influenza, patients who registered at the Mayo Clinic were advised to be vaccinated. From October 1 to May 1, 55,189 patients registered. Of these, 2,542 were vaccinated once, 1,030 twice, and 1,850 three times, a total of 5,422. A reliable morbidity and mortality rate for each thousand of the vaccinated and unvaccinated could not be determined because such a large percentage of patients remained in Rochester for too short a time.

It was thought that a study of the cases of influenza admitted to the hospitals might, however, be worth while. Of these, 749 were undoubted cases of influenza, and were analyzed from various standpoints. Fifty-nine of the patients were vaccinated once; twenty-four, twice, and fifty-seven, three times; while 609 were not vaccinated. The incidence of pneumonia and the deaths from pneumonia in these groups are

TABLE 10.—RESULTS OF PROPHYLACTIC INOCULATION IN PREGNACNY

		Incidence for 1,000 Persons									
		Disease					Deaths				
			Acute					Acute			
Groups	Total Number	Influenza	Edema of Lungs	Pneumonia	Empyema	Miscarriage	Edema of Lungs	Pneumonia	Empyema	Meningitis	Total Deaths	Mortality of Those Who Developed Influenza
Vaccinated 3 times	997	109.3	17.0	27.0	....	14.0	2.0	12.0	....	....	14.0	12 per cent.
Not vaccinated....	3,656	204.6	17.7	80.4	0.82	46.2	12.3	46.2	0.54	0.82	59.9	20 per cent.

tection. In a few cases no protection seemed to be afforded, but in most of these the vaccinated persons contracted the disease a long time after the inoculations. It is fully realized how difficult it is to judge just how much protection was conferred in many of these instances, and how much of the apparent protection was merely coincidental. But a careful study of the reports from 303 physicians, some of which were the result of careful observation, forces the conviction that real protection, especially against pneumonia, was afforded. In some of these instances most of the observations were made within six weeks to two months after the vaccine was given.

It was thought that the injection of large doses of a mixed vaccine might have some effect on certain chronic infections, especially of the respiratory tract. A summary of the reports shows that 961 persons with chronic bronchitis were benefited and that thirty-eight were made worse. The reports show that 127 persons with chronic sinusitis were benefited and four made worse. Improvement was noted in 121 persons having myositis and in 129 with arthritis, while in one of the former and in twenty-two of the latter the symptoms were aggravated. These figures are not considered to be especially significant but worthy of record. They are in accord with our own observations.

RESULTS OF PROPHYLACTIC INOCULATION IN PREGNANCY

The results of vaccinations in pregnant women as reported in the questionnaires are summarized in Table

recorded in Table 11. The average interval between the vaccinations and the onset of influenza was nine days in those vaccinated only once, twenty-six days in those vaccinated twice, and forty-five days in those vaccinated three times. The average temperature was more than one degree higher in the unvaccinated than in the vaccinated, and the average duration of fever nearly two days longer. The percentage incidence of pneumonia in those vaccinated three times was 21; in those not vaccinated, 57, while the percentage of deaths

TABLE 11.—RESULTS IN CASES OF INFLUENZA ADMITTED TO HOSPITALS IN ROCHESTER

Groups	Cases of Influenza	Incidence of Pneumonia	Deaths from Pneumonia, per Cent.
Vaccinated once..................	59	39	10
Vaccinated twice.................	24	95	12
Vaccinated three times...........	57	21	5
Not vaccinated...................	609	57	22

from pneumonia was 5 in the former group and 22 in the latter. The mortality from pneumonia of those vaccinated only once and those vaccinated twice is also well below that of the unvaccinated. The mortality figure in the unvaccinated is abnormally high because only the patients with relatively severe attacks were admitted to the hospitals.

5. Bland, P. B.: Influenza in Its Relation to Pregnancy and Labor, Am. J. Obst. 79: 184-197 (Feb. 19) 1919.
6. Harris, J. W.: Influenza Occurring in Pregnant Women, J. A. M. A. 72: 978-980 (April 5) 1919.

Rosenow-Sturdivant – JAMA – Aug. 9 1919 396-401; McCoy 401-4

The greater tendency to the development of pneumonia in influenza among the unvaccinated group as observed in this series is in keeping with the lower incidence of this complication (4.7 per cent.) in 11,325 cases of influenza in which the vaccine was given after the onset of the symptoms, as compared with the incidence (8.7 per cent.) in 41,788 cases in which the vaccine was not used. The average mortality in the cases in which the vaccine was used in treatment was 1.4 per cent.; in those not treated it was 2.1 per cent.

From these results considerable weight may be attached to the opinion of nearly all the 430 physicians who have used the vaccine and who have reported on this point, an opinion in agreement with our own observations, that is, that the attacks of influenza if contracted following vaccination are milder and of shorter duration.

SUMMARY

The immunologic and animal experiments reported[7] elsewhere indicate that the mixed vaccine used by us contained the important bacteria as they occur in influenza and the accompanying pneumonia, and that a relatively large number of strains of the green-producing streptococci which appear to have a specific relationship to the initial attack were included. The reports included results obtained under the most varied conditions, from many communities covering a wide range of territory. In some communities the mortality rate was excessively high, in others comparatively low. The number of persons inoculated is sufficiently large to make the statistical figures fairly accurate. The period of observation was from three to seven months. The incidence of influenza and pneumonia as reported to us is probably far from exact, but the percentage of error should be about the same in the vaccinated and unvaccinated groups. Indeed, if a difference exists, the number of cases reported among the vaccinated might be expected to be proportionately higher because, even though no protection was promised, the fact that influenza occurred after the vaccinations were taken would naturally lead to a higher percentage of reports to the physician who gave the inoculations. The average incidence of influenza and pneumonia in the group inoculated three times is about one-third that of the uninoculated group.

The average mortality rate in the uninoculated, as reported to us, approximates the mortality rate (5.4 per cent.) of sixteen large cities of the United States as given in *Public Health Reports* for February 7. The average mortality rate in the group inoculated three times is about one-fifth that of the uninoculated. A definite although a smaller degree of protection appeared to be afforded to those who took only one or two inoculations. From a study of a series of hospital cases of influenza it is found that the tendency to the development of pneumonia in the vaccinated is about one third as great as among the unvaccinated, and that the mortality in the former is about one fifth as great as in the latter. The number of completed vaccinations in pregnant women is not large enough to give exact figures, but the results indicate clearly that a definite degree of protection was afforded in this group of individuals.

It appears from all the facts at hand that by the use of a properly prepared vaccine it is possible to rob influenza of some of its terrors.

The preliminary results from the use of more than 500 doses of this vaccine suspended in oil, the immunologic studies and the results from the use of pneumococcus lipovaccine reported by Fennel[8] and by Cecil and Vaughan[9] suggest strongly that both the degree of protection and the duration of the immunity may be materially increased by the use of lipovaccine over that reported in this paper from the use of the saline vaccine.

STATUS OF PROPHYLACTIC VACCINATION AGAINST INFLUENZA *

G. W. McCOY, M.D.
Director, Hygienic Laboratory, U. S. Public Health Service
WASHINGTON, D. C.

When we consider the tragic experience through which the country and, indeed, the world, has passed during the last year, we realize that a great advance in preventive medicine would be made by the discovery of a prophylactic agent which would enable health authorities to control effectively epidemic influenza or the pneumonia that so often occurs as a complication. Perhaps at the outset it may be profitable to take stock of what we know about the etiology of influenza and the etiology and pathology of influenzal pneumonias.

OPINIONS AS TO ETIOLOGY OF INFLUENZA AND INFLUENZAL PNEUMONIA

Though the organism described by Pfeiffer in 1891 has long been known as the influenza bacillus, there really never has been convincing evidence of its relation to influenza, and the data that accumulated during the epidemic or epidemics here and abroad this past year have not contributed any confirmation to the view that this germ is the cause of the disease.

In this connection it should be borne in mind that it is quite possible that there are a number of organisms, varying greatly in pathogenicity, which are grouped under the name of Pfeiffer's bacillus. We have only to recall the great differences that exist in other groups, in which organisms having common cultural and morphological characteristics vary greatly in disease-producing properties, to realize that the rather vague limitations of what is called the influenza bacillus may cover a number of more or less closely related organisms.

French and English workers have claimed to have produced influenza by means of a filterable virus; this would, indeed, definitely eliminate Pfeiffer's bacillus; but we must bear in mind that attempts to produce the disease in man artificially in this country, by means of both filtered and unfiltered secretions, have in practically every instance been negative. Similar attempts by means of cultures of the so-called influenza bacillus have been negative.

7. Rosenow, E. C.: The Experimental Production of Symptoms and Lesions Simulating Those of Influenza with Streptococci Isolated During the Present Epidemic, Study II, J. A. M. A. 72: 1604-1608 (May 31) 1919. The Occurrence of a Pandemic Strain of Streptococcus During the Pandemic of Influenza, Study III, ibid. pp. 1608-1609.

8. Fennel, E. A.: Prophylactic Inoculation Against Pneumonia, J. A. M. A. 71: 2115-2120 (Dec. 28) 1918.
9. Cecil, R. L., and Vaughan, H.: Results of Prophylactic Vaccination Against Pneumonia at Camp Wheeler, J. Exper. M. 29: 457-483 (June) 1919.
* Read before the joint meeting of the Section on Pharmacology and Therapeutics, the Section on Pathology and Physiology and the Section on Preventive Medicine and Public Health at the Seventieth Annual Session of the American Medical Association, Atlantic City, N. J., June, 1919.

McCoy – JAMA – Aug. 9 1919 401-4

When we turn to the views on the etiology and pathology of influenzal pneumonia, we find a rather general opinion that the pneumonia is due to Pfeiffer's bacillus or to the secondary invasion by organisms of acknowledged pathogenicity, particularly the various types of pneumococci, especially those known as hemolytic, and, less commonly, Friedländer's pneumobacillus or the staphylococcus.

A few observers are inclined to the opinion that the original cause of the influenza, be it the influenza bacillus or another organism, is also an essential factor in the production of the pneumonia. This view would appear to be entitled to much respect, on account of the rather general opinion among pathologists that the pneumonia following influenza is generally of a type distinct from the pneumonias ordinarily encountered.

A number of interesting papers have appeared on the pathology of influenzal pneumonia, and a complete review of them would be valuable; but, for the present purpose, we may say that, in general, the pneumonias do not conform to those due to the organisms which are usually associated with pneumonia. Lack of definite areas of consolidation, the absence of the usual fibrinous pleural exudate, the extreme wetness of the lungs, and the blood-stained pleural fluid usually found bilaterally, in most cases serve to differentiate influenzal pneumonias from those ordinarily due to pneumococci, as lobar pneumonia. Emphasis is laid on this point because some workers have hoped that immunization against lobar pneumonia, which appears to be practicable, might prove of great value against influenzal pneumonia; but if the lung lesions of the two diseases are so different, one suspects there may be a material difference in etiology, and that this difference may be of such a nature as to make what appears to be a valuable prophylactic agent in one case of no use in the other.

Rosenow[1] calls especial attention to the fact that "the findings in the lungs, for example, in the so-called acute bronchopneumonia following influenza, are quite unique and are strikingly similar, irrespective of the species of microorganism present." This is quoted to emphasize the point that it is entirely possible that all of these lesions may be due to the primary cause of influenza, and that the various organisms which have been recognized in various cases and various places may really not reach even the dignity of secondary invaders, but may be looked on as leading a relatively saprophytic existence in the tissue damaged by the primary cause of influenza, whatever that may be. With this brief preliminary consideration of these important matters, let us consider the experience with prophylactic vaccination.

VACCINE FROM INFLUENZA BACILLUS AS A PROPHYLACTIC

In discussing this subject, we will give attention, first, to the results obtained from the use of a vaccine made from the influenza bacillus alone, or from other suspected etiologic agent, which aims, to be sure, to prevent the primary disease, and later to a review of the evidence with respect to vaccines which have been devised with the special object of preventing the development of pneumonia or of mitigating its severity.

A vaccine made from the influenza bacillus alone seems not to have appealed sufficiently to European workers to induce them to try it when the epidemic prevailed abroad. In this country, its use has been confined largely to New England. The early reports on this vaccine were very encouraging; figures were presented which, if taken at their face value, would convince any one of the efficiency of the agent; but, when these figures were submitted to careful analysis, much doubt remained as to whether the vaccine was of any service whatsoever. The chief source of error lay in the fact that the inoculations had been done during the progress of the epidemic, and that the case incidence among the vaccinated was compared with the case incidence in the general population or in the control groups from the beginning of the epidemic. Now, it is plain that if, after the epidemic is well under way, we vaccinate a portion of the persons in a population, the percentage of persons attacked will be smaller among the vaccinated than among the nonvaccinated, because a percentage of the total number of cases will have occurred before the vaccine is given. Not only does this introduce an error by counting in the control, or nonvaccinated group, cases that have occurred early, but also it leaves a select group to be vaccinated, wholly or in part, in which the percentage of susceptibles is smaller than in the original group of which they formed a part.

To make this clear, let us suppose that ten days after an epidemic started in a population of 1,000 persons, an admittedly worthless vaccine was administered to one half of those who at that time remained unattacked by the disease. Let us further assume that on the date of vaccination 20 per cent. of the population had sickened, leaving 800 well persons, of whom 400 were vaccinated. Since the hypothetical vaccine is worthless, the morbidity will be as great in the vaccinated as in the nonvaccinated group. Let us assume that to be an additional 20 per cent. Then the total morbidity in the vaccinated group will be 20 per cent. of 400, or eighty cases. The total morbidity in the unvaccinated, however, if we consider the entire period of the epidemic will be 20 per cent. of 1,000, or 200, plus 20 per cent. of 400, or eighty, which would make 280 cases.

Although the error is now sufficiently clear, we have seen reports which, on the basis of the above figures, if applied to this hypothetical worthless vaccine, make it appear to be a valuable prophylactic. The statement of these reports would be, in effect, that one half of the population was vaccinated, that among the vaccinated only eighty cases developed, while among the unvaccinated 280 cases appeared. Hence the obvious value of the vaccine.

We must also remember that a vaccine can scarcely be expected to exert any appreciable prophylactic effect before from seven to ten days after the vaccine is given, since a week or more is required for immunity to develop. A comparison is fair which considers, among both vaccinated and nonvaccinated, only cases that have occurred, say, ten days or more after the vaccinations are made.

When the influenza bacillus vaccine was submitted to such critical tests as the inoculation of approximately half of the individuals in institutions, or in other large groups, its failure became apparent. A few examples of this are worth citing. Hinton and Kane[2] were able to vaccinate about half of the patients at an epileptic

1. Rosenow, E. C.: Prophylactic Inoculation Against Respiratory Infections, J. A. M. A. 72: 31 (Jan. 4) 1919.

2. The Commonwealth, Bimonthly Bulletin, Massachusetts State Department of Health 6: 1-28, Nos. 1 and 2, 1919.

McCoy – JAMA – Aug. 9 1919 401-4

colony long enough before the disease became prevalent in the institution to justify the drawing of conclusions from their data. The vaccine used contained 800,000,000 organisms per mil, and a total of 2,000,000,000 were administered to each person. The results were as shown in Table 1.

TABLE 1.—EFFECT OF INFLUENZA BACILLUS VACCINE AS A PROPHYLACTIC

	Vaccinated		Not Vaccinated (Controls)	
	No.	Per Cent.	No.	Per Cent.
Number of persons	461	....	518	....
Cases of influenza	163	35.4	178	34.3
Deaths	28	17.0	24	13.5

On the basis of this experiment the authors reach the obvious conclusion that the vaccine was without value.

A similar test was made on the naval personnel at Pelham Bay Training Station; here a part of the individuals of a group were vaccinated, the remainder being held as controls. According to the latest available report,[3] 9 per cent. of the 554 inoculated persons developed the disease, and 5 per cent. of the 800 who had not been inoculated developed it.

Similar failure attended the attempts at immunization of men at the naval base at Paris Island, S. C. It was definitely shown that neither incidence nor severity was influenced by the vaccination. These observations were all on groups large enough to make the deductions of value.

A number of controlled vaccinations, in which influenza bacillus vaccine was used, carried out in institutions by the Public Health Service, gave the rather paradoxical result of showing an increased percentage of attacks among the vaccinated, but more deaths among the nonvaccinated. This result was obtained with a vaccine directed against the primary disease, not against the complicating pneumonia. The results are shown in Table 2. These figures illustrate the fallacy of giving much weight to the results of a small set of observations in work of this sort.

TABLE 2.—RESULTS OBTAINED BY INFLUENZA BACILLUS VACCINE IN INSTITUTIONS

	Vaccinated		Not Vaccinated (Controls)	
	No.	Per Cent.	No.	Per Cent.
Number of persons	484	....	842	....
Cases of influenza	153	31.6	223	26.4
Deaths	0	....	4	1.8

VACCINES FROM STREPTOCOCCUS AND OTHER ORGANISMS

Another series of vaccinations aimed directly against the supposed causative agent was that reported by Ely, Lloyd, Hitchcock and Nickson.[4] These workers believed that the epidemic was due primarily to a hemolytic streptococcus which could be detected in the blood and in the lungs. From the fact that the organisms with which these observers worked soon lost their chain-forming properties and, in some instances, the power to hemolyze promptly, they express some doubt as to whether they should be classed as streptococci, and they further assume that there are material differences between different strains. The results of the use of a vaccine prepared from organisms isolated from the cases were apparently most

encouraging, though none of the experiments was controlled in a manner that would definitely establish the value of the preparation. The work of these observers needs to be repeated before the results can be accepted for general application.

When we come to consider the evidence with respect to the vaccines especially designed to prevent the pneumonic complications of influenza, we find again such conflicting reports that one is somewhat bewildered.

The only papers from a foreign source that have come to my notice are those by Eyre and Lowe,[5] who used a mixed vaccine which contained the pneumococcus, the streptococcus, the influenza bacillus, *Staphylococcus aureus*, *Micrococcus catarrhalis*, *B. pneumoniae* and *B. septus*.

These authors believe, and indeed present rather convincing figures in their first paper[5] to prove their point, that the use of this vaccine produces lowered resistance, which may last for "from a few hours to two or three weeks," during which period the incidence of respiratory infections would be increased among inoculated groups.

The early experience of the English authors does not refer directly to the prophylaxis of influenza, but it is cited here to show that there may be an element of danger in the indiscriminate use of vaccines in the presence of a rapidly spreading epidemic like influenza in which naturally many persons in the "negative phase" would be attacked.

In a later paper,[6] the same writers report on the experience with vaccine in the epidemic in England in the autumn of 1918. Stress is laid on the necessity of preparing a vaccine from cultures but recently isolated.

The figures given and the facts presented by these writers are difficult of interpretation and permit of almost any conclusion that one wishes to draw from them, from the optimistic one that fatalities after influenza occur only among the nonvaccinated, to the pessimistic one that fatalities occur only among the vaccinated, though the authors believe the results were good. They frankly reiterate the opinion that for a short time following vaccination there is an increased incidence among the vaccinated, owing to temporarily increased susceptibility, but the writers consider that this risk is justified by the benefit that they believe may accrue later. As inoculations were performed largely during the prevalence of the epidemic, and as the controls appear to include persons who developed the disease prior to the vaccination, the alleged good results may be misleading.

THE POLYVALENT VACCINE OF ROSENOW

Rosenow[1] prepared a mixed, and, at least in part, polyvalent, vaccine from the various fixed types of pneumococci, pneumococci of Group IV, hemolytic streptococci, *Staphylococcus aureus* and the influenza bacillus, all of which had been recently isolated. This vaccine was adjusted to meet the bacterial flora encountered during the epidemic; thus, in a manner it may be said that it was designed to approach an autogenous vaccine, but was intended primarily for prophylactic purposes. Dr. Rosenow felt that this vaccine should be prepared for use in any community from the strains of organisms there prevailing, and that a vaccine adjusted to meet the needs of one local-

3. Notes on Preventive Medicine for Medical Officers, U. S. Navy bulletins, Nos. 50 and 51.
4. Ely, C. F.; Lloyd, B. J.; Hitchcock, C. D., and Nickson, D. H.: Influenza as Seen at the Puget Sound Navy Yard, J. A. M. A. 72 : 24 (Jan. 4) 1919.

5. Eyre and Lowe: Lancet 192 : 484-487.
6. Eyre and Lowe: Lancet 196 : 553-560.

McCoy – JAMA – Aug. 9 1919 401-4

404   PROPHYLACTIC VACCINATION—McCOY   Jour. A. M. A.
                                                                          Aug. 9, 1919

ity might not meet those of another. The figures given for protection are encouraging, but do not lend themselves to critical analysis.

Dr. Rosenow considers the immunity produced by his vaccine to be of relatively slight duration, as some persons were apparently protected during the first wave of the epidemic, but not during the second.

A vaccine, prepared essentially in accordance with Dr. Rosenow's formula, was used extensively in the Middle West with alleged good results, but it was not used until the epidemic was at, or beyond, the crest, and the records are not convincing. Vaccine prepared in the manner suggested by Dr. Rosenow should theoretically have a better chance for success than those we shall next consider, but the practical difficulties of preparing it from locally prevailing strains and adjusting it to meet the changing flora of the respiratory tract in a disease that spreads as rapidly as influenza are obvious.

A specimen of the vaccine which was being used in Illinois was tried in California, under rigidly controlled conditions, without success. The disease did not appear in the institution where the test was made until eleven days after the last injection, but, after the epidemic had swept through it, the results revealed that 37 per cent. of the vaccinated were attacked, against 28 per cent. of the controls, while 4.5 per cent. of the vaccinated population died, against 3.6 per cent. of the nonvaccinated. These are differences too small to be significant. Tests made in other institutions gave similar results, though we need not take the time to consider the details here.

There are several other reports of the use of vaccines prepared somewhat along the lines of Dr. Rosenow's, but the data are not presented in a manner to permit of analysis.

The only report we have on a vaccine directed against the influenzal pneumonias associated with the fixed types of the pneumococcus is that of Cecil and Vaughan,[7] whose work was conducted at Camp Wheeler and was directed primarily against the usual pneumonias of the camp. Apparently the antipneumococcus vaccine reduced somewhat the incidence of influenzal pneumonia among the vaccinated, though, to use the author's words, "influenza causes a marked reduction in resistance to pneumonia even among vaccinated men." These authors show clearly that the case mortality of secondary pneumonias was not reduced by the vaccination, contrary to the claim so often made, that the vaccine, when it fails to protect perfectly, at least leads to a milder type of the disease. Cecil and Vaughan believe that the results of their experiment with respect to pneumococcus pneumonia were obscured by the influenza epidemic; evidence that the prophylactic action of the vaccine employed against influenza was not striking, since the epidemic should have served to emphasize rather than obscure the results of the beneficial action of a really valuable prophylactic agent.

We must next consider, briefly, the stock commercial vaccines made from about the same organisms that went into the vaccine prepared by Dr. Rosenow. Concerning these there are no accurate figures. So far as I have been able to determine, the preparations have not been used anywhere under properly controlled conditions. What we have to consider are, chiefly, the enthusiastic reports of observers whose faith was bet-

ter developed than their judgment. A strenuous effort was made to secure the endorsement of the federal government for this form of prophylaxis against influenza. Under the direction of the Surgeon-General of the Public Health Service, careful investigators were sent to several communities from which glowing reports were received regarding the great value of stock vaccines, but in no case could the claims be verified. In this connection, we may trace the waning enthusiasm of one man who early in the epidemic reported that "immunization, using mixed vaccines, has proved beyond any question of doubt to be of great prophylactic value . . . why not extend this to all the people?" Ten days later, this man advised us that "we felt there was a strong possibility of it [the vaccine] preventing many cases. . . . At the present time we are not in a position to make any absolute and definite statement." So far as we know, the final reports from this source never have been published, though ample time has elapsed.

People wondered that those in positions of responsibility did not accept the first enthusiastic reports, adopt an attitude of optimism, and recommend the universal use of vaccination against influenza; but, in the light of present knowledge, there seems to have been some justification for an attitude of conservatism.

It must be clearly understood that what has been said above does not apply to vaccination against lobar pneumonia, using pneumococcus vaccine. The evidence on this is favorable, though perhaps the final word has not yet been said. It may be noted here that the very optimistic reports by Lister, who introduced vaccination against lobar pneumonia, are being called into question.[8] The rather startling suggestion is made by Fennel[9] that this antipneumococcus vaccine may be useful in combating epidemic influenza, but he admits the "information at hand is fragmentary and not to be seriously considered though possibly significant."

Though the evidence in respect to any vaccine that has been tried offers little to warrant hope that an effective agent has been found, we must not feel unduly pessimistic. The problem of vaccination in influenza is an extraordinarily difficult one. The etiology is uncertain, the influenza bacillus and the streptococci are poor antigens, and the epidemics are so far apart and so rapid in passage that the time to work out a prophylactic agent is very limited.

CONCLUSION

The general impression gained from uncontrolled use of vaccines is that they are of value in the prevention of influenza; but, in every case in which vaccines have been tried under perfectly controlled conditions, they have failed to influence in a definite manner either the morbidity or the mortality.

8. Johnson: Am. Med. 25: 149.
9. Fennel, E. A.: Prophylactic Inoculation Against Pneumonia, J. A. M. A. 71: 2115 (Dec. 28) 1918.

Making a Skilled Physician.—Hippocrates named six conditions necessary to become a skilled physician: Natural talent, instruction by a competent master, a place favorable to study, education begun in youth, love of work and long application. The first of these conditions is the most important, for where there is not a natural disposition it is useless to attempt to force Nature. Theory should be combined with practice. Want of experience begets either timidity or rashness. Timidity discloses impotence and rashness ignorance.—Tweedy, Brit. M. J. 2:598 (May 17), 1919.

7. Cecil and Vaughan: J. Exper. M. 29: No. 5, pp. 457-483.

Minaker-Irvine – JAMA – March 22 1919 - 847-850

represent every group of farm buildings within the area. At all stations at least one catch was made, while at several stations two or more catches were made on different dates. Table 1 gives the detailed information as to catches and types of mosquitoes caught. No attempt was made to catch any except *Anopheles,* but, as would be expected, a few *Culex* mosquitoes were included.

The total number of mosquitoes caught, by distance from point of liberation, may be seen in Table 2.

TABLE 2.—DATA AS TO LENGTH OF FLIGHT

0	399
¼ mile	148
½ mile	7,789
¾ mile	4,157
1 mile	1,942
1¼ miles	2,805
1½ miles	617
1¾ miles	158
2 miles	756
2¼ miles	248
2½ miles	814
Total	19,831

Examination of mosquitoes was made by adding a drop of solvent (alcohol, 3 parts; glycerin, 3 parts; chloroform, 1 part) to each mosquito placed on glass over a white back ground and by then observing evidences of the color by use of a small magnifying glass. At the time of examination for stain, observations as to the type and sex were made.

RESULTS

Of the total number examined, only ten were found showing evidences of stain, these all being caught on August 30, the first day of catching. Nine of these, all female *Anopheles,* were found on the screens of one house at Station 10, three fourths of a mile from the point of liberation, indicated on the chart by a concentric circle. One was found on the screen of a house at Station 15, one mile from the point of liberation.

Of the total of 19,831 mosquitoes, 19,238, or 97 per cent., were *Anopheles quadrimaculatus* and 597, or 3 per cent., *Culex.* But one type of *Anopheles* was caught, *A. quadrimaculatus,* confirming other observations that this is the one type of *Anopheles* found in this section during the summer months. Of the 19,238 *Anopheles,* 15,915, or 82.7 per cent., were female. While this percentage is that of the total, the percentage varied considerably for the various stations, and at one station in particular, Station 13, the reverse condition prevailed, as males predominated on one day.

In catching for staining, approximately four fifths of the mosquitoes were caught at Stations 5 and 9; and of the ten stained mosquitoes found, nine were caught at Station 10 or in the same general neighborhood. This brings up the question of the homing instinct observed by Carter, Le Prince and Griffitts.

At the stations in and near the ricefields, *Anopheles* was present in large numbers, and catching was carried on for not over one-half hour period at each station. As the distance from the ricefields increased, the number found decreased; and the time spent in a district increased, with a relatively lower catch.

From the results obtained it would appear that in this section at least a flight of 1 mile might be expected, but that with a fairly densely populated district there would be a dissemination of mosquitoes throughout the entire district.

CONCLUSIONS

1. Malaria has been eliminated from a typical ricefield district.

2. The question of flight of *Anopheles quadrimaculatus* may of necessity be regarded from two angles, that of experiment and that of observation. In one, the largest experiment of its kind ever undertaken in the United States, we have a record flight of 1 mile. In the other observation, there has been recorded continuously and on different occasions a flight of 1⅒ miles.

3. The use of 10 grains of quinin sulphate by mouth for sterilization of the blood of malaria carriers is evidently efficient for one malaria season if used actively over a period of thirty days.

4. The completely negative clinical history of the nineteen malaria carriers discovered on microscopic examination indicates, on the one hand, an immense difficulty in obtaining complete malaria control but emphasizes, on the other hand, the importance of the detection of the human carriers.

PROPHYLACTIC USE OF MIXED VACCINE AGAINST PANDEMIC INFLUENZA AND ITS COMPLICATIONS

AT THE NAVAL TRAINING STATION, SAN FRANCISCO

A. J. MINAKER, PH.G., M.D.
Lieutenant, M. C., U. S. N. R. F.
AND
ROBERT S. IRVINE, A.M., M.D. (SAN DIEGO)
Lieutenant, M. C., U. S. N. (T.)
SAN FRANCISCO

The fact that the recent influenza pandemic did not reach the Pacific Coast until about October 1, or more than a month after its appearance in the East, gave time to attempt a defense against it. The problems presented to Commander P. S. Rossiter, senior medical officer, of that period, were: (1) to prevent the entrance of the disease on the station, and (2) to prevent or lessen its spread and complications, should it appear among the personnel.

The U. S. Naval Training Station, being located on an island in San Francisco Bay, more than a mile from either San Francisco or Oakland, made an absolute isolation possible. This was maintained during the height of the epidemic, except for a very rigidly guarded supply boat making trips to San Francisco. To accomplish the second object, daily throat sprays of argyrol, 10 per cent., were administered to every person, and steps were taken to produce a prophylactic vaccine.

The reports available at the time from stricken camps and districts showed a great diversity of opinion as to the exciting cause, but there was general agreement as to the pneumococcus and hemolytic streptococcus being largely responsible for the fatal complications. The recent work of Cecil and Austin [1] at Camp Upton, confirming the observations of Lister,[2] had shown that a high degree of immunity can be produced against pneumonia by prophylactic vaccination.

1. Cecil and Austin: J. Exper. Med. 28: 19-41 (July) 1918.
2. Lister: South African Inst. for Med. Res., Pub. 2, 1913; VIII, 1916; X, 1917.

Minaker-Irvine – JAMA· – March 22 1919 - 847-850

Although there was difference of opinion as to the etiologic relationship of the influenza bacillus in this disease, and the possibility of conferring immunity against it,[3] a culture of B. *Influenzae* from a fatal case was obtained from the Rockefeller Institute to incorporate in a mixed vaccine.

After receiving the culture of B. *Influenzae* from the Rockefeller Institute, it was found most difficult to reproduce good growths with our ordinary human blood agar, prepared for meningococcic cultures. Therefore, other mediums were prepared and tested, such as streaked blood agar, laked blood agar (human) and rabbit's blood agar; but since the human blood agar titrated neutral to phenophthalein and gave a growth, much inferior to that of the rabbit's blood agar of the same reaction and percentage of blood (10 per cent.), and, furthermore, when it was observed that blood from different human donors gave variable growths, from barely perceptible to rather easily discernible colonies, and that the bacilli varied from the fine, minute, evenly stained rods to most bizarre forms, it was concluded that the human blood contained natural immune bodies in varying amounts.

It was found that with any of the foregoing methods in order to grow a sufficient quantity of bacilli quickly to make up vaccine for our needs (20,000 c.c.), a different medium was required. Following a suggestion of Professor Hall of the University of California, the human blood agar when cooled was cooked in a Freas dry oven at a temperature of from 100 to 115 C. or until it changed to a rich chocolate brown; in fact, it was found that even when this agar was apparently overcooked, luxurious growths were secured. Whether this result was due to the destruction of the natural immune bodies, or to a liberation of the hematin from the blood, or to both, remains to be settled. Suffice it to state that with this medium not only could subcultures be easily grown, but also primary cultures from lungs, sputum and postnares demonstrate the presence of B. *influenzae* in easily recognizable colonies. To obtain pure cultures of the pneumococci, human blood agar gave best results, while for vaccine, 2 per cent. glucose bouillon gave ample growths.

The streptococci were grown and gathered from blood agar, 15 per cent. human blood, centrifuged and washed (both washed and unwashed were tried with very little difference noted) and diluted in a 0.5 per cent. phenolized salt solution.

For the gram-positive bacteria the standardizing was done by using Wright's method and counting chamber; the influenza bacilli were counted by ratio with standardized pneumococci.

To arrive at a safe, though effective, dosage of the foregoing bacteria, it became necessary to ascertain if possible on laboratory animals the toxicity of each individually. For B. *influenzae*, the guinea-pig was used, first with dead, and later with live bacilli, neither producing any apparent serious effect in comparatively large doses (3 billion). This coincided with the results of Delius and Kolle's[4] experiments on laboratory animals.

For *Streptococcus hemolyticus*, volunteers were used, 60 million organisms producing no untoward symptoms. The report of Cecil and Austin covering

their studies in connection with pneumococcic vaccination of over 12,000 men demonstrated that no ill effects were encountered, that large doses were necessary to give full protection, and that the degree of immunity depended more on the dosage than the interval.

Based on the foregoing considerations, the final composition of the vaccine for each cubic centimeter was decided on as shown in Table 1.

TABLE 1.—COMPOSITION OF MIXED VACCINE

	No. of Bacteria
B. influenzae, Rockefeller strain........................	5 billion
Pneumococcus Type I, various strains..................	3 billion
Pneumococcus Type II, regular and irregular, various strains	3 billion
Pneumococcus Type III, one strain.....................	1 billion
Streptococcus hemolyticus, two strains................	100 million

These were sterilized separately for an hour at a temperature of 56 C., and then mixed with 0.5 per cent. phenolized salt solution to make the desired amount.

In addition to the foregoing vaccine as suggested by the experiments of Whitmore, Fennel and Petersen,[5] an attempt was made to prepare a lipovaccine: Definite quantities of each culture in the proportions mentioned were removed from plates, dried at 55 C. for one and one-half hours, and then triturated by hand under sterile conditions for eight hours, being moistened with ether from time to time. When completed, microscopic examination revealed a homogeneous mass with no bacterial forms.

To weighed portions of this powder, a sterile mixture of 10 per cent. lanolin in oil of sweet almonds was added and again triturated for three hours; each cubic centimeter of this mixture contained 2 mg. of the bacterial powder.

The effects of this mixture were first tried on a guinea-pig, 1 c.c. being injected with no serious results. Next, five members of the laboratory force were each inoculated with 1 c.c. Their reactions were slightly more severe than the sixteen referred to later, but none lasted more than seventy-two hours. The number of their leukocytes was increased from 4,000 to 8,000, and their serums agglutinated B. *influenzae* 1:200. The injection caused considerable local induration lasting about ten days, but there was no abscess formation.

OBSERVATIONS ON THE VACCINE

Owing to the fact that there were no reports at that time on the use of a mixed vaccine against pandemic influenza, 100 volunteers were given 0.3 c.c. as an initial dose, followed after three days by 0.6 c.c. and two days later by 0.8 c.c. However, before this was done, the temperature of each man was taken and recorded, the urine examined, and the blood from all was used to make a white and differential count. From sixteen men blood was drawn to make agglutination tests with B. *influenzae*, pneumococcus and streptococcus. Eight hours after the first inoculation the temperatures were again taken, with these results:

Before: 98.6 F., 90 men; 99. F., 8 men.
After: 98.6 F., 70 men; from 99 to 100 F., 18 men; 101 F. and over, 5 men.

The white and differential counts evidenced appreciable increase in the polymorphonuclear leukocytes, as illustrated by Table 2.

3. Scheller: Handbuch der pathogenen Microorganismen 5: 1292, 1913.
4. Delius and Kolle: Ztschr. f. Hyg. u. Infektionskrankh. 24, 1897.

5. Whitmore, E. R.; Fennel, E. A., and Petersen, W. F.: An Experimental Investigation of Lipovaccines, J. A. M. A. 70: 427 (Feb. 16) 1918.

Minaker-Irvine – JAMA – March 22 1919 - 847-850

The reactions recorded twelve hours after the first injection were: trivial, 40; moderate, 53; severe, 8. Trivial signifies headache, very often combined with giddiness and malaise; moderate, headache, backache, chill and slight rise of temperature; severe, all the foregoing symptoms intensified by higher fever,

TABLE 2.—WHITE AND DIFFERENTIAL COUNTS

Before		After	
White Count	No. of Men	White Count	No. of Men
6,000 to 8,000	40	6,000 to 8,000	1
8,000 to 10,000	56	8,000 to 10,000	47
10,000 to 12,000	3	10,000 to 12,000	48
		12,000 to 16,000	3
Differential Count		Differential Count	
Polymorphonuclear		Polymorphonuclear	
60 to 70 per cent.	54	60 to 70 per cent.	43
70 to 80 per cent.	46	70 to 80 per cent.	54

depression and general asthenia associated with multiple pains, in some cases sufficient to require medical aid.

The blood of sixteen of these men was secured for agglutination with B. influenzae of the type with which they were inoculated, with the results given in Table 3. Agglutinations with pneumococci and streptococci were unsatisfactory. There was no change in the urinary findings.

As it was considered that the results of the preliminary experiments were satisfactory, general inoculation began, October 12. The vaccine was administered subcutaneously at about the insertion of the deltoid muscle in doses of 0.5, 0.8 and 1. c.c. at three day intervals. In all, 11,179 persons were inoculated, composed of four distinct groups.

1. There were 4,950 persons in quarantine at the Naval Training Station, 171 being hospital corpsmen, transferred after a few days to duty in military and civilian hospitals for influenza cases.

2. At Mare Island Navy Yard there were 1,950 marines released after inoculation, ninety-nine hospital corpsmen on duty in the hospital, and forty civilian employees with unrestricted liberty in the adjacent cities.

3. At the Naval Training camp, San Pedro, Calif., there were 3,100 officers and men with liberty in Los Angeles and vicinity.

reports of inoculated persons during October and November, Table 4 was compiled. In discussing the results tabulated, we can safely omit from consideration the 4,950 men of the Naval Station because they were in quarantine during the height of the epidemic and therefore not exposed. No cases of pandemic influenza occurred during this period, and twenty-four days after release from quarantine, when there were still from 200 to 300 cases being reported daily in San Francisco, only fifteen cases of influenza developed in a personnel of 3,514. These fifteen cases were mild. There was no pneumonia and no fatality.

The inoculations of the 1,080 of the civilian population were completed October 16, which was twenty-one days after the epidemic began in San Francisco, and the incidence and mortality figures for the city represent the period of time, beginning with the inoculation and running until December 1, when the original epidemic subsided. They circulated freely in San Francisco and Oakland during the epidemic and in fifty-four instances assisted actively in the care of their stricken relatives, and apparently escaped the disease. Furthermore, the small number of this group who developed influenza had very light attacks.

The 1,950 marines were inoculated about October 20, about a week after the epidemic began, and were

TABLE 3.—AGGLUTINATIONS

Before Inoculation	No.	Five Days Later	No.
No agglutination at any dilution	2	No agglutination at any dilution	2
Agglutination at 1:200.	7	Agglutination at 1:200.	14
Sug. agglutination at 1:700.	2		
Sug. agglutination at higher dilutions.	0		

immediately released in Vallejo and San Francisco where the disease was at its height, and owing to the fact that statistical reports were not submitted to the Public Health Service, the personnel of the Mare Island Navy Yard seemed to furnish a fair comparison. Incidentally all of the severe cases developed within ten days after the last inoculation.

The low incidence of the disease in the inoculated persons can only be appreciated when we compare with it the morbidity and mortality of the large population with whom they associated at the same period. We

TABLE 4.—STATISTICAL DATA

Uninoculated Persons	Popula-tion	Influenza No. of Cases	Influenza Per Cent.	Mortality No.	Mortality Per Cent.	Inoculated Persons	Number	Influenza No. of Cases	Influenza Per Cent.	Mortality No.	Mortality Per Cent.
San Francisco and Oakland	625,000	33,065	5.3	3,035	9.2	San Francisco civilians	1,080	14	1.4	0	0.0
Mare Island Navy Yard	8,232	1,296	15.7	65	5.0	Marines at Mare Island	1,950	35	1.8	1	2.8
Nurses and attendants, San Francisco hospitals	550	186	33.8	4	2.1	Hospital corpsmen on duty in influenza wards	270	9	3.5	1	11.0
Los Angeles	600,000	9,124	1.5	612	6.6	Naval Camp, San Pedro	3,100	53	1.7	0	0.0

4. Finally, 1,040 civilian relatives and friends of the personnel of the Naval Training Station inoculated at our shore dispensary, living in San Francisco and vicinity, constituted the fourth group.

A careful record of all inoculated persons showed in the majority a moderate local induration, with some headache, general pains, and slight rise of temperature beginning about six hours after inoculation and abating within thirty-six hours. These symptoms were most marked following second injection. In no case did the constitutional symptoms persist after forty-eight hours.

RESULTS

By means of circular letters, personal investigations, official reports from localities, and from extended

also ask attention to the low incidence of disease of our inoculated hospital corpsmen detailed in military and civilian hospitals in San Francisco, in comparison with the nonvaccinated civilian nurses exposed to the infection under identical conditions.

The 3,100 men from San Pedro Naval Camp were inoculated about November 15, at which time the epidemic was in its recrudescence in Los Angeles and vicinity, and the figures given represent only the cases reported in Los Angeles during the period of twenty-four days following inoculation of the men.

Additional evidence that the men responded to the inoculation of the vaccine was furnished by serologic tests conducted with the strain of B. influenzae that had been used in their vaccine. On account of the men being transferred, it was impossible to follow the same group of men in all tests. Agglutinations were made with serum diluted from 1 : 50 to 1 : 400; but basing our opinion on our comparative experience, we felt that an agglutination in a dilution of 1 : 100 should be considered positive.

In Groups 3, 4 and 5, agglutination was also attempted in similar dilutions with a local strain of B. influenzae obtained from routine throat cultures on the station during the quarantine. The results are shown in Table 5.

TABLE 5.—AGGLUTINATION TESTS

	No. of Men	Days after Inoculation	Agglutinations Positive	Negative
Group 1	16	5	14	2
Group 2	39	30	33	6
Group 3	11	40	1	10
Local strain	11	40	0	11
Group 4	10	50	5	5
Local strain	10	50	0	10
Group 5	6	70	2	4
Local strain	6	70	0	6

CONCLUSIONS

The facts presented undoubtedly indicate that a noteworthy degree of protection against influenza and its complications was obtained by means of a mixed vaccine freshly prepared from predominating etiologic bacteria. These observations should also encourage further work along the line of immunity against pneumonia. To this end an attempt is now being made to regroup the Type IV pneumococcus with the object of adding it to a vaccine when needed.

ABDOMINAL COMPLICATIONS OF THE INFLUENZA EPIDEMIC AT CAMP CUSTER, MICH.

LYNN S. BEALS, M.D. (Buffalo)
Major. M. C., U. S. Army

WYNDHAM B. BLANTON, M.D. (Richmond, Va.)
Captain, M. C., U. S. Army

AND

DANIEL N. EISENDRATH, M.D. (Chicago)
Captain, M. C., U. S. Army

CAMP CUSTER, BATTLE CREEK, MICH.

The abdominal complications of the epidemic of influenza in October, 1918, present problems of interest in diagnosis and treatment. The clinical pictures varied so greatly that a grouping of the cases will be of value.

ABDOMINAL RIGIDITY AND TENDERNESS

The question frequently arose as to whether the boardlike rigidity and tenderness of one or both upper quadrants of the abdomen was due to acute abdominal affection or to muscle spasm from lesions of the chest.

Some of these cases were seen in the first twenty-four hours of the disease, before the physical signs of a pneumonia or of a pleurisy were sufficiently evident to make a positive diagnosis, all available methods, including the roentgen ray, being employed. The upper abdominal pain, with or without accompanying rigidity, which is seen in acute thoracic disease, has always been held to be reflex. Two cases of pneumonia following influenza showed at necropsy localized fibrinous subphrenic peritonitis of limited extent early

in the disease, and it seems certain that there is an actual pathologic basis for at least some of these cases of upper abdominal rigidity.

PAIN IN THE RIGHT LOWER QUADRANT

A number of patients were either admitted directly to the surgical wards or seen in consultation in the medical wards for pain in the right lower quadrant. Pain of a dull, aching character referred to the right lower quadrant was the most prominent feature. On examination there was only slight rigidity in a small number, and in the majority there was tenderness over the region of the appendix, but no rigidity. These abdominal signs and symptoms might ordinarily be diagnosed as appendicitis. However, it was repeatedly observed that the local abdominal signs disappeared in a short time; more rarely they persisted and increased in severity so that operation was deemed imperative. This group occurred in influenza patients, nearly all of whom later showed demonstrable signs of bronchopneumonia.

Another group, occurring during the epidemic, neither accompanied nor followed by pneumonia, was made up of a small number of fulminant cases of appendicitis. Operation seemed imperative and was performed under local anesthesia with good results.

PERITONITIS

Of 140 cases of bronchopneumonia following influenza coming to necropsy in all stages of the disease, six (4.2 per cent.) have shown acute peritonitis. Of the six cases, two manifested themselves as local inflammations in the upper left quadrant and were characterized by flakes of fresh fibrin adherent to the spleen and the contiguous surface of the diaphragm. The four remaining cases were generalized. One was extensive, 1,000 c.c. of thick greenish yellow pus being present in the abdomen. Another showed only a few cubic centimeters of pus, and, though generalized, the site of the greatest change was on the adjacent surfaces of the liver and diaphragm. In a third case there was no fluid, but a delicate coat of fibrin formed a layer over the surface of the stomach and the intestinal coils. A fourth case of generalized peritonitis will be referred to under subphrenic abscess. The fact that the process was twice localized to the upper quadrant, and once, while occurring generally distributed throughout the peritoneum, appeared most advanced over the hepatic surface, suggests an origin by direct extension through the diaphragm. In three cases there was a concurrent accumulation of pus on the corresponding pleural side of the diaphragm. On the other hand, a bacteremia was demonstrated in two of the cases during life, and in the heart's blood at necropsy of all except one (this patient had previously been embalmed). In every instance a hemolyzing streptococcus was recovered. In two of these cases pericarditis was an accompanying finding, and in one, jaundice was present. In addition to a bronchopneumonia, which was in most cases resolving, pleurisy was present. It seems certain, therefore, that with hemolytic streptococci in the blood stream and the accompanying involvement of other serous membranes, the peritoneal infection was hematogenous in origin and did not in all cases originate by the more difficult transdiaphragmatic route. In none of these cases was the appendix or gallbladder the site of any change except on the serous coat, as an incident to the general infection of the peritoneum.

GW McCoy, JAMA Vol. 71 No. 24, Dec. 14, 1918, p 1997

THE FAILURE OF A BACTERIAL VACCINE AS A PROPHYLACTIC AGAINST INFLUENZA

G. W. McCOY, M.D.
Director, Hygienic Laboratory
WASHINGTON, D. C.

V. B. MURRAY, M.D.
Assistant Surgeon, United States Public Health Service
AND
A. L. TEETER
Intern, Stanford University Hospital
SAN FRANCISCO

The necessity for accurate, controlled observations on preparations that are used as prophylactic agents for influenza is our reason for presenting the subjoined data.

The bacterial vaccine used in the present investigation was kindly furnished by Dr. F. O. Tonney, chief of the laboratory of the Chicago Health Department. While we are not intimately acquainted with the process of the preparation of the vaccine, we believe that it is an agent that should exhibit the immunizing properties, if any exist, of the micro-organisms used in its preparation.

Each cubic centimeter contains, approximately:

B. influenzae	500,000,000
Pneumococci Type I	500,000,000
Pneumococci Type II	500,000,000
Pneumococci Type III	500,000,000
Pneumococci Type IV	1,500,000,000
Streptococcus hemolyticus	1,000,000,000
Staphylococcus-aureus	500,000,000

Two or more strains of each organism were used.

The dose used was 0.5 c.c. at the first injection, 1 c.c. at the second and 1.5 c.c. at the third. The interval between the injections was forty-eight hours.

The persons vaccinated were patients at a state institution for the insane. Only patients of 41 years of age or under were vaccinated, as it was anticipated that if influenza appeared in the institution the great majority of cases would be in persons in this age group, and furthermore there was not sufficient vaccine at hand to provide material for a larger number of persons.

In each ward of the hospital a list was made of all patients aged 41 or under, and each alternate patient was vaccinated, the remainder being considered as controls. Each group numbered 390. The vaccination was completed November 15, and fortunately the institution remained free from influenza until November 26, when cases began to appear, although at this time the epidemic had almost disappeared from the community at large. The cases were clinically like those that have been observed elsewhere, and there was the usual percentage of severe cases and of cases with serious pulmonary complications, some terminating fatally.

The accompanying tabulation shows the results in the two groups up to Dec. 9, 1918.

INCIDENCE OF INFLUENZA AND PNEUMONIA IN THE VACCINATED AND THE CONTROLS

	Vaccinated	Not Vaccinated
Persons in group	390	390
Number developing influenza	119	103
Number developing pneumonia	23	17
Deaths	10	7

It appears clear from the evidence afforded by these observations that no protection was afforded by the vaccine.

The Last Word

There you have it! As documented herein, George Walter McCoy secures his place in medical infamy. His adverse legacy is confirmed with every unneeded death from influenza and/or influenzal-associated pneumonia, since 1918 and up to the present, a full century later.

McCoy may easily be viewed as the most harmful force in the history of American medicine. From 1915 to 1937, he was director of the PHS Hygienic Laboratory, which in 1930, when he was serving as Director, was renamed the National Institute of Health. As the first NIH Director (although an NIH chronology acknowledges three prior Hygienic Laboratory directors as preceeding NIH-directors), McCoy's perverted, misleading, pandemic perspective is now an integral part of the PHS and NIH historical record, abetted and even further twisted by a consumate patronizing apologist/hack, John Eyler, and enshrined as NIH gospel in an horrendous, phony, bogus faux-scientific 2010 article by Chien, Klugman (principal pneumonia researcher for the Bill and Melinda Gates Foundation) and Morens (Anthony Fauci's Senior Scientific Advisory).

God help us all.

#